Eating *for* Life

Eating *for* Life

Bill Phillips

HIGH POINT MEDIA

Empowering People Through Empowering Books

For information contact:

High Point Media, LLC
P. O. Box 16009
Golden, CO 80402
Tel: 303-273-2900
Fax: 303-273-2901
HighPointMedia.com

FIRST EDITION
ISBN 0-9720184-1-7

Designed by Craig Korn (VeggieGraphics.com)
Meal Photography by Dennis Lane (DennisLanePhotography.com)
Food and Prop Styling by Jacqueline Buckner (Food4Film.com)
Additional Photography by Craig Korn
Tableware and related accessories provided by:
     Peppercorn, Boulder, CO, Doris J. Houghland, owner (Peppercorn.com)
     Crate and Barrel, Broomfield, CO (CrateandBarrel.com)
     Pier 1 Imports, Boulder, CO (Pier1Imports.com)

Printed in the USA 🇺🇸

Join Bill Phillips online at EatingforLife.com

I am happy to dedicate this book to anyone
and everyone who, like me, loves food and
also desires to live a healthy life, in a fit body.

Giving Thanks

Creating this book for you has been so much fun!

I enjoy the process of discovering everything I can about nutrition and health. I love learning because it facilitates my passion to teach—to share with you the *right* way to eat so that you too can enjoy spectacular health and a rich quality of life!

The book you are reading right now has been a labor of love *and* a team effort. My sister and faithful friend, Shelly Phillips-Metz, helped me create this book and put each and every meal recipe to the test in the kitchen. Shelly, and her husband, Mike, helped prepare and taste test (along with her children Michelle, 19; Casey, 12; and my lovely mother, Suzanne) hundreds of recipes over the last year. Never before have I had the opportunity to enjoy so much delicious, nutritious food and such *quality* family time. Throughout this project, we created numerous new recipes, developed better ideas about how to eat right, *and* we grew closer as family, as friends and co-workers. We also each became healthier and more energetic throughout the process. The experience is priceless. Thank you, Shelly!

David Kennedy joined our Eating *for* Life team to help ensure that our meal recipes and plans, as well as the information which you'll discover in this book, reflect the latest scientific findings in terms of nutrition, fitness and health. David's patience, *focus* and attention to detail, as well as his collaborative efforts helping me write this book, are *greatly* appreciated!

Our Art Director, Craig Korn, has done a spectacular job in helping our team present this information to you in a pleasing, creative design. Thank you and well done, Korn!

Photographer Dennis Lane, as well as food and prop stylist Jacqueline Buckner, have made wonderful contributions. Thanks to them, this book looks darn near good enough to eat!

Also, assisting with this book, and virtually everything I've written over the past seven years, is Leigh Rauen, my word-processing magician, who helps transform my information and messages into the crisp, clean words, sentences and paragraphs you'll enjoy throughout this book.

Jim Nagle, my Manager and friend, has, as always, provided invaluable support, encouragement and guidance throughout the conceptualization and manifestation of Eating *for* Life. Thank you, Jim, for everything.

I'd also like to thank Melissa Martin, whose culinary expertise and good taste helped us fine-tune each Eating *for* Life meal. And to Brian Hersch, thank you so much for your insight and support. Thanks also to Suzanne Rosty and Lori Holton for all your help.

And last, but *certainly* not least, I would like to express my *sincere* appreciation to all of the great people who submitted recipes by email and letters and who have shared their transformation stories over the years. Your insight, real-world experience and success is an *inspiration*. To all of you who have made a change and share my passion to make a difference, thank you... ***thank you*** so much!

Contents

Introduction

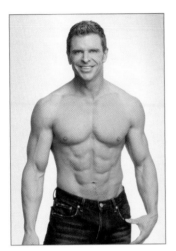

I *love* food.

What about you?

I enjoy *all* kinds of food. Everything from steak and potatoes to grilled chicken and brown rice to pizza, pasta, cheesecake, milkshakes and more!

Yet I *also* love fitness. Feeling healthy, energetic and strong is *so* very important to me.

These two powerful passions—food *and* fitness—may seem like natural-born enemies. After all, if you buy into today's diet dogma, food is the devil… and "diet," salvation.

Fact is, that is *not* so. Food is to fitness what sunshine is to flowers. What software is to hardware. What rocket fuel is to, well… *rockets*.

The two not only work together, they are *inseparable*.

I mean, come on, face it, you and I were born to love food. And we were perfectly fit when we stepped out of the womb and into this world.

Right?

So what happened?!

Well, somewhere along the way, wires were crossed, common sense lost and dollars found.

It's no mystery. The epidemic of obesity is not destiny. A "hiccup" in the magnificent waltz of evolution. That's all.

Complicated? No.

Curable? *Yes*.

The fact of the matter is, you *can* have your cake and eat it too, so to speak. Like myself, and hundreds of thousands of others, you can indulge your love for food *and* feed your fondness for fitness.

I *know* you can, because I'm doing it myself, and I've seen the mountain of success stories firsthand; a mountain so high, you need to see it to believe it! Living, breathing, eating, walking, talking, real-life examples of what is possible, even *probable*, when accurate information and heartfelt inspiration join forces. When *knowing* what to do is infused with the power to *do what you know*.

That, my friend, is what this book is all about. And *that* is where you'll find the surprisingly simple solutions to the struggles of so many… to find *true* fitness. To create peace of mind, in a *very* healthy body. And to enjoy the rich quality of life you were born with and deserve!

Make no mistake, the answers—*all* that you need to know—are not just "within" your grasp, they are *in* your grasp at this *very* moment. The answers, the solutions, the plan, the path… it's *all* yours in the pages of the book you are reading right here, *right now*. Eating *for* Life takes the guesswork out of eating right, once and for all. **I promise.**

And so, now, I *welcome* you to a new chapter in your life. And I *thank you* for allowing me to be your guide.

Very Sincerely,

Bill Phillips

Bill Phillips

P. S. If you have even half as much fun reading this book as I did writing it, we're both going to look back at this as a big success! ☺

Chapter 1

The Big Fat Problem

Houston, we have a problem.

Los Angeles, New York, Dallas, Denver, Detroit… you do too. In fact, America, you (we) *all* have a problem. A big one!

This year alone, more than 1,000 people will die, every single day, due to complications caused by being overweight, obese, out of shape.

Lost loved ones, friends who fall in their 40s and 50s, in the prime of their lives, extract a toll which, really, cannot be measured, monetarily. What is the price of *that* pain? Do you know? Does anyone? It's *high*, that's for sure. *Too* high.

Make no mistake, premature death is the most devastating debt that this epidemic of *preventable* ill-health is feeding.

If you're talking "dollars," the U.S. Department of Health and Human Services puts the price tag at $117 billion, this year alone. That's the health-care costs the government incurs.

When I step back and look at the big picture, what I see is not just 300,000 Americans dying each year, I see *millions* more living with low energy, poor self-esteem and confusion—conflicting thoughts about something which, in reality, is *not* complex at all. How to "eat right" is natural *intelligence*, which we are all born with. It's the result of thousands and thousands of years of natural selection, survival of the fittest, *evolution*.

Intuitively, you know how to eat right. In fact, deep down inside, that's all you know about food. However, on the surface, mixed messages get in the way. Big time! Consider that over $15 billion was spent on television food advertising last year alone—encouraging and enticing you to overeat the wrong foods, which does nothing to nourish your health and does a lot to feed frustration and the build-up of bodyfat.

All total, food companies spent over $33 billion last year to advertise their products. And, just 2.2 percent of that multibillion-dollar war chest went towards advertising truly healthy foods like fruits, vegetables and whole grains. Can you believe that?!

To make matters worse, mass media continually broadcast a stream of conflicting and confusing information. One day they compliment; the next day they criticize.

Yesterday's headline: "Low-Fat Diets *Cure* Obesity!" This morning's headline: "Low-Fat Diets *Cause* Obesity!" You know I'm not kidding, because I have no doubt you've seen these biased, bipolar reports too!

I'm not sure how or why this benefits the television stations, newspapers and magazine publishers, but it must. Otherwise, they wouldn't be so consistently inconsistent. It's almost as if they *want* to keep us uncertain and scratching our heads, if not pulling our hair out, searching for the answers.

It's overwhelming… the thousands of diet and nutrition books, millions of Internet Web sites, the advertising, the TV, radio, magazines, newspapers. And the most unfortunate thing about it all is that it interferes with you doing what *you* know is right. It keeps you from following your instinct and eating the way you could be, the way you should be, the way you would be if it weren't for all the misinformation and manipulation coming your way. The repercussions of it all are far from funny. And the statistics show it.

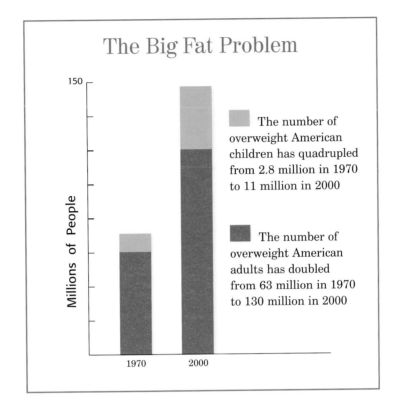

The Big Fat Problem

The number of overweight American children has quadrupled from 2.8 million in 1970 to 11 million in 2000

The number of overweight American adults has doubled from 63 million in 1970 to 130 million in 2000

Millions of People

150

1970   2000

Since 1970, the number of overweight American adults has increased from 63.2 million to over 130 million! Over 60 million of those adults are *so* overweight, the U.S. Department of Health and Human Services classifies them as obese, which is now "officially" a disease. Over that same period of time, the number of overweight American children (between ages 6 and 18) has quadrupled from 2.8 million to over 11 million! (*This* is my greatest concern!)

Not only are over half of all American adults now overweight and out of shape, but children are being affected faster than ever. In fact, according to the Centers for Disease Control and Prevention, if things don't change, one out of every three children born this year will eventually develop type-2 diabetes—a chronic illness that leads to crippling conditions, which include blindness, asthma, heart disease, depression and even death.

The bottom line is, we have a big fat problem. We really do. And *food* is at the core of it. To call it a problem is putting it lightly. An ominous, imminent threat, a catastrophe in process, a modern plague fueled by mis-information, mass marketing deception, individual, family, community and cultural denial. The end of the world? Not quite. But a damn good start!

There is no way to sugarcoat this issue… if you're not following a safe and sound, sensible approach to feeding your body, like the Eating *for* Lifestyle that I have very specifically prepared for you in this book, you may very well be eating for *death*. Most Americans are. And they are paying the price. In the short term with stomachaches, indigestion, headaches, after-noon energy slumps, moodiness and guilt. And, over the long term, contin-ually overeating the wrong foods always leads to self-destruction—a short life filled with days that seem to take forever.

But I'm not writing this book just to tell you about that. What I'm excited to share with you is the *good* news.

You see, hundreds of scientific studies and hundreds of thousands of real-world examples prove, beyond a shadow of a doubt, that we have the solu-tion. Quite simply, the "cure" is to follow your gut instinct. To reconnect with *your* common sense. To begin consciously, carefully and consistently Eating *for* Life. To feed yourself intentionally rather than accidentally.

Right here, right now and from this point forward, you too can begin Eating *for* Life. Start by asking *yourself* (not the media and *not* the mar-keters), before you put any food in your mouth, "Is this nourishing my health? Am I Eating *for* Life, or am I killing myself?" It's a simple question. Brutal, yes. But vitally important.

And if you're a parent, please ask yourself, "Am I poisoning my children, *or* am I helping them eat for life as well?" If you have friends and family and co-workers whom you care about and whom you see are suffering, help them discover how Eating *for* Life can save theirs.

Throughout this book, I will help you rise above the big fat problem. I will help you learn to listen to and follow your natural intelligence. And I will help you succeed.

Chapter 2

Fast-Food Frenzy

I believe in giving credit where credit is due. I also believe in placing blame where it's deserved. And when it comes to the big fat problem we just talked about, you simply cannot escape the fact that the fast-food industry deserves a supersized serving of condemnation.

Make no mistake, the modern meal made up of a burger, fries and soda is the gold standard of junk food. It's rotten. It's wrong. It's the opposite of Eating *for* Life.

A closer look at this fast-food classic reveals that it is saturated with trans fats, which have been shown to contribute to numerous diseases, including cancer. The burger, fries and soda combo is high in calories too, which feeds the build-up of bodyfat and eventually obesity. It's also low in vitamins and minerals, a poor source of protein and high in processed carbs, which scientific studies show may lead to the development of type-2 diabetes. And, it's so heavily spiked with salt and sugar that it is potentially addictive. Scientists have discovered that the combination of fat with salt and sugar has a powerful "neurochemical" effect on the brain, causing it to release natural opioids called beta endorphins that are similar to drugs like heroin and morphine. Just sinking your teeth into a fatty cheeseburger and salty fries releases a rush of those "feel good" neurotransmitters in the brain. In some people who eat fast food often, this response to the food can lead to addiction. (Do you suppose the fast-food manufacturers know about all that?)

Now, don't get me wrong—eating fast food, once in a while, is not going to make or break your efforts to be healthy and strong. However, the problem lies in the fact that eating fast food is a *daily* ritual for millions of Americans who get "hooked" on it. And when fast food is habitually consumed, not only does it contribute to the build-up of bodyfat, it has been linked to everything from bad skin complexion to eating disorders to poor heart health to obesity.

Another disturbing aspect about the fast-food business is that it's really not even about food. What they manufacture might look like, smell like, taste like the real thing, but it's *not*. It's fake food—pseudo food, which is virtually devoid of nutrition as we know it. We used to be able to identify real food because of its brilliant colors (like ripe fruits and fresh vegetables), its appetizing aroma, its texture and flavor. Not anymore! Thanks to colors created in chemists' beakers, artificial flavors developed by clever scientists and other food-synthesizing advances, fake food is almost undetectable.

And thanks to hypnotizing subliminal marketing strategies developed with the input of numerous psychologists, it's no wonder Americans have been completely duped into allowing the enemy not just within our borders but into our bodies.

Make no mistake, the frenzied lifestyle of eating behind the wheel, burger clowns and french fry playgrounds is feeding a multibillion-dollar business but starving people of basic and essential nutrition.

And for what? Money. That's it. It has nothing to do with nourishing American children and fueling the fast-paced lives of busy adults.

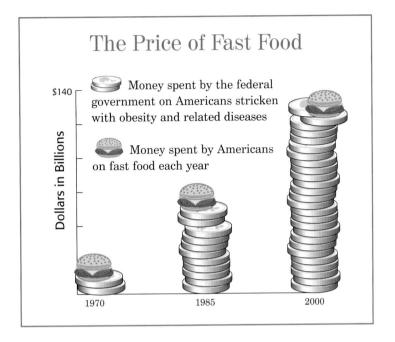

The Price of Fast Food

Money spent by the federal government on Americans stricken with obesity and related diseases

Money spent by Americans on fast food each year

Dollars in Billions

$140

1970   1985   2000

Consider the fact that in 1970, Americans spent $6 billion on fast food. This year, over $138 billion! (That's over a 2,000 percent increase in just over 30 years.) Since 1970, the number of fast-food burger drive-thrus has increased from about 2,000 to over 25,000. (That's an increase of over 1,000 percent.) Shocking really. Sickening too; literally and figuratively.

Not only have the billions of dollars spent on fast food skyrocketed, but the portion distortion has gone through the roof as well. The serving size of a soda, burger and fries has tripled over the past 30 years. They call it more "value," but it comes with a hefty price. Three times the fat, three times the sugar, three times the calories adds up to more than three times the ill-health effects. In fact, the price paid by the federal government to cover health-care costs related to overweight Americans has ballooned from less than $20 billion in 1970 to over $117 billion this year. (So much for the idea that fast food is any kind of bargain!)

Now, is fast food the *only* problem? No. As you'll soon discover, the so-called "diet industry" is feeding the dilemma as well. And, of course, each adult is responsible for his or her own decisions. However, over the last 30 years, Americans have had a heck of a lot of help making the wrong decisions when it comes to how they feed their bodies. And children are now the "primary targets" of fast-food promotions, which I have a big beef with.

When children are raised in this fast-food frenzy, they become victims of what this "business" is all about. And they can spend a lifetime suffering from the programming, conditioning and negative effects. It's been scientifically proven that the bad habits children develop with food make them more vulnerable to the ill-health effects of poor nutrition later in their lives. Knowing that, why would any parent allow their children to get hooked on fast food? *Why?*

So how do you steer clear of the fast-food frenzy? For starters, you can decide that you will *not* make the mistake of delegating something so important as your nutrition to an industry that is up to no good. That means not eating meals in your car; not eating out of Styrofoam containers; and not buying into the deceptive marketing message that fast food, good times and "happiness" go hand in hand.

As I see it, we must regain control of how we are nourishing and feeding ourselves. We must fire up our kitchens and begin preparing nutritious meals and feeding ourselves and our families the *right* way. The way it used to be, before the fast-food frenzy.

Chapter 3

The Dieting Dilemma

If you remember just one thing I share with you in this book, make it this: You *cannot win a fight with food*.

Unfortunately, millions of Americans don't know that. And there's a vast and ever-expanding "diet industry" which is convinced that it can convince you that there is indeed a way to finally and forever figure out how to fight food and win.

But the fact is, diets don't work. They can't work. Not now, not ever. Diets, all of them, are potentially dangerous, most always dumb and ultimately a dead-end street.

Eventually, anyone and everyone who is at all concerned with their health must learn how to *feed* their body, not how to starve it. This is what works in the long run.

As I see it, dieting is like going underwater and holding your breath. Eventually, you have to come up. And that's what dieting is like—it's like holding your breath underwater. Eventually you have to come to the surface, and when you do, you gasp for air and inhale all you can, so to speak.

It's that same way with trying to go without eating. No matter how strong your willpower is, eventually you'll give in, and you'll eat, sometimes even binge, gain weight and lose self-esteem.

The reality is that through tens of thousands of years of evolution, human beings have been "hardwired" to be vociferous eaters. In fact, way back when, those who could eat the most food, the fastest, and store the most bodyfat were the most "fit to survive" during that era. We are the descendants, the offspring, of these folks. And so, *we eat*. That's what we do. There is no getting around it. There is no stopping it.

What we need to do is work with our eating instinct and not against it. That's what I do. And I'm telling you, when you stop the struggle and you listen to what your body really wants, what it needs, what it's craving, and you *feed it* rather than fight it, you will be happy to discover that food and fitness can peacefully coexist. That gift we inherited also—natural selection wanted it that way.

Through this book, I'm *not* going to teach you how to diet; I'm going to teach you how to *eat*. There's a big difference. By learning how to eat, by learning how to feed your body, you'll be able to lose unwanted bodyfat, improve your health and lift your energy. You'll be able to *enjoy* food, which is *very* important to long-term success. Instead of fighting food, instead of it being a "guilty pleasure," it will become *pure* pleasure. At that point, I invite you to metaphorically take out a shovel, dig a six-foot hole, throw all the confusion, self-reproach, guilt, frustration... the entire dieting dilemma in it. Then, bury it and let it rest in peace as you move on with your life, enjoying food *and* a healthy, energetic, strong and lean body.

Please remember this: There is no diet "tricky" enough to override our hunger to survive. Consider that over the past 30 years, there have been over 10,000 diet plans published. Each supposedly offers the way to win the war against food and allow you to lose weight. But more than nine out of every 10 people who follow these plans fail to become healthier. And it isn't their fault. It's the diet that doesn't work, *not* the dieter!

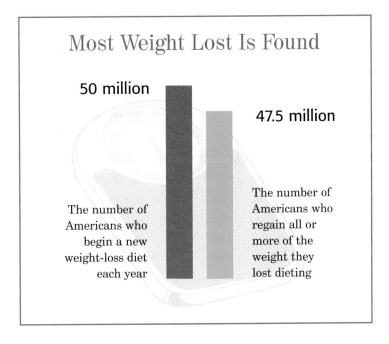

Most Weight Lost Is Found

50 million

The number of
Americans who
begin a new
weight-loss diet
each year

47.5 million

The number of
Americans who
regain all or
more of the
weight they
lost dieting

The reality that diets don't work is not just my personal opinion, it's a well-established fact. According to the Federal Trade Commission, the number of Americans who begin a weight-loss diet each year who regain all or *more* of the weight they lost is over 95 percent. Clearly, that is *not* the kind of success rate which is going to help us eventually solve this American health crisis—the big fat problem.

The dieting dilemma isn't limited to regaining lost weight; it's actually much more serious than that. You see, the vast majority of diets deprive your body of vital nutrients that are essential to good health and vitality. What I've discovered is that many people who diet suffer such low energy that they can't stick with an exercise program and oftentimes barely have the "get up and go" to even do their jobs.

Nutrient deficiencies also lead to immune system suppression and subsequently illness and disease. Everything from rapidly aging skin to headaches, irritability, anxiety and depression have been scientifically linked to the inadequate nutrition millions of dieters experience.

Another paradoxical aspect of the dilemma is that when you diet and "succeed" in losing weight, you fail in other ways. For example, scientific studies have shown that as much as half the weight lost on a diet is muscle and lean body mass. That means you are losing strength, agility, ability and you are getting "old" and frail. When you lose muscle, your metabolic rate goes down as well. This means you have to eat less in order to not gain the weight back, which, of course, virtually no one can do over the long term.

It's so obvious dieting is not the answer that, at times, I can't believe more people haven't woken up to this fact. That the diet industry continues to flourish (it's a $40 billion-a-year business), yet each and every year more and more Americans suffer the ill-health effects of being out of shape seems to confirm diets are not the answer.

Rest assured, there *is* a right answer, though. And now we know dieting is not "it." What is *it* is working with our natural evolutionary instinct, rather than against it. What is *it* is learning to satisfy cravings in a way that nourishes our bodies and minds; in a way that feeds muscle, starves fat, fortifies health and fuels energy.

Quite simply, the answer, the solution, is *not* a diet; "it" is *a lifestyle…* the Eating *for* Lifestyle.

Chapter 4

The Turning Point

As I see it, sometimes a problem is a good thing.

And sometimes, the bigger the problem, the bigger the opportunity it presents. Let me explain…

Life being what it is—imperfect, challenging, magnificent, interesting and full of unexpected surprises—forces us to *prioritize*. And part and parcel with that process is putting "little problems" on the back burner while we allocate available energy to first fighting fires that blaze the brightest.

And so, while America's health crisis has been simmering for several decades, it has only recently reached the boiling point—the flash point, where it can no longer be ignored and *must* be dealt with.

That's the good news. The big fat problem is front and center in the mindset of Americans today.

This is a great opportunity. It really is.

Now that we are *aware* of what's wrong, our collective energies can help make it right. And the fact that millions see and *feel* it, firsthand, adds to the sense of urgency that something has to change, *now*.

This high level of awareness and urgency is feeding the desire to change. That's empowering "will." That's definitely good. However, it's *not* enough. Let me explain…

I disagree with the popular saying, "Where there's a will, there's a way." Here's why: Having had the opportunity to work with thousands of people who desperately wanted to change, who had plenty of will, I witnessed something interesting, firsthand. What I saw was without knowing the *right way*, people with a powerful will were fired up, but yet very *frustrated*. That's because, despite their best efforts, they couldn't create a positive change—they couldn't manifest the turning point that they craved. Think of the frantic lab rat trying to escape a maze. Lots of effort, only to hit head on, one dead end after another. Eventually, exhausted. Rest assured, I don't want you to end up that way!

If you have the will (and I'm quite certain you do or you wouldn't be reading these words, in this book, at this very moment), I consider it my *responsibility* to show you the way. And make no mistake, I don't take that obligation lightly. I have dedicated my entire adult life to helping people make their way out of that maze—to break free, to escape the confinement of an unhealthy body and to discover what it's like to be liberated, healthy, strong and energetic again.

However, I can't do it alone. I can't do it for you. Consider that those who know the way, who have the knowledge, but lack the will, are the ones who epitomize knowing but *not* doing. They know what to do, but they lack the desire, the strength, the courage to change. They gave up at some point. They've settled. (Do you know people like this? I do!)

Here's something else I've learned: that will—that *desire*—can be fueled in a variety of ways. Some simply wake up one day, look in the mirror and say, "Enough is enough!" And *bam*… they have the will.

For others, it's a feeling that gradually builds over months, even years, until finally they reach the point where they are sick and tired of feeling sick and tired and are *willing* to do what it takes to make a change.

Some want to be better examples to their children—they don't want to see them fall into the same trap, suffer in the same way. That is a great reason, by the way!

In fact, any reason is a great reason, as long as it's *yours*. It might be to lose weight, but it might not. It might be to gain strength or to lower your risk of disease or to improve your mood and give you a boost of positive energy. Your reasons are unique to you. And it's those reasons that trigger your decision to make a change for the better—your decision to create the turning point in your health, your fitness, your quality of life.

As I see it, so many people in America today have the will, that if we can just clarify the way, there will be a great turning point. I feel that people have had enough of the fast-food frenzy, are fed up with the dieting dilemma and are ready to resolve the big fat problem. And I sense a "collective searching" for a way. The right way to transform this challenge into something extraordinarily good. I call this opportunity "The Great American Transformation." This is where our country can change from the most unhealthy modern nation in the world to the *healthiest*—where we go from worst to *first*. My goal is to do everything I can to help make that transformation happen within the next 10 years.

Make no mistake, such a change is possible—it *is* within our grasp. The fact that we have no choice but to change is feeding the fire, fueling the desire and is sharpening our focus on solutions.

And the turning point does not rely on any new federal regulations or policies. It doesn't have anything to do with developing a new food pyramid or fast-food lawsuits.

Fact is, the turning point starts right here, with *you* and *me*. It starts with our *will*. And it succeeds when we choose the *right way*.

Look, I know that scientists have searched far and wide, literally to the outer reaches of what the human mind is capable of comprehending, and they still can't unravel the vast mysteries of our human nature—why we do what we do.

Fortunately, we don't need to wait for all of those answers to make changes for the better and to create turning points in our own lives.

I know for a FACT that when it comes to making changes in our health, when you combine the force of will *and* the right way, you create success.

In a nutshell, that's the simple, basic formula that hundreds of thousands of people, no different than you, have followed to make dramatic, inspiring transformations in the way they look, the way they feel, as well as their health and the quality of their lives.

Yes, you can make it more complicated than that. You can dig deep and search forever for those emotional "issues," which you can blame for your bulging belly and widening waistline.

Oh… you're overweight and you "can't" change because deep down inside you have not been able to "resolve" your mixed feelings about the math test you cheated on in first grade?

Who cares?!

I mean, really, who has led a "perfect" life? Have you? Has *anyone?* I doubt it. In fact, as I see it, to be human is to be *imperfect.* If I carried around a pound for every unresolved "issue" of my life, I'd be as big as a Buick! But I don't, so I am *not.*

Rest assured, when you place the blame of your present condition on past circumstances, you disempower your future.

I'm not saying forget your past altogether. I believe in learning from the past and *moving on*. Focusing on a brighter, better future.

However, to move forward, we absolutely, positively need to accept the fact that *we do have the power to change*, and no one can take that away. The future is what we make of it… it really is.

So now, I ask, *do you have the will?* Do you have empowering reasons to make a change for the better? Are you ready to be part of the *solution* and not part of the big fat problem?

If so, congratulations! Your will and the Eating *for* Life way will create the turning point for you. And America too.

Chapter 5

Myth vs. Fact

Now you've reached the point where you're ready to move forward. You've learned a lot so far. You may very well be ready to create the turning point that we just talked about.

To help you move forward and succeed, I must warn you that your foremost enemy at this point is this: *uncertainty*. Time and time again I've seen people reach the point you're at now only to be turned away by confusion.

It's those mixed messages I told you about earlier. They create complexity, obscure clarity and cause second thoughts, which, far too often, lead to inaction. I don't want that nonsense to stop you. So, in this chapter, I'm going to help you separate myth from fact in order to protect and cultivate your confidence.

These myths leave such a sour taste in my mouth—they are so rancid and so much a part of the problem, I want to put them on a butcher block, slice them, dice them and then run them down the garbage disposal, where they belong. I want them out of your way. So let's expose and dispose of these myths right here, right now, once and for all.

MYTH: Foods that are good for you taste bad.

FACT: Good food can be delicious and nutritious.

My primary purpose in producing this book for you is to prove that your meals can and should be both delicious *and* nutritious. You'll know this to be true when you taste it and when you feel the positive, healthy, energy-enhancing effects of the foods, of the meals, of the treasure-trove of nutrition that you'll discover in this book.

I am determined to destruct the myth that "healthy food" is boring at first bite. I'm telling you, loud and clear, here and now, that you can and should look forward to a lifetime of enjoying food that is *both* nutritious and delicious. That's a fact.

MYTH: Eating right takes too much time.

FACT: You can create time by eating right.

You and I share the same amount of minutes in each day—1,440 to be exact. And we both must decide how to invest that time—how to make the most of it.

As I see it, far too many people simply spend time, rather than investing it. When you invest it, you produce a return that is even greater than what you put in—you actually *create* time. When you simply spend and squander time, you are wasting your most precious resource.

The fact I want to make crystal clear is that investing time in eating right—in nourishing your body—is virtually a sure thing. It pays back phenomenal dividends in terms of enhancing health and energy, which enrich your quality of life.

When you create the time to plan, prepare and enjoy delicious, nutritious meals—when you create time to make the Eating *for* Lifestyle yours, you will be very happy with the return on your investment. Give it a try, and you will see what I mean!

MYTH: You need to have a certain type of genetics to lose weight.

FACT: *Everyone* has the right genetics to be in great shape.

I'm often asked, "Do I need to have a certain kind of genetics to get in great shape?" My answer is, "Yes! You do need to have a certain kind of genetics—the kind of genetics human beings have!" You see, the Eating *for* Lifestyle produces predictable results in virtually every healthy adult. Recent scientific discoveries in gene mapping show that you and I are 99 percent identical in terms of our genetic fingerprint. And while certainly that 1 percent difference is conspicuous (different height, hair color, eye color, etc.), that does not mean that each person responds completely different to proper nutrition and regular exercise. As you can clearly see in the success stories beginning on page 345, that 1 percent difference makes each of our bodies look unique both before and after. However, you can also clearly see evidence of our "99 percent similarity" in the way we have each transformed ourselves.

MYTH: To lose fat, you need to take a diet pill.

FACT: You can lose fat without taking diet pills.

Over the last 10 years, I have helped literally hundreds of thousands of men and women collectively lose millions of pounds of bodyfat. And most didn't use any of these overhyped "miracle fat burners" that you see extensively advertised on television commercials, infomercials and in magazine ads. So my answer to the question, "Do I *have to* use a fat-burning supplement to get positive results?" is flat out, "No!"

What you do have to do is feed your body the right way. And you do have to make your health a priority in your life. You do have to plan to be healthy. You do have to set health and fitness goals, and you do have to focus on those goals daily. Eating right and exercising produces far greater results than using any diet pill. I challenge anyone to dispute that fact.

MYTH: It's too complicated to figure out how to eat right.

FACT: Feeding your body the right way is *not* complicated.

Through this book, you will become clear about how to eat the right foods, in the proper amounts and right combinations. You will know what to do and how to do it. You will clearly see that eating right is only complicated by those who try to make it that way. And you will discover that your intuition and common sense will guide your Eating *for* Lifestyle.

MYTH: If you exercise regularly, it doesn't matter if you eat right.

FACT: If you exercise regularly, it matters *even more* that you eat right.

Exercise *increases* your body's need for nutrients. And exercising a nutrient-deficient body actually creates worse nutrient deficiencies.

Make no mistake, for exercise to be effective and for it to help improve your health, you must feed your body plenty of protein, vitamins, minerals, essential fats, quality carbohydrates and drink ample amounts of water. Then you'll be able to build a stronger, healthier, leaner, better and more energetic body with each workout!

MYTH: Low-carb diets are the best way to lose fat.

FACT: Low-carb diets are *not* the best way to get in shape.

Low-carbohydrate diets, which are *so* popular today, are a razor-sharp, double-edge sword. Yes, they do help reduce weight; however, pounds are not all that are lost along with this extreme form of dieting, devised and popularized by the deceased doctor Atkins.

Fact is, low-carbohydrate diets are *not* the right way. As I see it, losing weight—simply taking up less space on the planet—is not the end-all, be-all of health and fitness achievement. My mission is and has been to help people transform their bodies—to help them gain strength, lose fat, feel younger and boost their energy levels. I've enjoyed helping hundreds of thousands of people achieve phenomenal results in that regard without "requiring" that they cut carbs out of their style of eating.

What I've seen is that the low-carb approach often leaves people lacking energy, losing strength, feeling frustrated, tired, irritable and, in some cases, severely depressed. Make 'em stand on a scale and record their weight in a research report, and you will find that they are indeed *down*. Open your eyes, open your heart, look, listen, feel… and you will sense that *down* is not just their weight… it is their state of being. Their level of living. And *not* a favorable one at that.

My intent is to lift people up. To help them lose bodyfat and gain strength and energy. And *that* is why eating right beats the living daylights out of "low-carb diets." That is a fact you can count on.

MYTH: Blood type determines which foods you should eat.

FACT: Basic, balanced nutrition is best, as long as your blood is *red*.

Beginning on page 345 of this book, you'll see before and after pictures and read success stories of men and women, from all walks of life, who have been following the Eating *for* Lifestyle. You'll notice that they've all experienced significantly improved health, while dramatically improving their physical condition. Fact is, I have absolutely no idea what their blood types are. I really don't. Nor do I know about the blood type of the hundreds of thousands of others who've succeeded when they began Eating *for* Life and exercising regularly.

It's a myth that obesity is caused by eating the wrong foods for your specific blood type. Obesity has a common cause (overeating the wrong foods and not getting enough exercise) as well as a universal solution (eating the right amount of the right foods and exercising). That's a fact you can take to the blood bank, I assure you.

MYTH: Once you reach a certain age, you can't get in shape.

FACT: You can improve your health and energy, at *any* age.

You can improve your physical fitness, boost your energy and even improve your mental performance at any age, when you start feeding your body the right way. See the success stories beginning on page 345 for proof!

MYTH: To be healthy, you just stop eating bad foods.

FACT: Your health is enhanced by eating the right foods.

There is so much emphasis in diet books on what not to eat and so much misinformation in the media about how "bad" food is for us I'm increasingly concerned that what's being overlooked is the fact that health is enhanced and our energy enriched by *eating* the right foods. Your body needs essential nutrients every day, and it's vitally important to understand that food is the ally, not the enemy.

MYTH: You should not eat for "emotional reasons."

FACT: You should enjoy eating, and it should be a pure pleasure!

The idea that you should not enjoy eating—that you should somehow find a way to eat that doesn't feel good is absolutely ridiculous.

I can't help but laugh when I hear these so-called "nutrition experts" insist, "Food should be used *only* as fuel for the body." That's like saying the only reason to have sex is to procreate. That's silly, and it's not realistic.

I wholeheartedly believe that you should enjoy food, and it should be a pure pleasure. There's absolutely no reason you shouldn't look forward to your meals and count on them to help you feel good. A delicious dinner can settle your nerves after a hectic day. A great breakfast can lift your mood and help you get ready to take on the day ahead. And a sweet, satisfying dessert can put a smile on your face. It does mine!

There's really no reason not to honor the tradition of making food a part of the process of celebrating holidays, birthdays and special occasions as well. I think it's perfectly fine to reach for a bowl of chicken soup when your body's aching and you're feeling under the weather too.

Through Eating *for* Life, you'll learn all about the right foods—the ones that are healthy and nourishing. And when you make those the mainstay of your meals, you can and will *enjoy* them. And you can eat to fuel your body, while *also* feeding positive emotions.

MYTH: To stabilize blood sugar, you have to stop eating carbohydrates.
FACT: Eating protein *and* carbohydrates balances blood sugar.

Today's carbohydrate confusion began years ago when we fell for the low-fat fad. When food manufacturers began removing fat from foods and replacing it with highly processed carbohydrates, our collective blood sugar went through the roof, and the problems began.

As it turns out dietary fat wasn't really the problem after all. However, in somewhat of a knee-jerk reaction, now the food fad is to cut carbs in an effort to bring blood sugar levels back into balance. Ten years from now, I guarantee we'll be looking back at this current craze and seeing some very serious side effects.

The fact is, cutting carbs is not the healthiest way to stabilize blood sugar levels. Carbohydrates are *essential* to eating right. The solution is to eat meals balanced with protein, quality carbohydrates and the essential fats your body needs.

You'll see 150 examples of balanced meals in this book. And I'm sure you'll get the idea. When you eat balanced meals consistently, you will find energy you might have thought you lost forever. And you'll lose body-fat you may have believed you were stuck with.

MYTH: In order to be satisfied, you need to eat large portions.

FACT: Quality, not just quantity, produces healthy satisfaction.

Our bodies crave *quality* nutrition, not merely massive *quantities* of food. So many people in America today have it completely backwards, though. They believe the more they eat, the better they'll feel.

Supersized portions at restaurants, fast-food chains and packaged goods at the grocery stores are obviously all playing into the myth that more is better. Yet so many people are stuffed but still "starving" for nutrition. The fact is, our bodies are satisfied by high-quality meals, not just big quantities of junk food.

MYTH: To make a change, you need to wait until you're all ready.

FACT: Don't wait until you're "ready." *Please*, do it *now*.

You need not wait until you are "all ready" to make a change in your style of living. Don't fool yourself into believing *now* is just "too soon." If you wait until everything is perfect in your life before you make a change for the better, you'll be waiting forever! Fact is, the time to do it is *now*. The longer you wait before you take action, the more you delay the rich rewards that are rightfully yours. Energy, strength, renewed health *and* decreased bodyfat... please begin feeding these benefits *now*.

Chapter 6

The Eating Right Recipe

"Eat right."

Each day, nutritionists, dietitians and diet doctors dish out this well-intended advice to clients, patients and those seeking the *right way* to reduce bodyfat and improve health.

Unfortunately, the well-intended admonition "eat right" has become a very obscure and ambiguous "prescription." I receive so many letters and emails from people who are confused about what it really means to eat right. "Is that low carb? Is that low fat? Does that mean joining a weight-loss clinic? What, when and how do I eat to 'eat right'?"

Good news: There is an answer. I call it the "Right Recipe." It has four primary ingredients. Each plays an important role in the overall process. And in this chapter, I'm going to teach you about each of these ingredients. Then I'll go on to explain how they all work together—in harmony—to form the Eating *for* Lifestyle.

So, if you're ready to learn what it really means to "eat right" once and for all, please review this chapter closely. I promise it reveals the *right way*.

The Right Recipe Ingredients

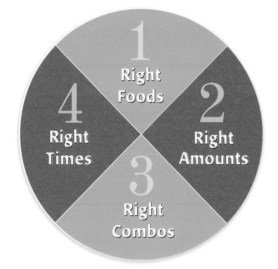

As you can see in the "pie chart" above, the four primary ingredients are: the Right Foods, the Right Amounts, the Right Combos and the Right Times.

That's it. That's all there is to it. When you combine these four ingredients, you absolutely, positively will have the Right Recipe to feed your body in a balanced, healthy, hearty, satisfying and effective way. You'll be able to gain energy, build strength, look and feel younger and reduce bodyfat.

As I walk you through an explanation of each ingredient in the Right Recipe, rest assured, I will not drag you through a complicated, convoluted and overly detailed dissertation of the many idiosyncrasies and trivialities of nutritional biochemistry. That's not my style.

As I see it, my job is to do the reading, the research, the reviews, then separate the wheat from the chaff, trim the fat and simply serve you the basic bottom-line facts. And that's what you'll find here.

That said, let's get down to business… let's learn what we need to know about the four ingredients that form the Right Recipe of the Eating *for* Lifestyle.

INGREDIENT #1: The Right Foods

The foundation of your success with Eating *for* Life begins with knowing which foods are right for you—which ones provide the high-quality, essential nutrition your body needs. In my book Body-*for*-LIFE, I called these the "authorized" foods, which are the ones that are a-okay to include in each of your daily meals. These foods get the green light because of the amount of nutrients they contain compared to calories. The best foods offer the most nutrients per calories. The technical term for these right foods is "nutrient rich and calorie compact." That is the opposite of "empty calories" or "wrong foods," which means they contain calories but little nutrition.

Right foods are healthy sources of the six nutrients that are *essential* to great health: protein, carbohydrates, essential fats, vitamins, minerals and water.

Just as every single one of the ingredients listed in each of the 150 very delicious and nutritious Eating *for* Life recipes featured in this book are absolutely essential for the meals to turn out right, the same is true in regard to these six essential nutrients and *you*. In order for you to "come out right"—in order for your mind to think clearly, your muscles to maintain strength, your body to metabolize fat efficiently and for you to enjoy great health and energy—you *must* feed your body the right foods, rich with ample amounts of essential nutrients.

Consider this statistic: Your body is made up of well over 75 *trillion* (75,000,000,000,000) cells.

Mind boggling, isn't it?

So is this: Within a year, each and *every* one of those cells will be completely *gone*. It's true!

You see, just as sure as the earth is revolving at this very moment, so too are our bodies—they're *always* moving, cycling and "re-creating." Life (yours, mine and everyone else's) is in a constant state of motion, even when you're just sitting there!

As sure as you're reading these words on this page, *right now*, each and every one of those 75 trillion cells is *de*generating and *re*generating. For example, our entire skin is "re-created" approximately every four weeks; our skeleton every three months; and our blood supply every four months. Every second of every minute of every day, your cells and mine are completely transforming.

Now, for this process to proceed in a healthy way—for all those new cells to be re-created the right way—it's vitally important that all the right raw materials and the essential nutrients are available when and where they are needed.

Problem is, far too many Americans aren't getting nearly enough of these nutrients. Scientific research shows most people are low on water, dangerously deficient in essential fats, undersupplied in quality protein and malnourished in many vitamins and minerals. This is not good. You see, even when nutrient deficiencies exist, new cells will still be created. Your body will do the best it can, in spite of the missing ingredients. The body is brilliant, and it can adjust and adapt to so many circumstances. But when it is starved of essential nutrients, day after day, its ability to re-create cells the right way becomes crippled. Over time, as your body's cells become unhealthy, so will you.

The signs and symptoms of this serious problem are often ignored: low energy, depression, insomnia, aches and pains and constant cravings for "something." The "new" you being created is an unhealthier version each and every day. But it doesn't have to be that way!

By eating right, you can feed the re-creation process and actually become a healthier new you beginning *now* and continuing *far* into the future. That's why eating the right foods that provide your body with all the *essential nutrients* it needs to keep the re-creation process going strong is so important.

Here's some essential information about essential nutrients you need to know before we go on to the next ingredient of the Right Recipe.

Protein

Protein is included in each Eating *for* Life meal, for good reason. It is an essential component of every one of those 75 trillion cells our bodies are made of. Protein is a *very* important nutrient; in fact, the word itself originates from the Greek word meaning "of prime importance."

Some of the very high-quality protein-rich foods that are ingredients in Eating *for* Life meals featured in this book include: chicken breast, turkey breast, lean beef, swordfish, orange roughy, salmon, tuna, crab, lobster, shrimp, lean ground beef, buffalo, eggs, cottage cheese, low-fat cheese, nutrition shakes and protein powder.

All of these foods offer complete proteins, which contain all nine of the essential amino acids: histidine, isoleucine, leucine, lysine, methionine, phenylalanine, threonine, tryptophan and valine. (By the way, knowing the essential amino acids by name, *plus* 2 bucks, will get you a cup of coffee at Starbucks!) The reason these amino acids are "essential" is because your body can't make them on its own, so they must be provided through the foods we eat.

The amino acids, derived from quality complete proteins, are the basic building blocks of muscle as well as a countless number of enzymes, hormones, neurotransmitters and antibodies. Also, when you eat meals containing quality protein, it supports your metabolism, helps stabilize energy levels through its effect on insulin and blood sugar and satisfies your appetite.

Now, although protein *is* of prime importance, it is only one of the six essential nutrients. And despite the proclamations of protein powder pushers, it is not in and of itself the panacea—it is not the "one key" that opens the door to increased muscle, health, strength and vibrancy.

Variety is as important as anything when it comes to protein. That's why I eat some chicken. I eat some turkey. I eat some beef. I eat some cottage cheese. And I eat eggs. And I drink my nutrition shakes, which are fortified with proteins derived from soy sources as well as whey.

The bottom line is, the right protein is not derived from just one source. Your body craves, intuitively, instinctively and very, very intelligently, a lot of sources of protein. Feed it, don't fight it. And, don't let protein pushers, who proclaim the power of their "source" to be superior to any other, to persuade and override your intuition.

The power of protein is in the variety, the satiety, the health-enhancing, muscle-strengthening effects, which are best derived from feeding your body with as many different quality right proteins as possible.

Carbohydrates

Carbohydrates, like protein, are essential to your health and are also included in Eating *for* Life meals. Among the foods that provide quality carbohydrates you'll find included in the 150 Eating *for* Life meal recipes are: brown rice, oatmeal, potatoes, yams, pasta, barley, apples, berries, oranges, whole-grain breads and pitas.

Carbohydrates are first and foremost a source of immediate *energy* for all of your body's trillions of cells. Carbohydrates also cause the release of insulin, a powerful hormone needed to help amino acids enter cells, which is very important. In that way, carbohydrates and protein work together, which is one of the many reasons I have included both in every meal.

In recent years, there has been a great deal of discussion and debate, amongst the diet doctors in particular, about the eminent evils of eating carbohydrates. And although I agree that the food supply in America, in particular that fast-food frenzy which I talked about in Chapter 2, is serving us a surplus of crummy carbs, that does *not*, I repeat NOT, mean that all carbohydrates are bad for you.

Other "experts" have alleged that you can draw the line between "good carb" and "bad carb" sources depending on whether they are refined, processed or what their score is on a scale called the "glycemic index." Once again, although I believe there is a morsel of truth to this, I don't think it's as literal—as black and white—as these diet doctors make it out to be.

For example, on several of the very popular low-carb diets, the authors fight that fruits, such as apples, are actually *bad* for you.

Come on… that's just silly!

If you have your nose stuffed so far up the scientific literature and lab reports that you determine something as natural, healthy and wholesome as an apple is to be a condemned carb and blamed for being part of America's big fat problem, then you have simply lost touch with reality!

Make no mistake, I am *not* going to tell you there are merely good and bad carbs and that they can be determined by a lab test, judging how fast or slow they are digested, how much or how little they, on their own, cause your body's blood sugar to rise and fall, and how much insulin levels are affected as a result.

The fact is, in the *real world* things don't work just like they do in the scientific laboratories. In the real world, I know for certain that what works, long term, is eating a *variety* of carbohydrates. And that's why I eat some brown rice, barley and oatmeal, which cause a relatively slow, steady release of blood sugar into my body. And I also eat ample amounts of apples, oranges, berries and other foods that contain carbs that provide quicker energy. But *variety* is the key!

This approach works! I'm living proof.

You know this already, *intuitively*. It's that common sense I've been talking about throughout this book. It's that natural intelligence we have inherited from our long-lost ancestors. We naturally reach for brightly colored fruits, which have been "kissed" by the sun and which literally contain particles of light energy, phytonutrients, as well as numerous vitamins and minerals, along with energy-rich carbohydrates.

Fact is, I recommend right carbs based on many factors, not simply on how fast they do or don't cause your blood sugar to rise or what their glycemic index is. For example, the carbohydrate foods that are included in the recipes featured in this book are there because they are *nutrient rich*. This not only makes them good for you, but it makes them taste good too.

You see, "good taste" is something we are all born with; something we inherited. And the desire to taste delicious, sweet and soft fruit is, once again, something we should *feed* and not fight.

So the bottom line is, the right carbs to eat for life include a vast variety and are not just selected solely on whether they are good or bad, quick or slow. Such classifications have been greatly exaggerated; they are counterintuitive and make the issue of carbs complex when, naturally, they should be a source of simple, sweet satisfaction.

Essential Fats

That's right, *essential* fats. I know that might sound and seem a little strange—the idea that any form of fat could be essential is quite foreign to most. For certain, the fact that fat fortifies and nourishes those 75 trillion cells within our bodies has been very well established for over 40 years. Unfortunately, that message has been lost in the marketing and media hype, which would have us believe bodyfat is simply a form of consumed fat from foods. Fact is, that is not so!

Bodyfat, that extra flub on your belly and buns, is not just there because you ate food with fat in it. The build-up of bodyfat is always a result of not following the Right Recipe. It's not simply a matter of eating something with fat in it. In fact, it's an established scientific certainty that the right fats, the essential fats, increase the metabolism of stored bodyfat and decrease fat production in the body.

So how could fat be essential in any way? It's because cell membranes, hormones, antibodies and enzymes all must have the "raw material" of certain essential fats in order for our DNA, our genetic blueprint, to fulfill its destiny and re-create the new you, the best you can be.

If you're malnourished in essential fats, which research shows over 95 percent of all Americans are, this process is compromised and certain deficiency symptoms begin to manifest themselves: dry skin, a depressed metabolism, mood disorders, decreased energy, dizziness and even memory loss.

You certainly don't need to know everything about the essential fats. Just remember that they, like the other nutrients included in Eating *for* Life meals featured in this book, are there for important reasons. Not just for flavor but because they are good for your health.

There are two particular types of essential fats in Eating *for* Life meals. These are ones that *cannot* be made by the body but are necessary for thousands of biochemical reactions to take place. These essential fats are called linoleic acid (sometimes called an omega-6 fatty acid) and linolenic acid (omega-3). In the ideal metabolism, linoleic and linolenic acid are the only dietary fats you need. These are found in healthy vegetable oils (canola oil, olive oil, safflower oil), fish oils (good fats in salmon, tuna, halibut, etc.) and in dark-green leafy vegetables, such as spinach. As long as you're eating ample amounts of these right foods every week, you will be getting the essential fats you need.

Now, there are *right* fats, and there are some *wrong* fats. Those which are bad for you include the *saturated* fats and the true dietary devil, *trans fats*, which are found in sick amounts in margarines, crackers, cookies and fast-food fries, burgers and so on. These fats have been proven to cause diseases ranging from cancer to diabetes to heart disease. They also are the fats that are the most likely to make you fat! We certainly want to avoid those fats, at least *most* of the time.

So the bottom line is, be sure to eat the essential fats your body needs in forms and foods such as healthy vegetable oils; fresh fish like salmon, albacore tuna and halibut; as well as dark-green leafy vegetables, such as spinach. That's what I do, and it works for me!

Vitamins and Minerals

All three of the nutrients I've talked about so far—proteins, carbohydrates and essential fats—need to be consumed daily in relatively significant quantities that are measured in ounces or grams. Scientists call these "macronutrients" (macro meaning large).

The other essential nutrients I'm going to tell you about now are consumed in very small quantities (often measured in milligrams). They're known as the "micronutrients" (micro meaning small). These are the vitamins and minerals. Although only small amounts of these nutrients are needed by the body, they serve a very important role in maintaining the proper biological functioning of everything from your muscles to your mind. Vitamins and minerals contribute to good health, muscle growth and proper fat burning by regulating the metabolism and assisting the biochemical processes that release and recharge energy from the food you eat. If you don't eat enough of these essential micronutrients to maintain proper levels, deficiency symptoms, which include muscle weakness, slow fat loss, connective-tissue deterioration and frequent colds and infections due to suppression of the immune system, just to name a few, will appear.

Vitamins are "organic" compounds, which means that they are produced naturally in both vegetables and animals, where they are found in abundant quantities. The main function of vitamins in the body is to help enzymes with reactions, including energy metabolism, protein synthesis, nutrient digestion and absorption, to name but a few of thousands of processes. Vitamins are essential—you cannot live without them. Literally.

Vitamins are either fat soluble or water soluble, depending on whether fat- or water-based molecules transport the vitamins through the bloodstream. Fat-soluble vitamins include A, D, E and K. Because these vitamins have an affinity for fat, they can be stored in both adipose (fat) tissue and in the liver, extending their effective life span in the body and strongly decreasing the chance of developing deficiencies. The water-soluble vitamins include all of the B vitamins and vitamin C; they aren't stored in the body for more than a few hours, so daily intake is a must.

Minerals are *in*organic in nature, meaning they are not produced by plants or animals. They can, however, be found in food sources, for example, iron in red meat, calcium in milk and potassium in bananas. Minerals are extremely important for your body to work right. They are essential for nerve cell communication, flexing muscles, fluid balance and energy production. Many minerals also serve as building blocks for body tissues, such as calcium and phosphorus for bones.

Minerals are referred to as either "bulk" or "trace" depending on the amount needed by the body. Bulk minerals include calcium, magnesium, potassium and sodium. Trace minerals, on the other hand, may be required in quantities as little as a few micrograms (that's just one one-thousandth of a milligram). These include minerals such as chromium, copper, iodine and selenium.

Within the Eating *for* Life meal recipes, you'll find vast amounts of vitamins and minerals in the form of fruits and vegetables, such as apples oranges, tomatoes, bananas, berries, broccoli and spinach. Also, right carbohydrates and proteins—whole grains, lean beef, chicken and nutrition shakes—provide rich sources of essential micronutrients.

Water

Water is so important to good health—consuming ample amounts is absolutely essential for fueling health and energy. Water covers approximately 70 percent of the earth's surface and makes up over 70 percent of our bodies as well. All living things rely on water to thrive, you and I included. It helps produce energy, detoxify our bodies, regulate body temperature, build new cells and lubricate joints, among thousands of other functions.

We naturally lose water every minute of every day, just through breathing. During the summer months, water losses are greater because body perspiration, which is used to cool our systems, evaporates faster in a hot environment. Caffeinated and alcoholic beverages are diuretics—they cause you to lose even more body water.

We generally lose about 10 cups of water per day. Unfortunately, most Americans, research shows, don't drink nearly that much. Consequently, many people are walking around in a chronic state of dehydration, which is *not good* to say the least. Water losses of one percent of your total bodyweight can impair functioning both mentally and physically. Losses of four percent can cause headaches, loss of energy, muscle weakness and irritability. Losses of seven percent can be fatal. Serious? You better believe it is! But it is easily prevented.

Don't wait until you're thirsty to drink water, or you'll give back less than what you really need. It is essential that you replenish your water losses daily.

It's not a discussion topic for good company, but watching your urine may be the best way to tell if your body's properly hydrated. Dark, gold-colored urine is a sure sign you're low on fluids. Drink enough water to aim for light-yellow or, better yet, almost clear urine. The average person needs at least 10 cups of water per day. People who exercise regularly need even more. I drink water from dawn to dusk and then some. I drink 16 ounces of bottled or filtered water first thing in the morning and another 16 ounces during my workouts. All total, I drink almost a gallon of water each and every day, and I drink an extra cup of water for each cup of coffee or diet soda I drink during the day. I suggest you do the same.

INGREDIENT #2: The Right Amounts

Now that you know which foods are right—which ones are high in nutrients, convenient and taste good—it's time to move on and discover the right amounts of the right foods you should eat in each meal.

Fortunately, you don't have to become a calorie counter nor do you need to meticulously monitor the carbs or fat grams of each and every food to know if you're eating the right amount. What works well is to gain an understanding of the importance of *portions*.

You don't need to get out a calculator to figure out if you're on target with the right portions of right foods included in each Eating *for* Life meal. In fact, the information you need to know is transmitted to you at 186,000 miles per second! That's the speed of light. And that's how fast the answer to the question, "Is this the right amount of food for me?" is reflected.

So what is a portion?

Well, a portion is an amount of right protein roughly equal to the size of the palm of your hand. For example, a chicken breast about the size of the palm of *your* hand is a proper portion of chicken for *you*.

A portion of a right carbohydrate is an amount roughly equal to the size of *your* clenched fist. For example, a baked potato about that size is the right amount for *you*.

The right amount of a serving of vegetables is approximately what you might imagine you can hold in the cupped palm of your hand. For example, a portion of steamed broccoli could be a little or a lot, depending on your appetite, really. You see, with vegetables, like those included in the Eating *for* Life meal recipes in this book, you have a lot of leeway—you don't have to limit yourself to a certain amount, and you certainly don't have to force-feed yourself a certain serving size.

What I do, generally, is eat a portion of protein and a portion of carbohydrates in each of my daily meals, and in two of these meals, I include a serving of vegetables (my favorites are broccoli, steamed spinach and zucchini). Sometimes I'll eat a little serving of vegetables, and sometimes a lot, depending on my appetite… depending on what I'm intuitively craving. Once you too begin the Eating *for* Lifestyle, you'll get the hang of it.

Eating the right amounts of the right foods in each meal is important. I've discovered that people eat too little amounts just as often as they do too much. The critical component is eating the right amounts of the right foods. When you do this, you become more connected with what a satisfying meal actually feels like. You're not hungry or stuffed. Your appetite and cravings are satisfied. Your energy is fed.

Be forewarned: Eating too little or overeating the right *or* wrong foods in one meal will throw your energy off for hours later in the day. For example, eating too little for breakfast may manifest in overeating dinner or dessert. And the contrary… a breakfast binge may mean missing midmeals and abruptly interrupting energy, as well as physical and mental performance throughout the day. When I say eating the *right amounts* of the right foods is vitally important to your success with the Eating *for* Lifestyle, I'm not kidding at all!

And, as I've already explained, eating the right amounts is not complicated or inconvenient. You just must simply know what to do!

INGREDIENT #3: The Right Combos

Now that you know about the right foods *and* the right amounts, it's vitally important to understand the right *combinations*.

Quite simply, what you do is choose a portion of protein and carbs, and include that in *each* of your Eating *for* Life meals. For example, chicken breast (protein) and brown rice (carbohydrate). And in at least two of your daily meals, include a portion of vegetables. An example of this would be a dinner with a chicken breast, brown rice and *broccoli*. Throughout the 150 meal recipes featured in this book, you'll see an array of ways to combine protein, carbohydrates and vegetables.

Combining the right foods in the right amounts not only calms your cravings, but it also helps feed your muscles by providing both the amino acids from protein, along with carbohydrates, which help "shuttle" that protein into cells. Scientific studies and real-world results reveal that eating a portion of protein along with the right amount of carbs provides a synergistic effect—carbs help protein fulfill its destiny, so to speak.

Rest assured, the Right Recipe ingredient of combining protein and carbs in each meal is based on sound, scientific research. For example, in a recent study published in the *Journal of Nutrition*, researchers found that balancing protein and carbohydrates stabilizes blood sugar and insulin (the purported benefits of the low-carb diets) and tended to decrease body-fat, cholesterol and reduce the risk of type-2 diabetes.

In another study reported last year in the journal *Physiology and Behavior*, a team of Swiss researchers reported that by balancing protein and carbs in each meal, you could benefit not only your muscles but your *mind*. Balanced eaters experienced *better* overall cognitive/mental performance compared to test subjects who ate meals that were not balanced.

In yet another study published in the *European Journal of Clinical Nutrition*, scientists cited, once again, that eating a balance of protein and carbohydrates and essential fats in each meal resulted in greater feelings of energy and lower levels of fatigue. They determined that balanced meals promote stable energy and greater endurance.

In another scientific study, this one published in the journal *Medicine and Science in Sports and Exercise*, researchers reported that in test subjects who exercise, consuming a post-workout meal with *both* protein and carbohydrates resulted in better moods—enhanced feelings of strength and confidence. That's good news because the more optimistic you are, the more likely it is you will continue to eat right!

More proof for the pudding: Scientists have also shown that people who eat a balance of protein and carbohydrates have better digestion and absorption of nutrients and a higher "thermic effect" (fat-burning effect) from each meal. On top of all that, studies show that meals balanced in protein, carbohydrates and essential fats help people like you and me control our appetite.

I could go on and on, but rest assured, the results of research in the realm of traditional science, as well as reams of real-world results, absolutely and positively support the Eating *for* Life recommendation of combining protein and carbohydrates in each meal. This advice, although it goes against the grain of the popular low-carb diet dogma, provides a basic, balanced and in my opinion the *best* approach to making the most of each and every meal.

INGREDIENT #4: The Right Times

Okay… now you know that eating the right foods, in the right amounts, in the right combinations are three of the essential ingredients in the Right Recipe. And the fourth and final ingredient, that's eating at the *right times*.

Q: What are the right times?

A: *Six times a day is the right way!*

It's true!

What about the old adage that "three square meals a day" is best?

Well, that nonsense is *not* based on anything even remotely related to good health or sound nutrition. The expression "three squares" comes from centuries ago when serving crew aboard warships gave the gunners three daily meals served on square wooden platters—meals that consisted of salty, half-rotten meat and crusty old biscuits. I think you also get three square meals a day in county jail, but I don't know for sure.

Anyway, the fact of the matter is, your body, my body, *everybody's* body works better when we eat the right foods, in the right amounts, in the right combos, not three but *six times per day*.

Eating six meals a day creates a "metabolic environment" that supports your energy and muscle metabolism, while helping you burn bodyfat. Study after scientific study has shown this to be so. For example, a recently published report in the *European Journal of Clinical Nutrition* cites that people who ate six times a day had a faster resting metabolic rate than those who ate just three meals daily. As you may very well know, your metabolic rate is the pace at which your body burns fat and food energy to keep you going strong. This study showed eating meals frequently throughout the day allows you to burn fat more efficiently. That's good!

Researchers at Georgia State University recently arrived at the same conclusion. They found that those who ate just "three squares" a day had, on average, a higher percentage of bodyfat than those who ate *six* times per day, leading the researchers to cite that the idea of eating three square meals is best is *downright wrong*. (I agree, by the way! ☺)

Another way eating six complete meals a day helps you lose bodyfat is by allowing you to maintain lean muscle. Remember, muscle not only helps you look leaner but also makes your body more metabolically active. Muscle burns calories even when you are just sitting there. Fat does not.

Numerous studies have shown that eating frequent meals increases fat loss while helping you keep your muscle. One recent report studied physically active people who ate the *same* amount of food each day but in a different number of meals. The people who ate only two meals a day lost about *twice* the muscle and *half* the fat as the people who ate six meals a day. In other words, the weight lost by those eating six meals was primarily bodyfat, while those eating just two meals lost mostly muscle.

When you eat meals every few hours, you'll have more energy; you'll also have less hunger and cravings, as was demonstrated in yet another recent study where it was shown that people who ate two large meals a day, given the same food choices as those eating six meals a day, consumed an average of 27 percent more food.

As I see it, eating one big meal causes your blood sugar to spike, then crash. Research shows that this "nosedive" in your blood sugar strongly stimulates hunger. So at your next meal, you're more likely to get to the table ravenously hungry, which, of course, can cause you to eat too much. But with six balanced meals per day, you never get to that point of ravenous hunger. At meal time you feel a little hungry; then you eat; you feel full—you feel *satisfied* until your next meal.

Another study published recently in *The New England Journal of Medicine* showed that in as little as *two weeks*, people who ate frequent, portion-controlled meals as opposed to three large meals (containing the same total amount of food) reduced their "bad" cholesterol levels by nearly 15 percent, reduced their cortisol levels (the "stress" hormone that contributes to belly flub and many other side effects) by more than 17 percent and reduced insulin levels by almost 28 percent.

There's more... a scientific study reported in the *European Journal of Clinical Nutrition* shows that eating "compact," balanced, nutritious meals every two to three hours throughout the day increases your metabolism, allowing you to burn more fat. When your daily food intake is eaten in a small number of large meals, there is an increased chance to become overweight.

Yet another study revealed that eating often helps your blood sugar and insulin levels stay strong and steady. When insulin levels spike, fat storage starts, blood sugar drops and energy levels plummet. Six meals per day do away with the highs and lows of blood sugar and insulin, as demonstrated in a recent study which clearly shows blood sugar remains much more constant and insulin levels stayed much lower in the six-meal-a-day group than in the two-meal group. That's good.

I could go on and on. Another study published in the *International Journal of Obesity and Related Metabolic Disorders* found that when you eat frequent meals throughout the day, it helps control the appetite.

Again, a study published in the *American Journal of Clinical Nutrition* reported that people are most successful at losing fat and keeping it off when they eat numerous meals throughout the day.

Had enough?

I have!

The bottom line is, when you eat every few hours, when you work *with* your body instead of against it, you'll not only look better but I'm certain you'll just flat out feel better too… *a lot better.*

Right Recipe Wrap-up

So there you have it—the Right Recipe. What it really all boils down to is this: When you eat the **right foods**, in the **right amounts**, in the **right combos**, at the **right times**, you simply cannot go wrong!

Got it?

Good!

Chapter 7

Have Fun and Feel Free

Now that you've learned the specifics of Eating *for* Life and you know about the right foods, right amounts, right combinations and the right times to eat, here's what I want you to do next…

Forget all that stuff!

That's right, put it out of your mind. Not every day. Just one day a week. Let me explain…

I've discovered that the healthiest people, with the healthiest eating habits, enjoy eating "fun foods" that are not necessarily the most nutritious, from time to time. I'm the same way. And so I have designed the Eating *for* Lifestyle to accommodate this natural pattern. Blending both common sense and science in a way that makes Eating *for* Life even more effective *and* enjoyable.

So what I'm asking you to do is to follow the Eating *for* Lifestyle, as I've described in this book, six days a week. And on the seventh day, I ask that you *eat whatever you want,* whenever you want, in whatever amount and combination you so desire. I call this your "free day."

On that one day a week, if you want to eat waffles with whipped cream, all covered in maple syrup for breakfast, that's fine. If you crave lasagna and bread with butter for lunch, go for it. If you want a thick pepperoni pizza with double cheese for dinner, be my guest. A piece of apple pie with ice cream for dessert… sounds good to me!

Do this and don't worry about it, *please*.

There are two physiological benefits to purposely eating extra once a week: It boosts fat burning *and* it helps you control your appetite. You see, when you make a significant change in your eating habits and cut out the junk food, the saturated fat and the high amounts of sugar, it may set off that thousand-year-old encoded alarm inside your brain—the one telling you to *eat more*. (Remember, way back when, those who could eat the most food, the fastest, and store the most bodyfat were the most "fit to survive" during that era.)

Sensing the change and not knowing that there isn't a famine around the corner, your body may begin to limit production of a hormone called "leptin." Leptin is one of many feedback systems your body needed to help keep it from starving in the old, old days. Strong leptin production equals a strong metabolism. Diminished leptin production, on the other hand, makes your metabolism go down and your appetite go up. That is not what we want!

Knowing that science shows the more leptin levels fall, the more your appetite rises and also being aware that response is forged from tens of thousands of years of evolution, we can be certain it's better to *feed it* than fight it. When you do, a message moves from your belly to your brain and says, "It's all good!" In a nutshell, this is how and why eating extra once a week stimulates your metabolism, supporting your efforts to lose unhealthy bodyfat, while it also helps you gain control over cravings.

Now, there are also numerous psychological benefits to the free day. For starters, people find they can live without some of their old favorites like unhealthy desserts, candy bars and burgers and fries *most* of the time *if* they know they can eat them *some* of the time. This really helps people stay on track and keep a *positive mindset*. And that is so important. No one wants to play a game he or she can't win. You don't want to set yourself up for failure. You don't want to create standards you can't meet. If you say, "I'm not going to eat another chocolate chip cookie from now on," and if *you* happen to like chocolate chip cookies, well, then you're setting the table for failure, so to speak. So let's not do that, okay?

Another benefit of the free day is that it creates *freedom*. Freedom from unrealistic rules, as well as freedom to make decisions for yourself. That's important because I've discovered most people are willing to draw some lines and create a framework for their eating, as long as there's an element of freedom that remains. And so I don't tell you what to eat... *you* decide for yourself. Even on your six Eating *for* Life days of the week you decide what to eat.

The free day also helps create openness, honesty and self-respect. You see, all healthy people have needs and cravings that should be *expressed*, not suppressed. Everyone I've ever met has a few "favorite foods." For me, it's double-cheese pepperoni pizza, Krispy Kreme doughnuts (the glazed ones) and carrot cake with rich cream cheese frosting. For others, it's fries and cheeseburgers or ice cream and chocolate. And for others, it's something altogether different.

Each person has his or her own favorites. Some remind them of warm moments from their childhood. Other favorites are driven by identity, region, heredity and gender. Anyway, I encourage you to eat some of *your* favorite foods on your free day, even if they are not highly nutritious. This advice goes against the grain of today's popular diet dogma, which makes eating those foods completely off limits and creates rather than resolves problems.

What I've noticed is people on diets "sneak eat" their favorite foods, and when they do, they often serve up a side dish of shame and a tall glass of guilt. This is unnecessary. With Eating *for* Life, no foods are forbidden. None! Some we only indulge in once a week, but we *never* say never... *ever*!

So please, don't deny that you have favorite fun foods, and don't pretend that your appetite for those foods is nonexistent. When you stuff those cravings down, look out! They may manifest in the most unusual places! Make no mistake, it's best to eat some of your favorite foods once a week. It's healthy, natural and normal.

Got it? Good!

Okay, now there are two types of free days: *planned* and *unplanned*.

An example of a planned free day, for me, is if I know I'm going to a Denver Broncos football game on Sunday with my brother and we intend to "get into it" and eat hot dogs, nachos, those giant pretzels and hope for overtime so we have time for popcorn and peanut M&M's as well.

As far as when you should plan your free day, that's up to you. Some set aside every Sunday to eat whatever they want. Your free day doesn't have to be the same day every week. Oftentimes, you might plan it for a special occasion. For example, Thanksgiving—there's no question, that's a free day on my calendar. So is my birthday. I don't know about you, but I really like the tradition of eating birthday cake. (I love German chocolate cake with coconut frosting!) I think most people do. It's fun, and it feels good. (By the way, what do people who follow a low-carb diet all the time eat on their birthday… a brick of Brie with bacon and candles on it? Yuck. And *boring*.)

Here's an example of an *unplanned* free day: On my last trip to New York, I got stuck at the airport with a delayed flight, missed two meals and arrived at the hotel after a *long* day to find they didn't clean out the "mini bar" like I asked them to ahead of time. Fatigue and hunger took over for a few minutes, and I lost "full awareness." When I came back to, I found a pile of crumbs and a few empty bags of Chips Ahoy and Oreo cookies, along with one-half of a broken Pringle sitting in the bottom of the can. *Oops!* Hey, it happens. Fortunately, not all that often. But when it does, I go to my journal and simply cross out my Eating *for* Life plans for the day and write "FREE DAY!" Then, if I was planning for a free day on Sunday, I simply follow the Eating *for* Lifestyle that day instead. Follow me?

This is how to utilize the free day when, despite your best efforts, your day doesn't go as planned and you end up eating wrong. This helps add flexibility and practicality to Eating *for* Life. Remember, it's what you eat *most* of the time, not some of the time, that feeds success.

Having had the opportunity to help so many thousands of people begin Eating *for* Life, I've noticed that, at first, their free days become feasts. However, what they discover is when you eat right, six days a week, and then you pig out once a week, I mean really go for it, it hurts. Stomachaches are the rule, rarely the exception. And this becomes a learning experience. Psychologists call it "aversion therapy." Kind of like when parents catch their kids with a pack of cigarettes, which they might puff on at school to try to look cool, and the parents actually "make them" smoke a few. They turn a little green, become just ill enough that cigarettes no longer seem cool; in fact, they seem disgusting.

And this is why free days tend to become self-regulating, self-limiting and part of the overall solution, not part of the problem. They teach you to manage your food intake. And this is something I point out to those who initially are concerned that their free days will be so out of control, it will cause them to gain fat, even if their six Eating *for* Life days are right on track. I haven't seen that become a real issue, long term. So don't worry about it. Even I've learned there are only so many Krispy Kreme doughnuts I can eat before I make myself absolutely, positively sick and sorry. You will too!

Some people find that on their free days they have one big meal, like a brunch with pancakes, an omelet, bacon and orange juice, and then they don't feel like eating the rest of the day. That's fine. You don't have to force-feed yourself. The point is to eat what you *want*. No more, no less. It's your free day. Do what you wish. If you eat a big lunch and don't feel like eating a big dinner, that's okay.

I've also discovered that free days help remind you of what it was like when every day was free day, so you are aware of what you're getting away from—the *ill* feeling and the energy drain created by overeating.

By the way, the afternoon of your free day is a great time to do your grocery shopping for the upcoming week. Your appetite will be completely satisfied, so the urge to buy tempting but unhealthy foods will be stuffed.

Another thing you will discover is that as you begin to learn how to plan, prepare and cook many of the Eating *for* Life meals that are featured in this book, you'll find yourself enjoying new favorite foods that are healthy and balanced with protein and carbohydrates. For example, sometimes on my free days, I'll eat Chicken Enchiladas (page 114) or Spaghetti and Meatballs (page 89), and my "freedom" is expressed by simply serving seconds, sometimes even thirds. I'll eat a little more of these healthy foods for fun, for satisfaction. But I don't make myself sick to my stomach, like I used to when free day meant a free-for-all.

With Eating *for* Life, I never feel like I'm sacrificing or suffering or starving. And I'm never bored. I enjoy eating right six days a week, and I also enjoy eating my favorite fun foods every week. And I am able to stay healthy and strong.

The free day has been one of the keys to my maintaining this approach for over a decade. It's not something I do for just a certain amount of time. It's my lifestyle. And I think it will be for you as well.

The important thing to remember is that your free day is *yours*. Have fun with it and feel free to be yourself. And, please, feel right about it because, in more ways than one, it's good for you!

Chapter 8

How I Put It All Together

So now you know all about the Eating *for* Lifestyle. You've learned what it really means to eat right. You know how to break free from the fast-food frenzy. We've separated myth from fact and have covered a great deal of information. Now it's time to put it all together—to see Eating *for* Life in action. So I'm going to show you how I personally apply the Eating *for* Lifestyle. I'll walk you through a typical day and show you what I eat, when, where and why. I'll also share a little insight, as well as a few of the valuable lessons learned along the way.

Ready? Then let's do it.

My Eating *for* Life day starts at *night*. Each evening, I invest just a few minutes planning what I'm going to eat the following day. I write it down in a journal or on an Eating *for* Life meal plan, like those shown on pages 330 to 337 of this book. Planning my meals is one of the *very* good habits that feels natural to me since I've been doing it for so long. It's easy because I have such a "consistent variety" to what I eat. It's not exactly the same every day, but there is a pattern and predictability to it.

Fast forward to sunrise. When I awake on weekdays, I'm eager to start moving, so I do. First, I drink a 16-ounce bottle of water to help hydrate my body. Then I throw on an old T-shirt, a pair of workout shorts and slip on a beat-up pair of Nikes, trot downstairs to my kitchen, have a quick cup of coffee, grab another 16-ounce bottle of water (to drink while I exercise) and scoot on over to my home gym for my morning workout ritual.

If you've read my book Body-*for*-LIFE, you know I work out first thing in the morning on an empty stomach. I don't eat before I exercise because I know, and scientific studies show, that I'll burn more fat for fuel (rather than blood sugar/glucose) during a workout on an empty stomach than I would if I had just eaten before.

My workout routine is very basic. Three days a week, I do 20 minutes of aerobic exercise. In the summertime, I'll often jog and sprint, doing interval training outdoors. In the winter, when I'm at my home in Colorado, I exercise indoors, usually performing my 20 minutes of aerobics on a recumbent stationary Lifecycle. When I'm at my home in Maui, summer or winter, I'll walk, run and jog on the beach to start my day.

Scientific studies have shown that even 20 minutes of exercise in the morning helps boost the metabolism so my body burns fat faster throughout the day. Also, morning workouts help me control my appetite. This is something else scientists have confirmed in recent years.

I also lift free weights three days a week, doing basic exercises like the bench press, shoulder press, biceps curls, triceps extensions, lunges and dumbbell squats for the legs, and a few sets of abdominal crunches for the midsection. (No, I don't train my abs every day… it's a *myth* that the more you work the midsection, the leaner it gets.)

Make no mistake, basics are best when it comes to strength training. The same 36 exercises I featured in Body-*for*-LIFE are really all you need to know to enjoy great benefits from weight training. Those were the best strength training exercises 30 years ago. Those will be the best exercises 30 years from now.

It's not hard to learn how to lift weights, but I'll tell you what, if you push yourself, every one of those darn workouts is hard! Afterwards, it's really a great feeling, though. You see, not only does a good morning workout help get the blood pumping and wake my ass up, it has also been proven to increase the body's natural "feel good" neurotransmitters, including the beta endorphins. That's one of the body's most powerful, natural good-mood enhancers. It's what joggers are referring to when they talk about the "runner's high." However, you don't have to be a long-distance runner to enjoy the positive effects of endorphins released secondary to exercise. You can get those juices flowing by simply getting up and getting going! And the more you "exert" yourself, the more you'll enjoy the "afterglow" effects of exercise and activity.

My morning workouts help set the tone for my whole day, and they give me something positive I can count on no matter what.

Anyway, after my exercise, I get showered, dressed, attempt to do something with my hair (although it doesn't always show), and then I head for the kitchen.

Typically, I give it an hour between finishing my workout and when I eat my breakfast. This is another way I'm able to extend my exercise efforts. You see, scientific studies have shown that if you don't eat for an hour after you work out, your metabolism is revved up and you'll burn even more fat for fuel.

For breakfast I usually have four pieces of cold, leftover Domino's pizza and a couple cans of Pepsi. (Just kidding… and making sure you're *still* with me here!)

For real, on the weekdays, my breakfasts are super simple—I usually have a nutrition shake, which is balanced in protein and carbohydrates and fortified with vitamins and minerals. This is no surprise to those of you who've followed my work over the years. I've been hooked on nutrition shakes since I helped start the healthy food company called MET-Rx back in the early 1990s. I used MET-Rx daily for years, and then I switched to Myoplex, a similar product developed by a company called EAS, which

I owned from 1995 to 1999. Although it has been over four years since I turned EAS over to a new management group, I still use Myoplex nutrition shakes, even though I have to stand in line to buy them at health-food stores like GNC. It's worth it, though. I like the way I feel after drinking a nutrition shake. I'm satisfied but not stuffed. And I know that I've nourished my body with the nutrients it needs—quality protein, essential carbohydrates, vitamins, minerals *and* water.

I don't skip breakfast, but I do rush through it. I know I can feed my body what it needs with a nutrition shake, which I make in the blender and takes me all of about, oh… *a minute.*

On the weekends, I'll have an omelet, whole-wheat toast, coffee and water for breakfast. Or a breakfast burrito or the Egg-Cellent Enchilada recipe (page 223).

Okay, so far so good… a sound night's sleep, water, coffee, a workout and a healthy Eating *for* Lifestyle breakfast. Always a great start!

When I get to work in the morning, I really get to work. Focus, focus, focus! Even when I'm writing a book about food, like this one, the last thing I'm thinking about throughout the morning is eating. And so I have to remind myself to eat my morning midmeal by scheduling it at 10:30 a.m. on my day planner.

Now, with Eating *for* Life, it's important not to think of these midmeals as snacks. Snacking is generally unconscious munching and crunching on something that is usually not nourishing.

Chips, crackers, candy… they offer very little nutrition, and what most people don't realize is they *stimulate* the appetite and increase cravings. *Ugh…* keep that crap away from me!

My morning midmeal consists of another nutrition shake or a portion of cottage cheese mixed with Yoplait fat-free yogurt. (I eat a lot of that stuff. I like almost all their flavors: vanilla, blueberry, strawberry, peach… yum! I think you could mix a cup of dirt in that Yoplait yogurt and it would still taste good to me!)

Between breakfast and lunch, I drink another 16-ounce bottle of water. You won't see me carrying around a bottle of water, though—I don't sit and sip—I "chug" big bottles of water like college freshmen do bottles of beer.

Lunch… that's my third Eating *for* Life meal of the day, and I typically eat that at 12:30 p.m. A turkey sandwich with lettuce, tomato, mustard on whole-wheat bread. That, and a 16-ounce bottle of water, is very simple and satisfying to me. So is a chicken breast, brown rice and broccoli. I bring lunch with me or pick it up at the local deli. Quick, nutritious. And I'm back to work. I rarely go out for lunch. Waste of time. But that may just be the way I see it. I'm moving fast, and I want to get things done.

Unlike my morning midmeal, which I typically have to be reminded of, my *body* reminds me to eat by midafternoon. So at 3:30 p.m., I'll have either another nutrition shake or another serving of yogurt and low-fat cottage cheese or an apple with cottage cheese. And another 16-ounce bottle of water. Now it takes me all of about three minutes to eat my afternoon midmeal, but I can tell you, this may very well be the most underrated meal of the day.

If I miss this meal, if I don't feed my body with a balance of protein and carbohydrates in the afternoon, I begin to lose focus, feel tired and that cuts into my work performance.

On the rare days that I miss my afternoon midmeal because of poor planning on my part, or meetings that ran overtime, or delayed airline flights, etc., I find that not only do I lose energy in the afternoon, but I'm also setting the table for a setback that evening. You see, like many people, I have the potential to binge eat at night. To get ahold of a box of cereal, crackers, cookies or ice cream late in the evening and just go hog wild. It happens once in a while. And when it does, the next day I look back at what "triggered" the binge, and almost every time it was a result of missing my afternoon midmeal. So be forewarned. Don't miss that afternoon midmeal!

Dinner… *ahhh*, dinner… my favorite meal of the day. The meal that I truly invest time to enjoy. To sit down, catch my breath, relax and divide the "go-go" part of my day from an evening of rest and relaxation. Over the last year, throughout the process of producing this book, most evenings our family gets together, and we enjoy the dinner recipes that you'll find beginning on page 79 of this book. I've enjoyed every single one of those meals. Most, several times. Among my favorites are the Chicken Pomodoro (page 183), Grilled Salmon (page 84), Spaghetti and Meatballs (page 89) and Chicken Enchiladas (page 114).

I have hearty portions for dinner. In fact, dinner is my biggest meal of the day. I don't stuff myself like a Thanksgiving turkey, but I love to leave the table fully satisfied. I know diet dogma dictates that dinner should be your smallest meal or that you shouldn't eat after 6 o'clock in the evening and other nonsense. That might look good on paper, but in the real world, it's not practical. It's just not. And I don't expect you to follow any silly rules like that. I encourage you to *enjoy* your dinners. Really make them special. Invest the time to plan and prepare, to cook and share the experience with family and friends. Sit down, relax and *eat* for goodness' sake!

When I'm at my home in Maui, I usually go out to dinner at sunset. And I order a meal very much like you'll see in the dinners featured in this book. A fresh piece of fish (seared Ahi and salmon are my favorites), a portion of brown rice or pasta, steamed spinach or broccoli and sparkling water.

One of the keys to eating right when you go out to restaurants is remembering the Right Recipe: the right foods, the right amounts, the right combinations and the right times. When you keep those four ingredients of Eating *for* Life in mind, you can almost always find something on the menu that will work for you. And if you don't see it on the menu, simply explain to the waiter or waitress what you need. More and more, you'll find food servers who are familiar with Body-*for*-LIFE and the Eating *for* Lifestyle, and they will be happy to help you out.

At restaurants, it's important to ensure you have the right amounts before you dig in. You might have to "scale down" the portions, especially the carbohydrate. And sometimes, especially for women, dinner is so big it's a "double portion," which means you can ask to have part of it boxed up, *to go*, even before you start eating, and just like that, tomorrow's lunch is already planned and prepared!

Okay… so a couple hours after dinner, I virtually always have dessert. It's my sixth Eating *for* Life meal of the day. Like midmeals, my desserts are different in that they are balanced with protein and carbohydrates *and* healthy. Dessert is fun, satisfying and provides nutrients that help my body and mind relax, recover, rebuild and renew overnight. Among my favorite desserts are Banana Cream Pudding (page 206), the Anyday Sundae (page 197) and Carrot Cake Muffins (page 211) or, *another* nutrition shake.

So that's how I put it all together. That's a typical Eating *for* Life day for me. As you can see, I exercise in the morning. I eat six meals. I drink a lot of water. I eat relatively small, easy-to-prepare, quick-to-consume meals for my breakfast, morning midmeal, lunch and afternoon midmeal. I enjoy each of those meals, but I don't necessarily sit down, celebrate and get too worked up about them. Dinners, on the other hand, I really look forward to, and I *savor*. And desserts—they really are the icing on the cake of a great day of Eating *for* Life.

Now that's typically how it goes for me six days a week. And usually, Sunday is my free day—the day I don't work out; the day I eat pretty much whatever I want. That might mean doughnuts or a danish and milk for breakfast, but not always. It might mean pizza or pasta for lunch. But only sometimes. It might be eating a hot dog and nachos at a ball game. And/or it could include a big plate of lasagna at my favorite Italian restaurant and apple pie with ice cream for dessert. On my free day, I really don't have a pattern. Sometimes I eat a lot. Sometimes I don't. I pretty much just follow my gut instinct.

By the way, if I have free day foods around the house on Sunday, like oatmeal cookies, doughnuts or Twizzlers, I make sure I get rid of them when free day fun time is over. And I often do my grocery shopping for the week after I've eaten a free day meal or two. That way my cravings are virtually nonexistent and going to the supermarket doesn't feel like I'm trapped on Temptation Island. When I'm full and satisfied, I simply stick to my Grocery Guide (like the one on pages 339 to 344).

My kitchen cabinets and pantry are very "clean." Over the years, I've learned that if I don't want to wear it, I simply don't buy it at the grocery store—I don't allow it into my home. Chips, cookies, ice cream, sugary breakfast cereals… none of that stuff looks good on me! And so I don't keep it around. It's much easier to do the *right thing* if you put yourself in the *right situation*. And a refrigerator, kitchen cabinets and pantry stocked only with the right foods makes it easier to do the right thing. At least it does for me.

So how is this working out for me? Well, at 38 years of age, I'm not doing too bad at all. My bodyfat stays between 6 percent and 7 percent, year-round. My cholesterol, triglycerides, blood pressure and blood glucose levels are all in the *very* healthy range. And I am stronger than I was 10 years ago. Overall, I'm holding up very well. All that in spite of the fact that 10 years ago I was 20 pounds overweight, already had high cholesterol and I looked like a mess! Felt like one too!

On the following page, you'll see what I look like *now* and what I looked like 10 years ago, before I knew how to put it all together. You'll notice that under the "way I was then" photo is an example of how I used to eat. And under the photo of me now, you'll see how I follow the Eating *for* Lifestyle.

I hope you find this information helpful. If you do, be sure to review the two dozen other "success stories" I've prepared and am presenting in Appendix A of this book, which starts on page 345. I learn a lot from the real-life examples of people who've succeeded in transforming their bodies and lives for the better. I think you will too.

Of course, not every day goes as planned. Sometimes I miss meals. Sometimes I overeat. Sometimes I under eat. And when that happens, I simply make a note of it, vow to do better the next time, put it behind me and *move on*.

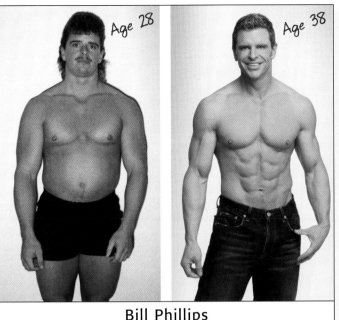

Bill Phillips

Age 38 • Golden, CO • Author/Entrepreneur
I've Maintained a 20-Pound Loss of Bodyfat for Over 10 Years

BEFORE TYPICAL DAY'S EATING:

8:00 a.m.	2 bowls of Wheaties with milk
12:00 p.m.	1 box macaroni and cheese
5:00 p.m.	Apple, banana and a quart of Gatorade (before working out)
7:30 p.m.	2 big platefuls of pasta, 1 chicken breast, iced tea
9:30 p.m.	2 bowls of Cheerios, 3 cups milk

AFTER TYPICAL DAY'S EATING:

7:45 a.m.	Cappuccino nutrition shake
10:30 a.m.	Strawberry nutrition shake
12:30 p.m.	Turkey sandwich, water
3:30 p.m.	Cottage cheese and an apple, water
6:30 p.m.	Baked chicken parmesan, pasta, spinach, water
9:00 p.m.	Banana cream pudding, water

Favorite Eating *for* Life Meal: Mom's Chicken Enchiladas (page 114)

Favorite Free Day Food: Warm oatmeal-raisin cookies and a glass of ice-cold milk!

Toughest Eating Obstacle Overcome: I did not know how to eat right back then. I was taught to "carb up" each day. I did that. And I got fat! Once I learned about balancing protein and carbs, and eating the right amounts six times a day, I achieved the results I was striving for.

Current Exercise Routine: I do 20 minutes of aerobics, first thing in the morning, three days a week, and I lift weights three days a week, first thing in the morning, on alternating days.

Favorite Benefit of the Eating *for* Lifestyle: What I love most about my experience with Eating *for* Life is sharing what I've learned with others!

I don't follow the Eating *for* Lifestyle "perfectly." No one does. Remember, it's what you do most of the time, not some of the time, with this style of eating that creates long-term, positive results.

I want to emphasize that although teaching people about health and fitness is something I enjoy, I am far from obsessed with it. I simply have developed a daily routine of eating and exercise that works. It requires a minimal investment of time and energy. And it's not at all complicated.

So all in all, what the Eating *for* Lifestyle does for me is provide a basic, balanced, scientifically safe and sound, practical approach to eating right. One which is "imperfect," flexible and *realistic*.

Following the Eating *for* Lifestyle feeds my mind, so I can work hard and stay focused. It nourishes my muscles, so I have energy to work out and the essential nutrients needed to recover and renew. It is simple to follow, so I don't have to constantly count calories or look for "hidden carbs." It's also a way I can feed my emotions—a way I can allow food to lift *or* soothe my mood.

Also, Eating *for* Life is not a "head trip." I don't have to become self-absorbed in ethereal explanations of why I eat what I eat and what that means about my "inner self." Rest assured, I'm all for self-awareness and self-actualization, but I also do my best to *not* make things more complicated than they need to be.

Eating *for* Life also just flat out feels good and *tastes* good too! There are an endless variety of foods that I can choose from, which keep me from getting bored (the downfall of many dieters). The way I eat doesn't exclude me from any social occasions or interactions, like holiday celebrations or dinners out with friends.

All in all, it's just a good, smart, fun way to eat and a very respectable and responsible way to care for myself.

There you have it—that's how I put it all together. And now, it's *your* turn to give the Eating *for* Lifestyle a try. I guarantee it will work for you, like it has for me and literally thousands of others.

Chapter 9

Questions and Answers

QUESTION: Bill, have you ever tried the low-carb diet?

ANSWER: I have. When I did, within two weeks, my muscles got so small, so fast, that people asked if I was getting sick. I not only looked like it, I *felt* like it. I was so weak I could barely lift weights and so tired by the middle of the day that I could hardly read or write.

And, irritable… *oooph!*

Man oh man, you did *not* want to be around me at that time.

And the icing on the cake of the low-carb approach (and in actuality, there would be no icing because it has sugar in it, and there would be no cake unless it were made out of beef, bacon or cheese) is that I would feel like an absolute retard when I'd go out to dinner or to my mother's or sister's house for a meal and I'd have to try to explain why I was just eating meat.

I could go on and on, but the bottom line is, low-carb diets *suck* if your priorities include being strong, *energetic* and mentally "there."

QUESTION: Do men and women need to eat different foods?

ANSWER: The basic fundaments of nutrition for men and women are the same. Eating the right foods. Eating six meals a day. And consuming the proper portions (women's portions most always being smaller than men's).

The difference between men and women from a nutritional standpoint mirrors the basic differences between men and women from a hormonal standpoint. Scientific studies have shown that women can benefit from slightly greater amounts of certain vitamins and minerals, such as folic acid, iron and calcium, which support metabolic processes that are unique to women because of their levels of estrogen, progesterone, etc.

Men can benefit from additional amounts of minerals, such as zinc and magnesium, as well as slightly higher amounts of B vitamins, all of which support healthy testosterone levels and thus, protein and fat metabolism.

QUESTION: Do I need nutrition shakes to follow Eating *for* Life?

ANSWER: Nutrition shakes can help if your days are so busy that you can't consistently find time to plan and prepare six healthy whole-food meals that are rich with essential nutrients and balanced in protein and carbohydrates.

I've utilized nutrition shakes, just like I have chicken, brown rice and broccoli, as mainstays of my Eating *for* Lifestyle, for many years. Nutrition shakes offer a very favorable and desirable advantage in terms of quality and convenient nutrition. They're also not expensive.

They provide an abundance of vitamins and minerals and other important nutrients, which means that I don't have to take a bunch of vitamin pills and capsules, morning, noon and night, to ensure that my body has each and every essential nutrient it needs to feed muscle metabolism, good health and *energy*.

I also really enjoy the taste of nutrition shakes and the way they fill me up without making me stuffed. You may or may not like them too. That is really up to *you*.

QUESTION: How many calories should I consume each day to follow Eating *for* Life? And what percentage of those calories should be from protein, carbohydrates and fat?

ANSWER: With Eating *for* Life, you don't have to count calories, but that doesn't mean calories don't count. They do.

As you may very well know, and as most experts are most certain of, when you weigh in the weight loss/fat loss of various feeding styles, there's no denying that to burn stored bodyfat for fuel, you absolutely have to create a "caloric deficit."

With Eating *for* Life, when you apply the four ingredients of the Right Recipe, without counting calories, results happen. This is because the Eating *for* Lifestyle is very satisfying. It's nutrient rich and very low in empty calories. Its effectiveness is primarily a result of satisfying survival instincts and empowering intuitive impulses, rather than fighting against them.

What this amounts to is that your cravings, your appetite, your hunger, your body's needs for nutrients are all being taken care of by eating the right foods, in the right amounts, in the right combinations, at the right times. And all of this happens, very naturally, almost effortlessly, once you get the hang of it. And this style of eating, this lifestyle, becomes habitual. And that usually takes about a month.

Anyway, in terms of calories, I don't encourage people to count them, but I have very meticulously and carefully analyzed the issue. Long story short, I can tell you that if you look at the two weeks' worth of examples of Eating *for* Life meal plans, which begin on page 330, for women, the average calorie intake per day is right around 1,545. For men, the average is right around 1,925 calories. Of those calories, approximately 38 percent are protein, 44 percent carbohydrates and 18 percent fat.

Now those are real-world numbers. That's not some fantasy or fictional formula, which cannot be replicated in the real world. There's no magic to any particular percentages of protein, carbohydrates and fat. There isn't.

There is, however, a balance. And that isn't something that you can or should determine daily. It's something that's more accurately measured weekly, even monthly.

You see, people don't become overweight because of how many calories they ate one day. And they don't develop nutrient deficiencies in that way either. What I do is assess where people are by week, by month and even three months at a time.

If you would like to know the nutritional profile of each and every Eating *for* Life meal recipe featured in this book, visit Eating*for*Life.com and click where it says "Nutrition Stats." It's *all* there for you.

One last bit of insight on this topic... the vast majority of the hundreds of thousands of people who've experienced extraordinary transformations following Eating *for* Life have no idea how many calories they're eating each day, much less the percentage of food from fat, protein, carbs. They are simply "tuned in" to their intuitive eating instincts. And nutritional analysis, statistics, carb and calorie counts are of very little concern. What really matters—what counts—for them, and me, is results. How we look, feel and how well we are living.

QUESTION: I know you've helped thousands of people transform. What are the average results? Specifically, what can I expect if I follow this Eating *for* Lifestyle *and* work out?

ANSWER: Well, for each person, the results happen at a slightly different rate. That's because while, for the most part, virtually every human is essentially the same, we are "custom designed" in certain ways. The obvious being height, skeletal structure and the color of our hair, eyes and skin.

Also unique to each of us is our metabolic rate. It's a fact that some people do burn fat faster than others. Some people can eat more without gaining weight. This, like other unique characteristics, has to do with the specific adaptations and genetic traits that helped our ancestors survive for literally tens of thousands of years before you and I showed up. Even with my Body-*for*-LIFE Program, which includes the Eating *for* Lifestyle described in this book and an exercise routine, the results vary.

For example, in reviewing specific case studies of 10 women, each the mother of two children, each 36 years of age, each who followed the program to the letter, for 12 weeks, all experienced positive results. On the upper end of the spectrum, one woman reduced her bodyfat by 37 pounds while gaining seven pounds of lean, firm, healthy muscle.

On the other end of the spectrum, one woman reduced her bodyfat by eight pounds while gaining two pounds of lean body mass. And the other eight women you would find somewhere in between. The test subjects on average lost over 17 pounds of fat in just three months, while gaining an average of 6.5 pounds of firm muscle. Men averaged 25 pounds of fat loss over 12 weeks while gaining muscle size and strength.

For specific examples and role models, review the two dozen success stories beginning on page 345. Find a transformation which inspires you and aim for that kind of change. If they can do it, so can you!

QUESTION: Do I really need to exercise? Can't I just eat right?

ANSWER: Make no mistake, exercise is very important to achieving optimal results from eating right. And it's not just because when you exercise your body burns more calories. Exercise has many other benefits. Doing just 20 minutes of aerobic exercise, three days a week, can help you control your appetite by increasing the levels of neurotransmitters that cut cravings.

For example, when a type of neurotransmitter called beta endorphins are low, at a subconscious level, and occasionally at a conscious level, we don't feel all that good. When you're not feeling good, not only will you be less optimistic, less productive, less fun to be around, you may also have a hard time controlling cravings for foods, specifically foods that contain sugar and fat. That's because eating those foods immediately increases the level of beta endorphins and lifts your mood. Unfortunately, you only get temporary relief, and often the slight lift in your mood is quickly followed by another change—a negative one—where you feel guilty about eating something that you know isn't good for you. This can become a vicious cycle. Fortunately, there's a healthy solution. And that's where physical activity comes in.

Numerous scientific studies have shown that when you jog, get on the stationary bike and pedal away, or even get outside and go for a brisk walk for at least 20 minutes, or lift weights, at least three times a week, your beta endorphin levels go up. And this helps you control your appetite.

Make no mistake, developing healthy ways to control your appetite is one of the most important keys to succeeding in the short and long term with Eating *for* Life.

QUESTION: Bill, what should I eat for the holidays?

ANSWER: Whatever you want! Really. It's so silly to try to cut calories or carbohydrates or follow some other stupid dieting technique on holidays like Thanksgiving, Christmas, the 4th of July, Labor Day or other special occasions like your birthday.

I just make those days free days, and I eat whatever the tradition calls for. Like on Thanksgiving, I eat as much turkey, mashed potatoes and stuffing covered with gravy, cranberry sauce and pumpkin pie as anyone else. It's my free day. It's my day to eat whatever I want and to do so *without* guilt!

Don't underestimate how much guilt—how much self-reproach—can eat away at the confidence you need to make a change for the better.

Trying to "diet" on holidays… don't even talk to me about it! And don't you even think about it! Remember, it's what you do *most* of the time, not some of the time or on special occasions, that makes or breaks your efforts to live a good life in a great body!

Relax, *lighten up*, and you just might! Okay?

QUESTION: Is it okay if I follow your Eating *for* Life but adjust the recipes so they're low carb?

ANSWER: Well, first things first, *you* can do whatever *you* want!

But, in terms of what I recommend, I suggest that if you're following the low-carb diet, that you follow it as strictly as you can. In that case, I'd suggest you pick up one of Dr. Atkins' books and utilize the recipes and meal plans he suggested, before he died.

My experience has been that when you "crossbreed" health, fitness, weight-loss and nutritional theories that are as different as Eating *for* Life and Atkins, you don't create an evolutionary "hybrid," you form a mutated mush of extra nothing. So please, go with one or the other. Don't mix and match. Okay?

QUESTION: What if I'm not losing fat but I'm eating six meals a day and balancing my protein and carbohydrates?

ANSWER: Okay… here's how you "troubleshoot" with Eating *for* Life. You start by going back to the four ingredients of the Right Recipe, which I thoroughly explained in Chapter 6. Then you ask and answer the following questions:

Am I eating the *right foods?*
Am I eating the *right amounts?*
Am I eating the *right combinations?*
Am I eating at the *right times?*

What I've discovered is that people can become their own coach and counselor when they regularly (for example, once a week) ask and answer those questions.

When I can feel some fat building up on my belly, I typically find *two* "problem areas." It starts by missing one of my midmeals (by not eating at the right times), and then the trouble manifests by overeating (eating the *wrong* amounts—eating too much) at dinner and/or dessert.

Once I'm aware of what's wrong, I can make a conscious decision to make it right by better planning and preparation. And in just a week, I am back on track.

Remember, the Eating *for* Lifestyle is not perfect. It's not something I follow perfectly, but it is a very *forgiving* way of feeding yourself.

With the way our modern lives have become so hectic, it's not hard to get sidetracked from time to time. Fortunately, with the Eating *for* Lifestyle, it's easy to get back on track.

Remember to ask yourself those four questions about the Right Recipe. Perhaps even keep a journal, and ask and answer them in writing, once a week. This really helps me, and it may very well work for you too!

QUESTION: How can I ask you more questions about Eating *for* Life?

ANSWER: If and when you have more questions, *please* ask me for the answers. You can do so by visiting the "Q&A" section of Eating*for*Life.com or by writing to me at Eating *for* Life, c/o Bill Phillips, P.O. Box 16009, Golden, CO 80402.

I promise that I, along with the entire Eating *for* Life team, including our researchers and culinary experts, are committed to giving you the highest level of care and support. We will do *everything* we can to help satisfy your appetite for accurate answers to any and every question you might ask. We may not *always* know the precise response—there may not always be a "right answer" to every question, but we will do our best to help you, guide you and *encourage* you, to the fullest extent of our abilities.

Rest assured, *we are here* to help you succeed! We are standing by, ready, willing and able to support your efforts to become leaner, stronger, healthier and happier! ☺

Chapter 10

Countdown to Cooking

I don't buy into a lot of clichés and sayings. You know, the pop culture quasi philosophies, "Just do it." "Rock on." "Have a Coke and a smile." Yeah... *whatever*.

However, as I prepare to present this final chapter of your Eating *for* Life guide to great nutrition, there's one saying which rings true that I'd like to share with you. It goes something like this...

"If you give a man a fish, you feed him for *a day*. But if you teach him *how* to fish, you feed him for a *lifetime*."

You've heard that before, huh? I thought so.

What I think that centuries-old message means is: A quick fix *fails fast*. But practical knowledge *always lasts*.

With that in mind, the contribution I want to make is to *empower you* with the knowledge and confidence you need to take care of yourself, now *and* far into the future.

I feel very strongly about this. As your guide, my deep-down desire is for you to become *independent* rather than dependent on me, or anyone else.

As I see it, far too many people in America today are forced to have others feed them because they simply don't know how to feed themselves. The vast majority don't know how to "fish." And so this very important part of a healthy style of living is delegated to entities where making money is the main motive—where your fitness takes a back seat on the bus but your financial contribution to these multibillion-dollar enterprises' bottom line flies first class. Make no mistake, it's time to order up a change for the better instead of settling for second servings of the same old slop which is causing the big fat problem.

Having read the words I've written and assimilated the information I have served you thus far in the first nine chapters, I know that you *know* what to do. You know about the dieting dilemma, the fast-food frenzy, and you're also aware of the four ingredients of the Right Recipe. So now it's time to give you the final countdown to cooking so you can *apply* this information and begin to enjoy greater health, reduced bodyfat, higher energy and a richer quality of life.

The first thing I want to emphasize is that *anyone* can learn to cook, and virtually everyone should. It's a sorry sign of the times that many people consider cooking an unusual and even rare talent. The fact is, cooking, being able to prepare your own meals and *feed* yourself and your family, is a very rewarding skill and one that you can succeed at from the get-go. Especially with the Eating *for* Life meal recipes, which await your arrival, just eight pages from now!

I can tell you from firsthand experience that Eating *for* Life meal recipes are indeed as delicious as they are nutritious. By design, the vast majority are *very* easy to prepare. In fact, you don't have to be a chef or culinary expert to make these meals magnificent... you simply need to plan, prepare and then patiently follow the directions that are provided for each and every meal recipe.

Next, I want you to know that even though most people bite into the misperception that they don't have time to cook, the reality is we *all* do.

The idea that fast food is so much more "convenient" than home-cooked meals is a notion that isn't worth its weight in salt. I'm well aware of how valuable time is. But the myth that eating fast food, ordering takeout or going to restaurants, night after night, somehow saves you time is fiction, a fallacy, it *is* false! The fact is, it requires *less* time to cook the vast majority of nutritious, delicious Eating *for* Life meals presented in this book, in the comfort of your own home, than it does to call for a pizza and wait for it to be delivered.

When I began preparing Eating *for* Life, I knew that convenience, practicality and time efficiency all needed to be in favor of this healthy way of nourishing your body, your mind, your emotions. And all that, *it is*.

Another reward of the Eating *for* Lifestyle, which you will quickly discover, is that it is something special you can share with others—your spouse, your children, family and friends. Not one of them will ever shun a well-prepared, delicious, nutritious Eating *for* Life meal that you serve them. You'll know you're sharing a healthy style of living, of nourishing the body the right way, which is important to you. However, all they may recognize is that you're feeding them a meal that looks good and tastes great.

What a wonderful thing that is about Eating *for* Life meals—they're so rich with nutrition and based on such sound, scientific principles of eating right that they're good for children and adults alike. Unlike extreme diets, such as those that exclude entire healthy food groups, Eating *for* Life serves up balanced and nutritious meals, which intuitively appeal to virtually anyone and everyone.

Few things are as gratifying as planning, preparing and then serving an Eating *for* Life meal, which results in rave reviews at the dinner table without your even boasting about its nutritional strength. I want you to experience that feeling. I really do.

But before you start cooking, please review the following final countdown, which has been carefully prepared with the input of my sister, Shelly, who has worked hundreds of hours in the kitchen to help me with this book.

Countdown to Cooking

Six...

At this stage, consider reorganizing or "transforming" your kitchen. Make it an area that is focused on food. A place for you to keep the essential appliances and utensils for meal preparation. An area where there is a place for everything and everything is in its place.

Consider clearing away the countertops and moving stacks of mail and the kids' homework to another area.

Then, open your cupboards and drawers and organize the pots, pans, long-handled spoons, spatulas and other utensils so they are neatly stored and are within easy reach.

Take stock of your kitchen equipment and tools. Decide what, if anything, you need to add (see the list of Kitchen Essentials on page 391).

Also, invest time to rid your pantry and refrigerator of old, stale stuff, and take time to toss food that is not good for you and that is *not* part of your new Eating *for* Lifestyle. Clear out the old to make room for the new!

You'll feel great when you complete your kitchen makeover! And you'll be ready for the next step.

Five...

Now, begin to review the Eating *for* Life recipes featured in this book. Notice that each is a meal that includes the right foods (ones that are high in nutrients and low in empty calories) and the right combinations of protein and carbohydrates. Each meal recipe has been specifically designed for the Eating *for* Lifestyle.

Take your time and enjoy your recipe review. Look for dinners, desserts, breakfasts, lunches, midmeals and nutrition shakes that appeal to your particular preferences. When you're ready, begin to make selections. Decide which meals you will make first, and then, following the example meal plans on pages 330 to 333, record your own custom menu on the blank meal plans, beginning on page 334.

Since dinner is my favorite meal of the day, I plan my dinners first, then desserts, breakfasts, lunches and midmeals. (That's why I've placed the Eating *for* Life meal recipes in that order in this book.)

I can't emphasize enough how important it is to plan your meals ahead of time. When you plan, you can prepare. You set the table for your success. That will not only help you eat right, it will reduce stress. There will be no more last-minute, desperate decisions of what's for dinner, and then either settling for fast food or wasting precious time and energy with a mad dash to and through the grocery store, when you deserve to be dining, resting, relaxing and nourishing your health.

Four...

Once you have made your meal plan, refer to the recipe ingredients to gather your grocery list, using the very thorough grocery guide, which begins on page 339.

Now, when you're following the Eating *for* Lifestyle, you'll be determining the right amounts of protein and carbohydrate right foods by the portion sizes. Remember, for proteins like chicken, fish and beef, that's an amount roughly equal in size to the palm of *your* hand. And for carbohydrates like a potato, yam, brown rice and pasta, a portion is roughly equivalent to the size of *your* clenched fist. As you'll discover, those are easy standards to follow, once you get the hang of it.

However, when you're grocery shopping, most proteins, like chicken breasts, you'll be buying by the *ounce*. And so, to help you out, here are some "quick conversions" for you. For me and most guys, a portion of chicken breast is about 5 ounces. And for most gals, it's about 3 ounces. Typically, the proper portion for women will be about 30 to 40 percent smaller than it is for men.

That's why, when it's necessary to list an ingredient like chicken, fish or beef, the amount of that ingredient needed to make "4 servings" is an average between the right portion for men and women.

Notice that many of the recipes call for portions of certain ingredients, usually the protein and carbohydrates. When the recipe calls for "4 portions chicken breast (about 1 lb)," that is the *average* for four people. Your portions may be a little more or less, depending on what the *right amount* is for you and those you will be serving.

When a recipe calls for fish (other than canned tuna), the average portion is 6 ounces in consideration that most fish has some skin and bones, and also loses more weight as it cooks. If "4 portion-size potatoes" are listed, simply consider who you will be feeding and choose the proper portion for each person.

Now remember, Eating *for* Life is not "perfect." And it's not necessary for it to be absolutely precise. Approximating portions is perfectly fine.

Three...

Okay... now we're really getting somewhere. Having made your meal plans, and your grocery guide in hand, it's time to invest in the market—to head for the grocery store and stock up on your inventory.

If you've planned a week's worth of meals in advance, you can save a great deal of time by doing all of your grocery shopping once a week as well. A helpful hint is to go to the store on Sunday, in the afternoon, after you've eaten a few free day meals and cravings are under complete control.

Many people find that in the past, since they had no plan, they were drawn into the supermarket maze—led down one aisle of temptation after another, where you are at the mercy of multimillion-dollar merchandising and marketing manipulation. Luring you, tempting you and virtually trapping you. Almost without even being aware of it, you find yourself standing at the check-out aisle with a cart full of crap that is destined to end up being stored *not* in the kitchen but on *you*—as bodyfat in the belly, hips, thighs, as well as inside the body, slowly but surely clogging arteries and eventually creating catastrophe. A great deal of the nutritional damage that's being done in America today begins in the grocery store. When you have no plan, no list, no grocery guide, your odds of getting it right are slim to none. But that won't happen to you! Not anymore.

All you need to do is follow your grocery guide from one area of the supermarket to the next, just as it's laid out on the form that begins on page 339. Start in the produce section, filling your cart with fruits and vegetables, then making a beeline for the deli counter. (Ignore those Doritos and Oreos sticking out from the end aisle, which almost block your way!) Then move on. Imagine you are on a *mission!* You are not bumbling, browsing and then buying unhealthy, highly processed and also highly profitable foods.

Get in, get what you need and *get out*. Got it? Good!

Two...

After selecting Eating *for* Life meals that appeal to your particular preferences, invest a few minutes of your valuable time to read and review the recipes. You'll notice that each provides you with standard information including the *preparation time* and the *number of servings*.

Rest assured, we have tested the preparation time of all 150 Eating *for* Life recipes. One of the things I'm sure you'll notice is that it doesn't take all that long to make meals that look and taste *magnificent!* For example, even the more elaborate dinners, like Chicken Pomodoro (page 183), take only 30 minutes. And hearty Spaghetti and Meatballs (page 89) requires an investment of only 40 minutes. Shrimp Scampi (page 167), 25 minutes.

Breakfasts, lunches and midmeals require even less of an investment of your precious time. For example, Golden Pancakes (page 220) take only 15 minutes. Midmeals and nutrition shakes can easily be prepared in as little as 3 minutes!

Keep in mind that everyone works at a different speed and that you'll probably get faster after you've made a meal a time or two. The preparation times were tested in well-organized kitchens using some "already readied" foods such as boneless, skinless chicken breast, shredded cheese and prewashed baby spinach leaves.

Depending on your kitchen, ingredients, appliances and even the elevation you live at, your preparation time can vary a little.

Each recipe also lists the number of servings it makes. Servings can be adjusted to meet your needs—the number of people you are feeding plus "planned-overs." Remember, planned-overs are extra servings of meals that you prepare for the next day's lunch or freeze, then thaw, for fast premade future dinners.

Most recipes can easily be cut in half or doubled (tripled or even quadrupled) just by dividing or multiplying the amount of each ingredient. If you are doubling (or more), the preparation time will usually be a little longer as you will have more food to chop and slice. The actual cooking time will usually be a little longer too. If the recipe calls for sautéing or stir-frying, you might find it easier to do it in batches. (If you overload a skillet, it can take a long time to cook.)

Likewise, if you are preparing less servings than the original recipe, preparation time may be a little shorter. In either case, use the original cooking time as a reference point and monitor the food closely for the desired results.

As for baking time for muffins, brownies, cheesecake and casseroles like Chili Rellenos and Turkey Bacon Quiche, it is best to make the full recipe.

Remember that this is a learning process and your cooking skills will improve over time—that's all part of the fun and the feeling of pride you enjoy when you become better and better!

One...

Now it's time to prepare your planned meal. You are officially "cooking" at this point.

A few basics as you begin: Wash and dry your hands, before and after handling food; change the towels and dish cloths every day; thoroughly rinse fresh fruits and vegetables before eating or using in recipes; be *sure* to wash cutting boards, knives and all utensils after every use, especially after handling raw chicken, turkey, meats or fish; don't put any ready-to-eat foods on a surface where raw chicken, turkey, meats or fish have been prepared; and after you cook, be sure to refrigerate or freeze planned-overs as soon as possible.

With all the above given its due consideration, move forward... open this book to the recipe that you'll be preparing, read it through and leave it open for reference. Then line up all of the ingredients on your kitchen counter, in the order you will use them. You'll notice that the order in which the ingredients are listed is the order they will be used in the recipe.

Then, follow the directions to prepare each meal. These directions have been developed carefully, after a great deal of testing, and I can guarantee you will find the results quite satisfying.

Now while the food is cooking, set the table, literally, with nice plates, silverware, glasses, napkins, etc. When you serve great food on a well-set table, it's even better!

When your Eating *for* Life meal is ready, serve *and* savor it. Sit down, relax and begin to enjoy the rich rewards of the Eating *for* Lifestyle. ☺

* Rest assured, when you begin planning, preparing and cooking, you'll have questions. The good news is, we have answers. Visit us at Eating*for*Life.com and we'll help you!

Dinners

Zesty Italian Chicken

Chicken marinated in Italian dressing
over fettuccine and fresh spinach

Servings: 2
Preparation Time: 50 minutes

INGREDIENTS

2 portions chicken breast (about $\frac{1}{2}$ lb)

$\frac{1}{4}$ cup fat-free Italian dressing

2 portions fettuccine (about 4 oz uncooked)

1 cup low-fat pasta sauce

2 cups baby spinach leaves

2 Tbsp reduced-fat Parmesan cheese, grated

—— Tasteful Tip ——

*To bring out even more flavor in this delicious recipe, plan ahead and marinate the chicken overnight or while you are at work. Simply place the Italian dressing and chicken breasts in a large Ziploc® plastic bag, and squeeze it a bit to make sure the chicken is coated with marinade. Then, place the bag on a large plate and **refrigerate.**

DIRECTIONS

1 Marinate chicken breasts in Italian dressing for at least 30 minutes prior to cooking.*

2 Preheat grill to high. Prepare fettuccine according to its package directions.

3 Place marinated chicken on hot grill and cook for about 6 minutes; turn and grill for about 6 more minutes, until no longer pink in the center.

4 In a small saucepan, warm pasta sauce over medium heat.

5 Divide spinach leaves between two separate plates. Layer portions of warm fettuccine and grilled chicken breasts over spinach leaves.

6 Top with pasta sauce and Parmesan cheese, serve and enjoy! ☺

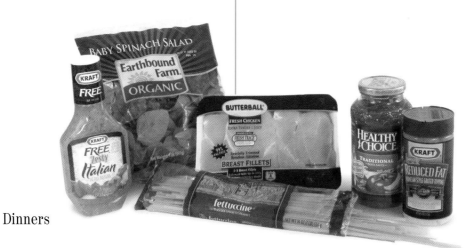

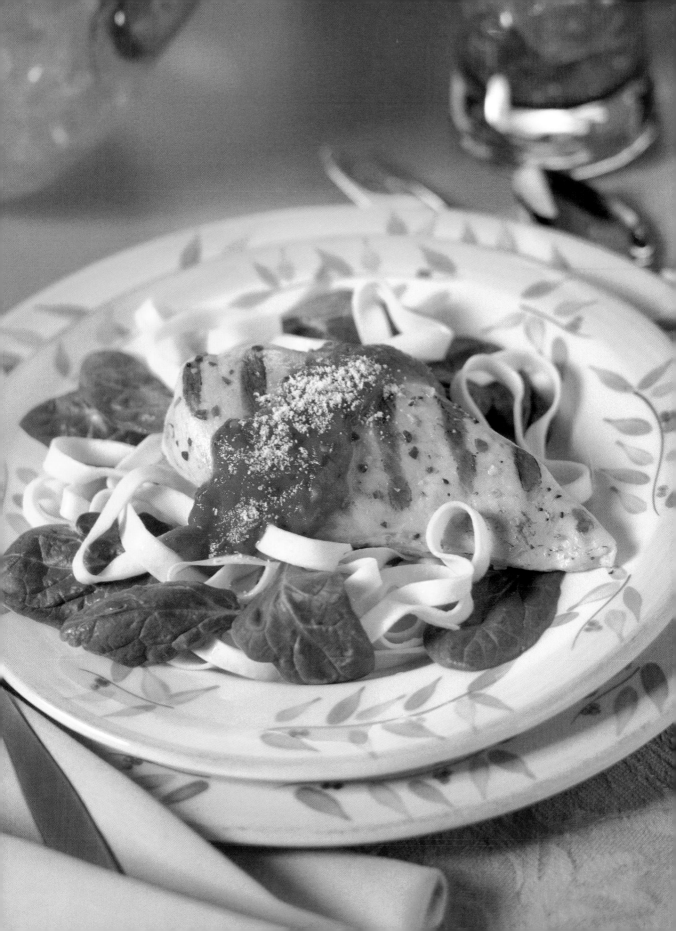

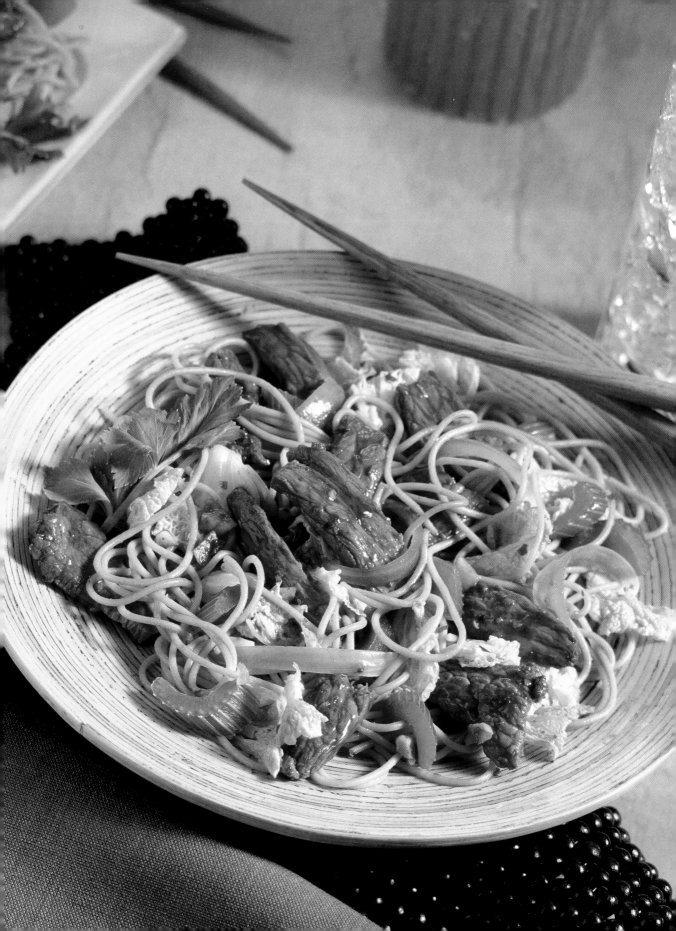

Asian Beef Stir-Fry

Peppered steak strips with oriental-style vegetables and noodles

Servings: 4
Preparation Time: 30 minutes

INGREDIENTS

4   portions spaghetti (about 8 oz uncooked)

4   portions lean steak (about 1 lb)

⅛   tsp crushed red pepper flakes

3   cloves garlic, minced

1   onion, sliced

4   celery stalks, sliced

1   head napa cabbage, shredded

½   cup lite soy sauce

———— Tasteful Tip ————

When selecting the cut of beef for stir-frying, look for a naturally lean cut, such as top sirloin, top round, top loin or flank steak, which are bursting with bold beef flavors!

DIRECTIONS

1 Prepare spaghetti according to its package directions; drain and set aside.

2 While the spaghetti is cooking, slice steak lengthwise into 2-inch strips. Cut crosswise into ⅛-inch-thick slices.

3 Lightly coat a large skillet or wok with cooking spray. Over medium-high heat, stir-fry red pepper flakes and garlic for 1 minute.

4 Add the steak strips to the skillet, stir-fry just until no longer pink, approximately 2 minutes. Remove the steak from skillet and set aside.

5 Lightly recoat the skillet with cooking spray. Stir-fry onion and celery until tender, approximately 5 minutes. Add cabbage and cook until crisp-tender, approximately 2 more minutes.

6 Return steak to the skillet. Add cooked spaghetti and lite soy sauce; mix gently and heat thoroughly.

7 Divide into 4 portions, serve and enjoy! ☺

Grilled Salmon

Sweet-baked yam and salmon fillet
on a bed of sautéed spinach and mushrooms

Servings: 2
Preparation Time: 50 minutes

INGREDIENTS

2   portion-size yams

1   lemon, halved, divided

2   portions salmon fillet (about 12 oz)

2   tsp olive oil

8 oz fresh mushrooms, sliced

1   bag (5 oz) baby spinach leaves

—————— Tasteful Tip ——————

To keep the salmon fillet from sticking to the grill, place a small amount of olive oil on a paper towel and lightly coat the grill *before* preheating it.

DIRECTIONS

1 Preheat oven to 450° F.

2 Place yams on a baking sheet and bake until tender, about 45 minutes.

3 After yams have baked for about 25 minutes, preheat grill to medium.

4 Squeeze half the lemon over salmon fillets and brush with olive oil. Place salmon on grill and cook until opaque throughout, about 5 minutes on each side.

5 While salmon is cooking, lightly coat a large skillet with butter-flavored cooking spray and place over medium-high heat. Add mushrooms and sauté for 3 minutes. Add spinach and sauté until wilted, about 3 more minutes.

6 Place a portion of salmon on a bed of spinach along with a portion-size yam on each plate. Squeeze remaining lemon over salmon and spinach. Serve and enjoy! ☺

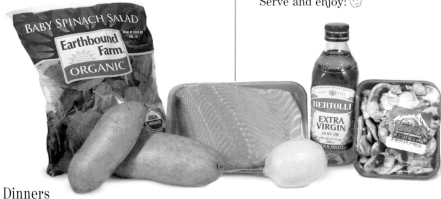

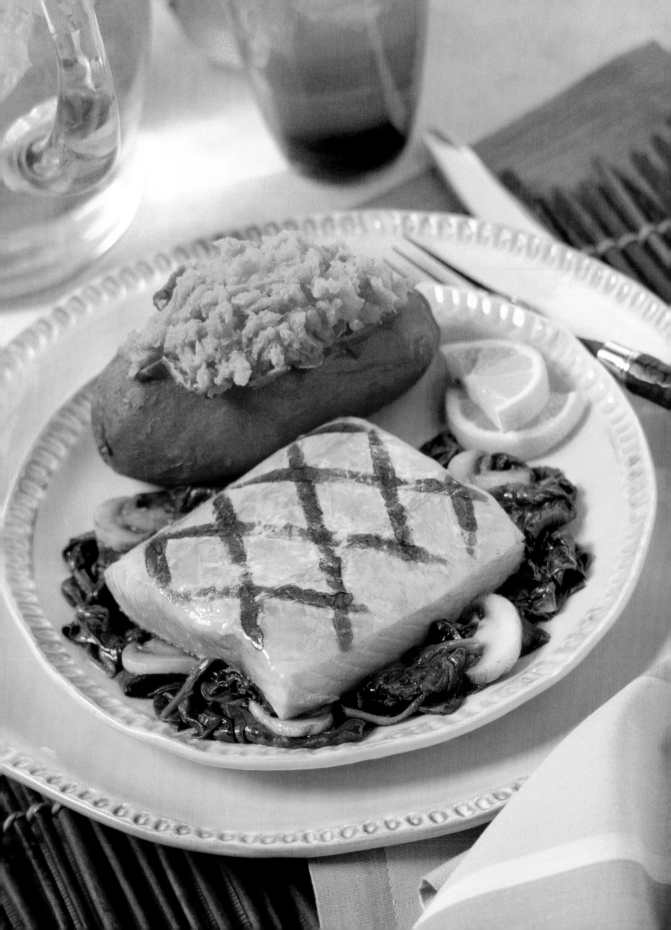

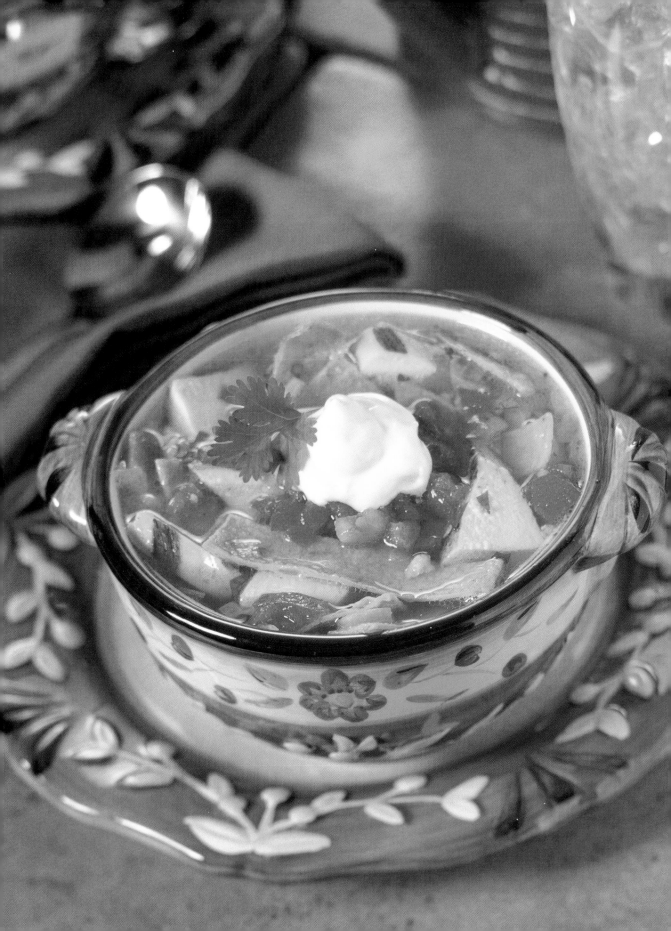

Santa Fe Chicken Soup

Spicy chicken in green chili broth
with crisp tortilla strips, salsa and sour cream

Servings: 4
Preparation Time: 55 minutes

INGREDIENTS

⅓ cup brown rice (uncooked)

4 portions chicken breast (about 1 lb)

1 lime, halved

2 tsp taco seasoning

6 corn tortillas

1 Tbsp olive oil

1 clove garlic, minced

½ onion, chopped

1 can (4 oz) diced green chilies

6 cups fat-free, reduced-sodium chicken broth

4 Tbsp salsa

¼ cup fat-free sour cream

2 Tbsp cilantro, chopped

——— Tasteful Tip ———

Santa Fe Chicken Soup is a delicious and nutritious "planned-over." Consider making extra servings and storing them in portion-size (about two cups) air-tight Tupperware® containers; refrigerate for use in one or two days, or freeze for up to two months. (Store without the tortilla strips and garnish.) Microwave to reheat for quick lunches and dinners.

DIRECTIONS

1 Cook brown rice according to its package directions. While the rice is cooking, place chicken breasts in a shallow dish; cover with lime juice, and lightly coat both sides with taco seasoning. Then place chicken on a hot grill and cook for approximately 6 minutes on each side. Let the chicken cool slightly, then cut it into strips and set aside.

2 Preheat oven to 350° F and cut corn tortillas into ½-inch strips, then place them on a baking sheet. Bake for about 15 minutes or until they are crispy, then set aside.

3 While the tortilla strips are baking, heat olive oil in a large pot over medium heat. Add garlic and onion; sauté until the onion is transparent, about 8 minutes.

4 Add cooked rice to the pot and sauté for 3 minutes. Add green chilies and sauté for 2 more minutes. Then pour fat-free chicken broth into the mixture and bring it to a boil. Add sliced chicken and reduce heat to low. Simmer for about 25 minutes.

5 Place a few baked tortilla strips in the bottom of bowls, and spoon about a fourth of the soup into each. Garnish each bowl with a few more tortilla strips, a spoonful of salsa, fat-free sour cream and cilantro. Serve and enjoy! ☺

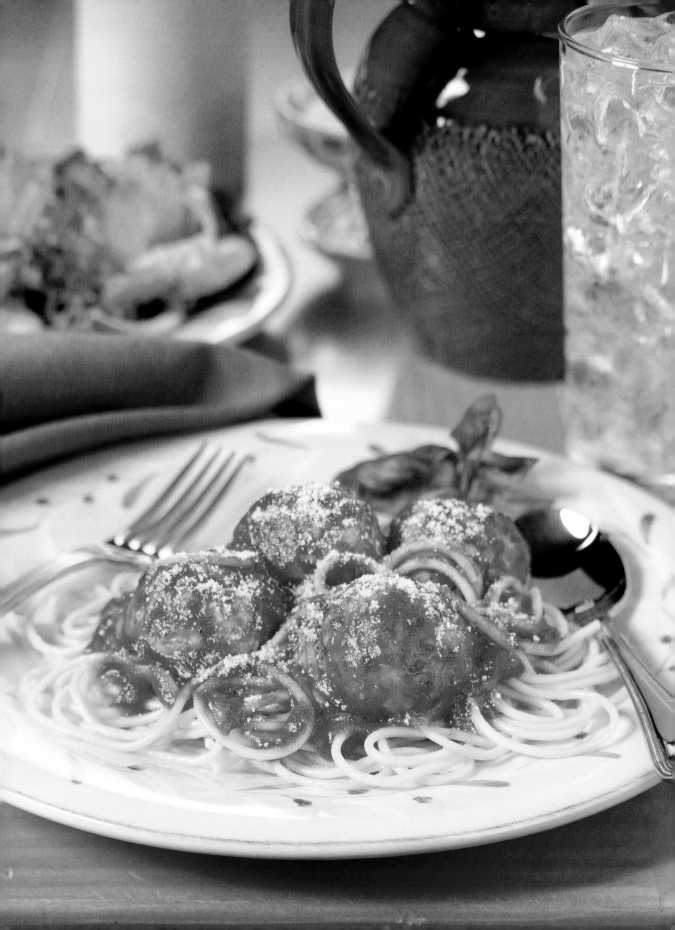

Spaghetti and Meatballs

Hearty turkey meatballs in a rich Italian tomato sauce over traditional spaghetti

Servings: 6
Preparation Time: 40 minutes

INGREDIENTS

6 portions lean ground turkey (about 1 1/2 lbs)

2 egg whites

1/2 cup dry breadcrumbs

1/4 cup water

1/2 onion, finely chopped

2 cloves garlic, minced

1/4 cup fresh parsley, minced

2 tsp dried basil

1 tsp ground black pepper

3 cups low-fat marinara pasta sauce

6 portions spaghetti (about 12 oz uncooked)

1/4 cup reduced-fat Parmesan cheese

DIRECTIONS

1 Preheat oven broiler.

2 In a large mixing bowl, combine turkey, egg whites, breadcrumbs, water, onion, garlic, parsley, basil and black pepper. Mix ingredients thoroughly and then shape into 1 1/2-inch diameter meatballs.

3 Arrange meatballs on a baking sheet and place under broiler for 10 to 12 minutes, turning occasionally until they are browned on all sides.

4 In a large saucepan, combine pasta sauce and cooked meatballs. Simmer over low heat until warmed thoroughly, about 20 minutes.

5 While the pasta sauce is simmering, prepare spaghetti according to its package directions.

6 Place a portion of spaghetti on each plate, cover with a portion of meatballs and pasta sauce, then top with Parmesan cheese. Serve and enjoy! ☺

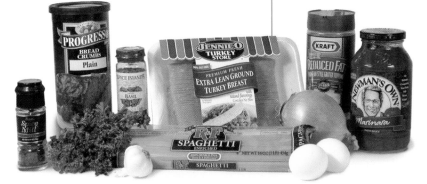

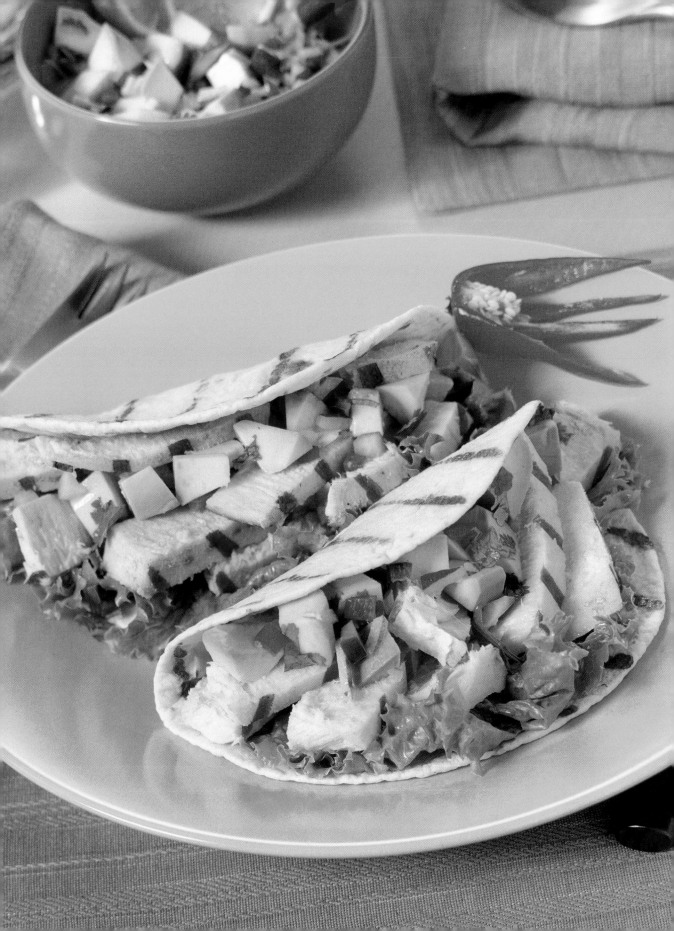

Grilled Fish Soft Tacos

Tangy avocado salsa and grilled fish in a warm flour tortilla

Servings: 4

Preparation Time: 35 minutes

INGREDIENTS

1 Tbsp olive oil

4 limes, halved, divided

5 cloves garlic, minced, divided

2 tsp ground cumin, divided

4 portions swordfish or tuna (about 1½ lbs)

1 ripe avocado, peeled, pitted and diced

¼ red onion, minced

2 jalapeños, seeded and minced

2 Tbsp fresh cilantro, chopped

8 (6-inch) flour tortillas

8 lettuce leaves

DIRECTIONS

1 Preheat grill to medium.

2 Combine olive oil, juice of 3 limes, 4 garlic cloves and 1 tsp cumin in a shallow bowl or pie plate. Then add fish to this marinade and let it soak up the flavors for 15 minutes at room temperature, turning once after about 7 minutes.

3 While fish is marinating, in a separate small mixing bowl, stir together the remaining lime juice, garlic and cumin with diced avocado, onion, jalapeños and cilantro.

4 Place marinated fish on hot grill and cook for approximately 5 minutes, turn and grill for approximately 5 more minutes, until opaque throughout. Place cooked fish on a cutting board, let it cool slightly, then slice into thin strips.

5 While the grill is still hot, place tortillas directly on it and grill them for about 30 seconds on each side.

6 Place two tortillas on each plate. Put a lettuce leaf in each tortilla, fill with a portion of grilled, sliced fish, and top with tangy avocado salsa. Fold the tortillas over, serve and enjoy! ☺

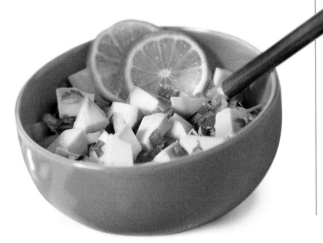

Homestyle Turkey Meatloaf

*Lean ground turkey in a traditional meatloaf style
with mashed potatoes and fresh green beans*

Servings: 6
Preparation Time: 1 hour, 15 minutes

INGREDIENTS

1 1/2 lbs lean ground turkey

1 onion, chopped

4 egg whites

1 cup salsa

3/4 cup old-fashioned oats, uncooked

1 pkg Knorr® Vegetable Soup mix

1/4 tsp ground black pepper

1/2 cup ketchup

6 portions red potatoes

2 lbs green beans

3/4 cup skim milk

2 Tbsp Butter Buds

—— Tasteful Tip ——

Meatloaf makes a great "planned-over." Consider making an extra loaf and freezing it. Cool it completely, then cover tightly with plastic wrap. Overwrap it with aluminum foil, and store it in the freezer for up to two months.

DIRECTIONS

1 Preheat oven to 350° F.

2 In a large mixing bowl, combine ground turkey, onion, egg whites, salsa, oats, soup mix and black pepper. Press mixture into 9" x 5" loaf pan and spread ketchup over top. Bake in preheated oven until meatloaf is no longer pink in the center and juice is clear, about 60 minutes.

3 Approximately 25 minutes after putting the meatloaf in the oven, cut potatoes into 1-inch chunks. Place cut potatoes in a large saucepan, cover with cold water and bring to a boil over high heat. Reduce heat to medium and simmer until tender, about 20 minutes.

4 Cut stems off green beans and place in a large saucepan with 1 inch of water in the bottom. Heat to boiling over high heat; reduce heat and simmer, uncovered, for 6 to 8 minutes or until crisp-tender; drain.

5 Remove meatloaf from oven and let sit for 5 minutes before slicing.

6 Drain the potatoes and return them to the pan. Mash while adding skim milk a little at a time. Add Butter Buds and mash vigorously until potatoes are light and fluffy.

7 Place a portion of meatloaf and mashed potatoes along with about a cup of green beans on each plate. Serve and enjoy! ☺

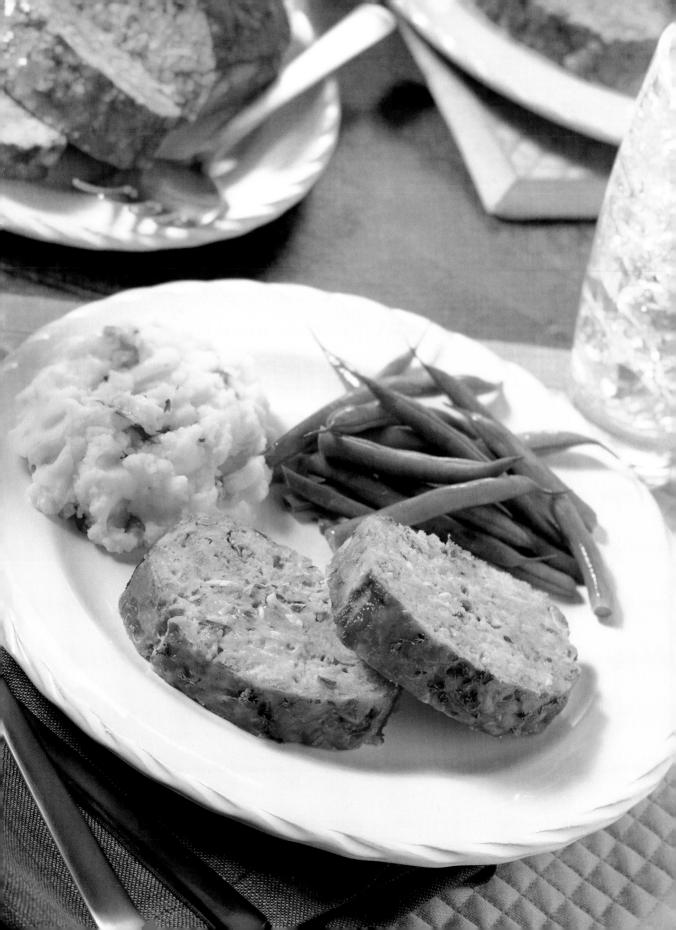

Mediterranean Halibut

*Lemon-seasoned halibut fillet, cooked "campfire style"
with cannellini beans, fresh tomato and basil*

Servings: 2
Preparation Time: 25 minutes

INGREDIENTS

- 2 sheets (12" x 18" each) heavy-duty aluminum foil

- 1 can (15 oz) cannellini beans, drained and rinsed

- 3 Roma tomatoes, diced

- ¼ cup fresh basil, sliced

- 2 portions halibut fillet (about 12 oz), skin removed

- ½ tsp lemon-pepper seasoning

- 1 lemon, sliced

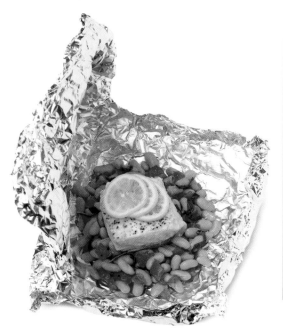

DIRECTIONS

1 Preheat grill to medium-high. Fold foil sheets in half lengthwise to crease, then unfold. Lightly coat the foil with cooking spray.

2 Divide beans into 2 portions and spoon onto foil in the center of the right half. Layer each with half the diced tomatoes and sliced basil. Place a portion of halibut fillet on top. Sprinkle halibut with lemon-pepper seasoning and top with lemon slices.

3 Fold foil over the top of the halibut, leaving room for air circulation. Close packet by double folding the 3 open foil edges.

4 Place foil packets on grill and lower cover. Grill until halibut is opaque throughout, about 14 minutes.

5 Use tongs to remove foil packets from grill. Open packets carefully and spoon contents onto plates. Serve and enjoy! ☺

——— Tasteful Tip ———

This flavorful meal can also be prepared in the oven. Simply place sealed foil packets on a baking sheet and cook in your oven at 450° F for about 18 minutes.

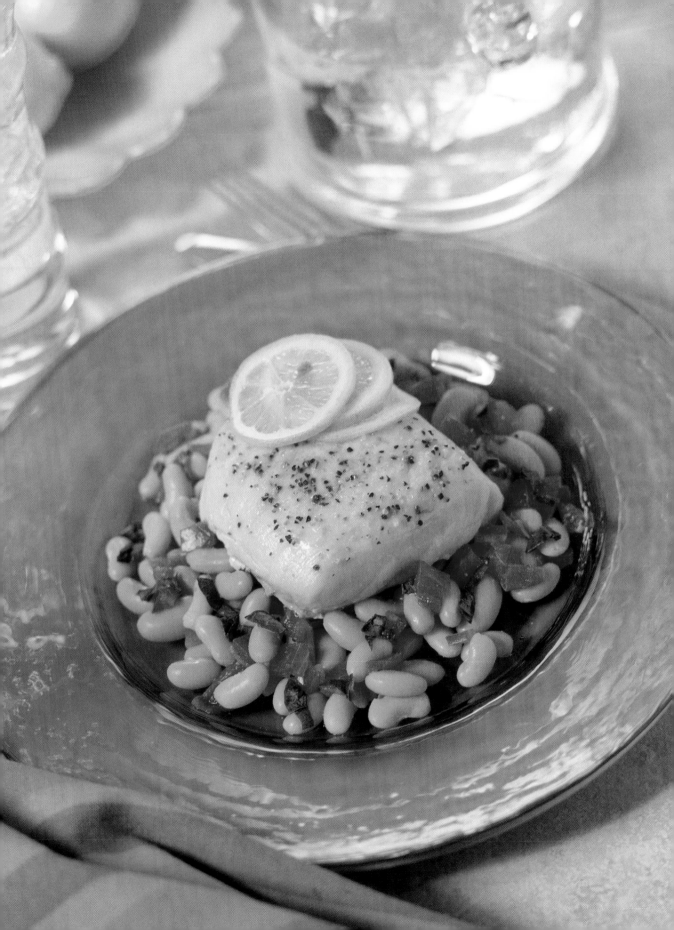

Lettuce Wraps

Crisp iceberg lettuce around a Chinese-spiced
stir-fry with ground turkey and crunchy water chestnuts

Servings: 4
Preparation Time: 30 minutes

INGREDIENTS

1   bag (12 oz) soybeans with pods (edamame)

4   fresh shiitake mushrooms

7   stalks napa cabbage

1   lb lean ground turkey

$\frac{1}{2}$ onion, chopped

2   Tbsp hoisin sauce

1   Tbsp lite soy sauce

$\frac{1}{4}$ tsp five-spice powder

1   (8-oz) can sliced water chestnuts, drained

12 large leaves iceberg lettuce

—— Tasteful Tip ——

These lettuce wraps taste even better when you add "dipping sauces" such as Chinese hot mustard, lite soy sauce and chili sauce. Simply spoon a little bit of one or more of these sauces on top of the stir-fry, or roll the lettuce wrap up and try dipping it into the different sauces for added flavor and fun!

DIRECTIONS

1 Prepare soybeans according to package directions.

2 Remove and discard stems from shiitake mushrooms. Then chop the mushroom caps. Chop napa cabbage keeping leaves and stems separate.

3 Lightly coat a wok or skillet with cooking spray and place over medium-high heat. Add turkey and then stir-fry until no longer pink, about 3 to 4 minutes. Remove turkey from the wok and set aside.

4 Lightly recoat the wok or skillet with cooking spray. Add chopped cabbage stems and onion; stir-fry until tender, about 2 minutes.

5 Stir in hoisin sauce, soy sauce and five-spice powder. Add cabbage leaves, mushrooms and water chestnuts; stir-fry for about 1 minute. Add cooked turkey back into the skillet and stir-fry until well combined and heated through, about 2 more minutes.

6 Place 3 lettuce leaves and a fourth of the soybeans on each of 4 plates. Divide stir-fry mixture into 4 portions. Then divide each portion into thirds and spoon into the lettuce leaves. Serve and enjoy! ☺

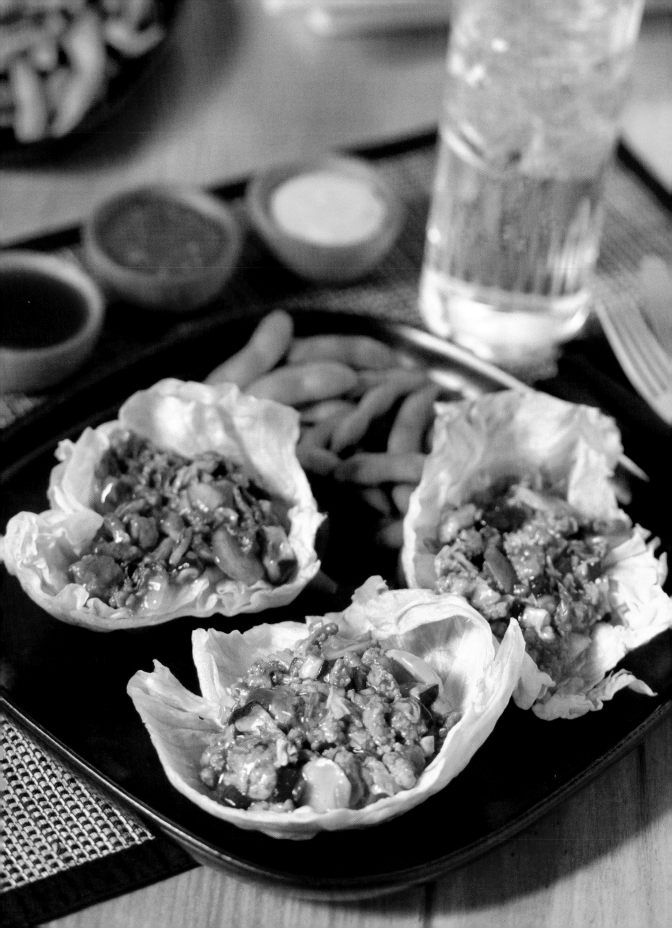

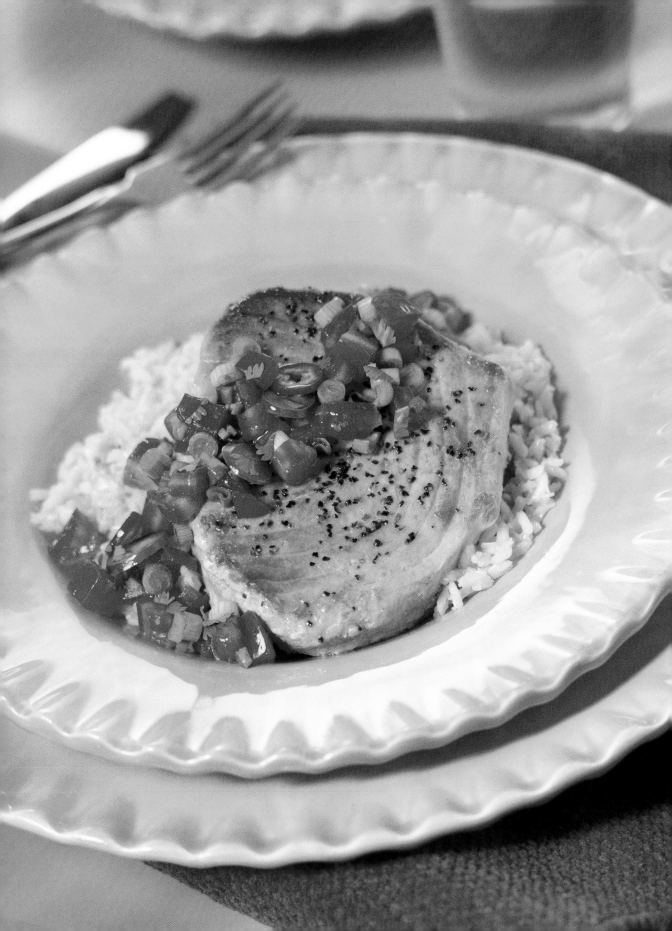

Pico de Gallo Seared Ahi

Tender tuna steak with Roma tomato,
cilantro and lemon over brown rice

Servings: 2
Preparation Time: 45 minutes

INGREDIENTS

2 portions brown rice (about ½ cup uncooked)

3 Roma tomatoes, diced

3 green onions, sliced

1 lime, halved

1 jalapeño, seeded and sliced

1 Tbsp fresh cilantro, chopped

2 portions tuna steak (about 12 oz)

1 Tbsp olive oil

¼ tsp freshly ground black pepper

1 lemon, halved

—— Tasteful Tip ——

You will discover that the flavor of fresh fish, when properly prepared and seasoned, will take on many wonderful varieties! It's only "fishy" if it's not fresh or if it is improperly prepared.

DIRECTIONS

1 Prepare brown rice according to its package directions.

2 In a medium bowl, combine tomatoes, green onions, lime juice, jalapeño and cilantro to make "Pico de Gallo." Cover and refrigerate to let the flavors blend.

3 Preheat a large skillet over high heat. Brush both sides of tuna steaks with olive oil and season one side with black pepper. Add steaks to hot skillet, pepper-side down. Sear for 2 minutes, then turn steaks and reduce heat to medium. Loosely cover skillet with foil and allow steaks to cook 5 minutes for rare, 7 minutes for medium.

4 Spoon a portion of rice onto each of 2 plates and top with a portion of tuna steak. Divide Pico de Gallo equally atop each piece of tuna. Finish with a squeeze of fresh lemon. Serve and enjoy! ☺

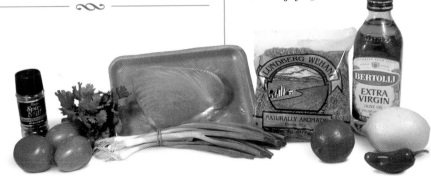

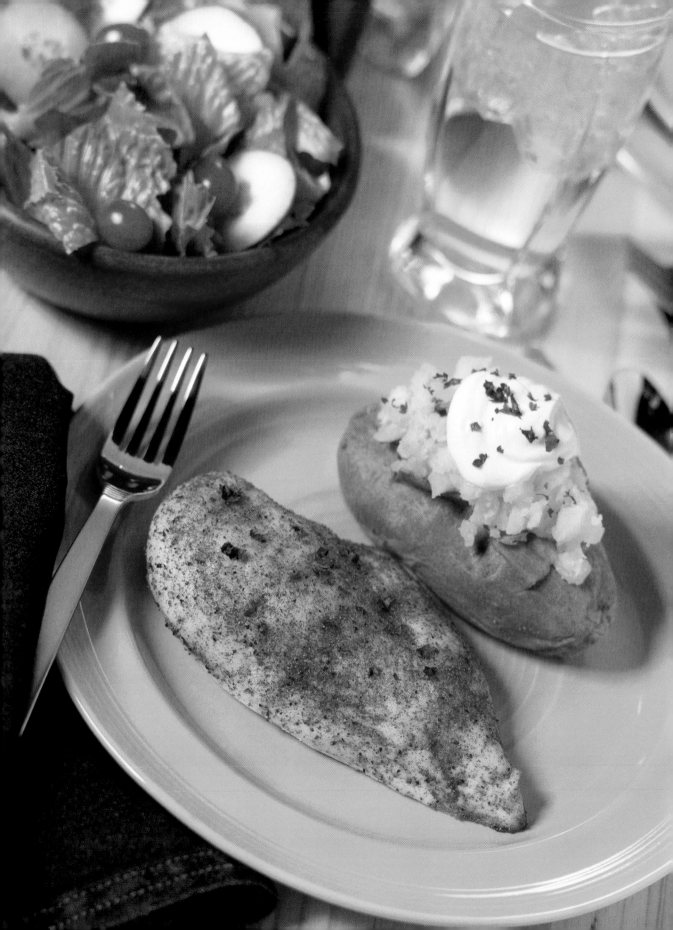

Rotisserie Seasoned Chicken

Roasted chicken breast, baked potato and fresh garden salad

Servings: 2
Preparation Time: 50 minutes

INGREDIENTS

2 portion-size potatoes

2 portions chicken breast (about $^1/_2$ pound)

1 tsp McCormick® Rotisserie Chicken seasoning

2 cups romaine lettuce, chopped

$^1/_2$ cucumber, sliced

$^1/_2$ cup grape tomatoes

1 Tbsp olive oil

1 Tbsp balsamic vinegar

2 Tbsp Butter Buds®

2 Tbsp fat-free sour cream

1 Tbsp fresh parsley, chopped

DIRECTIONS

1 Preheat oven to 450° F.

2 Wash and dry potatoes, then pierce several times with a fork. Place directly on bottom oven rack and bake until tender, about 45 minutes.

3 After potatoes have baked for about 25 minutes, lightly coat an 8" x 8" baking dish with cooking spray. Coat chicken breasts with rotisserie seasoning and place in baking dish. Bake on middle oven rack, until no longer pink in the center, about 20 minutes.

4 In a large mixing bowl, combine lettuce, cucumber and tomatoes. Then drizzle with olive oil and balsamic vinegar, toss to coat. Divide into 2 serving bowls.

5 Place a portion of chicken and a portion-size potato on each plate. Slice open the potatoes and top with Butter Buds and sour cream. Sprinkle parsley over potatoes and chicken. Serve and enjoy! ☺

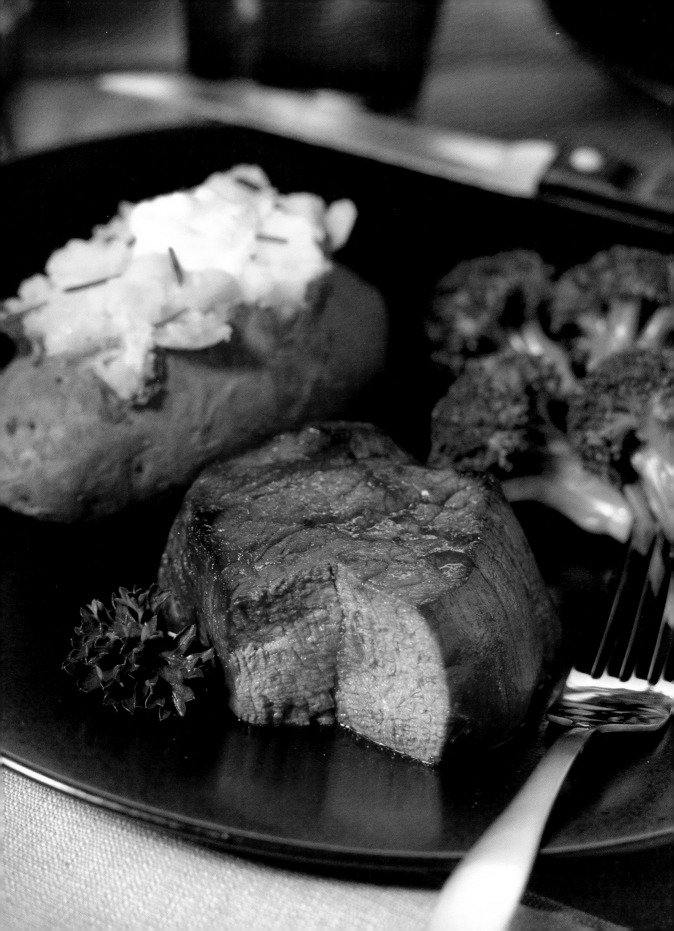

Filet Mignon

Broiled tenderloin steak, a baked potato and steamed broccoli

Servings: 2
Preparation Time: 50 minutes

INGREDIENTS

2 portion-size potatoes

2 portions filet mignon (about $1/2$ lb),
   2 inches thick

1 tsp ground black pepper

$1/2$ lb broccoli florets

1 Tbsp Butter Buds®

1 Tbsp chives, sliced

$1/4$ cup light sour cream

—————— Tasteful Tip ——————

Filet mignon is arguably the most tender and flavorful cut of beef. Unfortunately, it's also the most expensive. And, it does have more fat and calories, ounce for ounce, than other kinds of steak. Still, it is delicious and packed with quality protein, B vitamins and creatine. All in all, it's a-okay to eat this meal and savor the flavor! (Just don't eat it every night.)

DIRECTIONS

1 Preheat oven to 450° F. Wash and dry potatoes and pierce several times with a fork. Bake directly on oven rack until tender, about 45 minutes.

2 After potatoes have baked for about 30 minutes, move them to bottom rack of oven and preheat broiler.

3 Lightly coat a broiler pan with cooking spray. Sprinkle filets with ground black pepper on both sides and place on the broiler pan.

4 Broil filets 3 inches from heat source for 4 minutes. Turn filets and cook about 3 more minutes for rare, 5 more minutes for medium and about 7 more minutes for well done.

5 While the filets are cooking, fill a medium saucepan with about 1 inch of water and place over high heat. Add broccoli and bring to a boil. Cover and steam until crisp-tender, about 7 minutes.

6 Place a portion of filet mignon, a portion-sized baked potato and a serving of broccoli on each plate. Slice potatoes open and top with Butter Buds, chives and a dollop of sour cream. Serve and enjoy! ☺

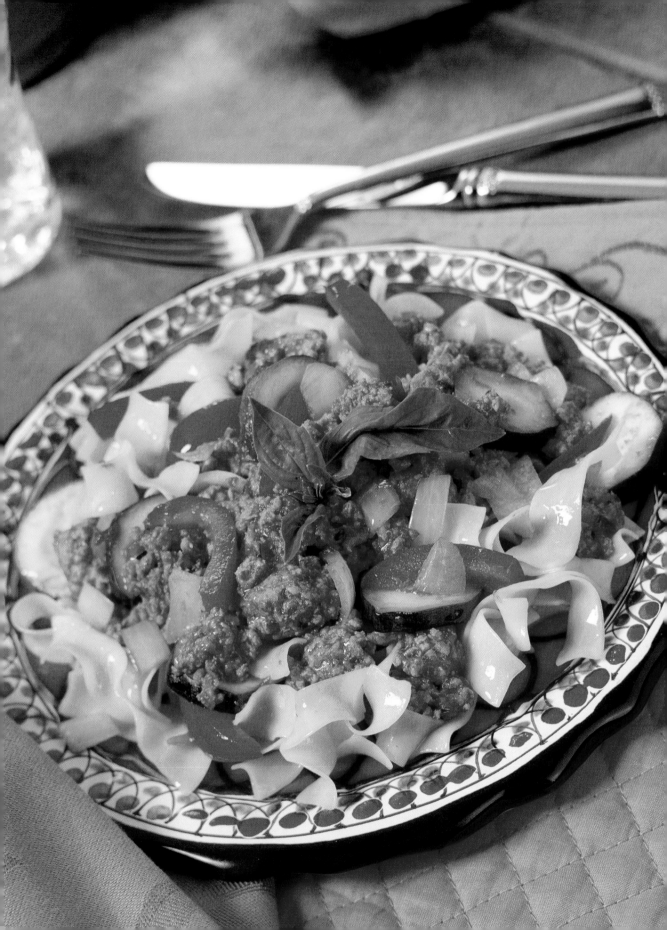

American Turkey Goulash

*Tomato-basil sauce with lean ground turkey,
sautéed red bell pepper and zucchini over noodles*

Servings: 4
Preparation Time: 30 minutes

INGREDIENTS

4   portions egg noodles (about 8 oz uncooked)

1   onion, chopped

1   red bell pepper, sliced

1   zucchini, sliced

4   portions lean ground turkey (about 1 lb)

2   cups tomato sauce

2   Tbsp fresh basil, chopped

2   Tbsp red wine (optional)

DIRECTIONS

1 Prepare egg noodles according to package directions.

2 Lightly coat a large skillet with cooking spray. Over medium-high heat, sauté chopped onion for 2 minutes. Add bell pepper to the onion and sauté for another 2 minutes. Add zucchini and sauté for 2 more minutes. Remove vegetables from the skillet and set aside.

3 Add ground turkey to the skillet and sauté until no longer pink, about 10 minutes.

4 When the ground turkey is done, return vegetables to the skillet. Add tomato sauce, basil and red wine (if desired). Cook, stirring occasionally, for 5 minutes or until heated through.

5 Place a portion of noodles on each plate and top with a portion of turkey mixture. Serve and enjoy! ☺

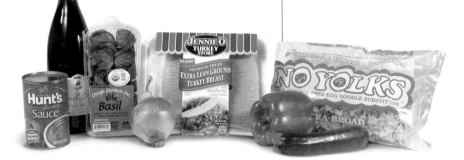

Caribbean Chicken Salad

Grilled chicken on a bed of vegetables and fruit,
topped with honey-Dijon dressing

Servings: 4
Preparation Time: 30 minutes

INGREDIENTS

- 4 portions chicken breast (about 1 lb)
- 2 tsp McCormick® Montreal Chicken seasoning
- 1 bag of baby romaine salad
- 1 bag romaine salad blend
- 1 cucumber, sliced
- 1 red onion, sliced
- 1 cup radishes, sliced
- 1 red bell pepper, diced
- 2 tomatoes, diced
- 1 can (11 oz) mandarin oranges, drained
- 1 can (8 oz) pineapple tidbits, drained
- ½ cup reduced-fat cheddar cheese, shredded
- ½ cup lite honey-Dijon salad dressing

DIRECTIONS

1 Preheat grill to high. Season the chicken breasts on both sides with the Montreal seasoning. Then place chicken on hot grill and cook for approximately 6 minutes; turn and grill for approximately 6 more minutes, until no longer pink in the center.

2 While the chicken is cooking, combine the baby romaine salad, romaine salad blend, cucumber, red onion, radishes, red bell pepper and tomatoes in a large mixing bowl and toss.

3 Divide the salad between four plates. Top each with one-fourth of the mandarin orange slices, pineapple tidbits and shredded cheese.

4 Place the cooked chicken on a cutting board, let it cool slightly, then slice into ½-inch strips.

5 Top each salad with a portion of chicken. Pour honey-Dijon dressing over salads. Serve and enjoy! ☺

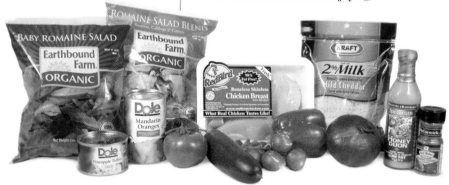

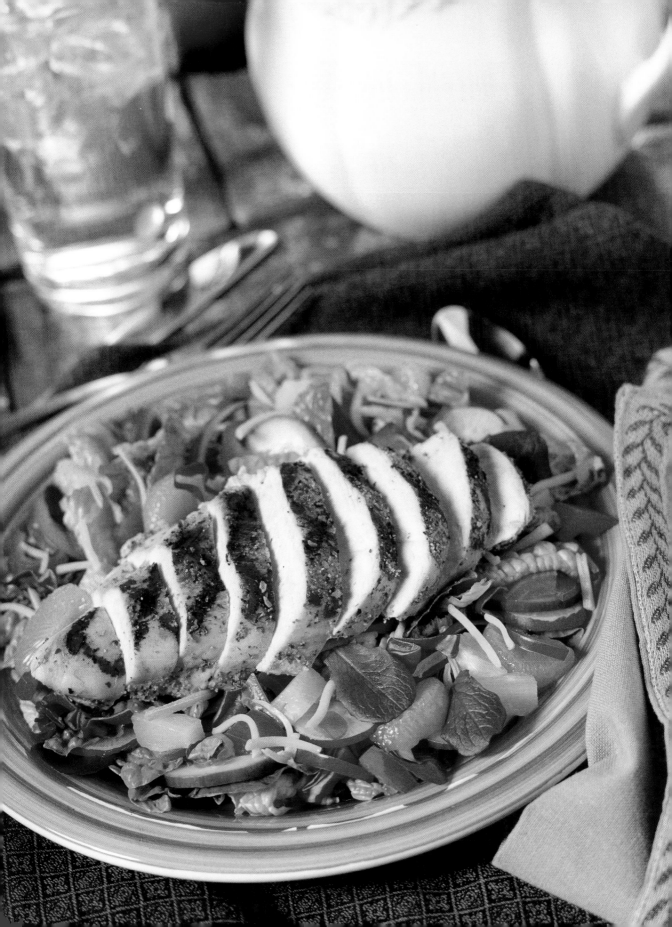

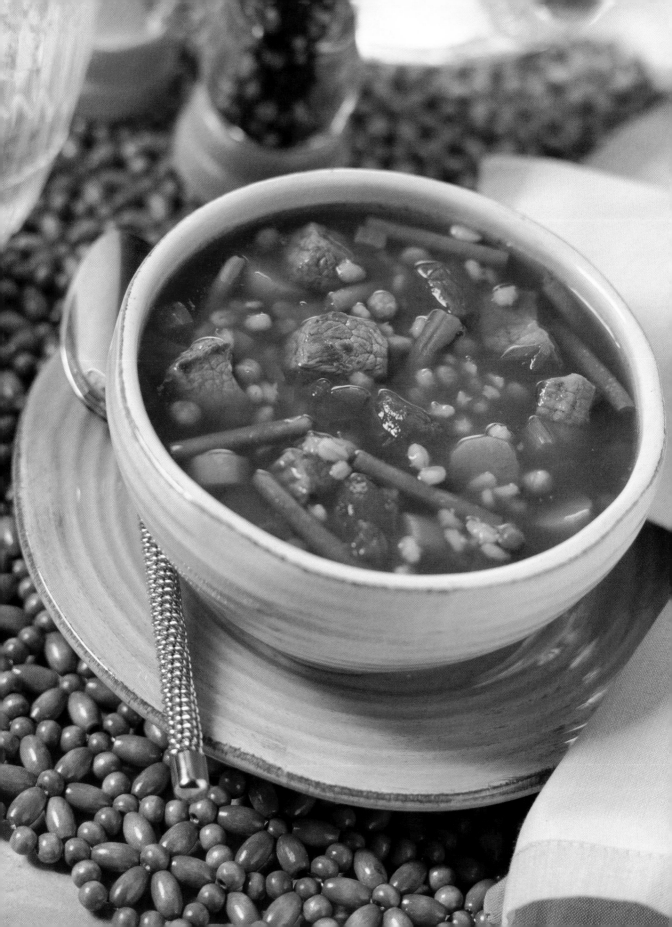

Beef and
Barley Soup

Savory vegetable soup simmered with
braised beef and pearl barley

Servings: 6
Preparation Time: 1 hour, 15 minutes

INGREDIENTS

1 Tbsp olive oil

6 portions top sirloin (about 1 1/2 lbs),
  cut into 1-inch cubes

4 cups low-fat, reduced-sodium beef broth

1 cup water

1 onion, chopped

1 stalk celery, sliced

1 carrot, sliced

1 tsp dried oregano

1/4 tsp ground black pepper

2 cloves garlic, minced

1/2 cup pearl barley

1 bay leaf

10 oz frozen green beans

1 can (14 1/2 oz) diced tomatoes

10 oz frozen green peas

DIRECTIONS

1 In a large pot, over medium-high heat, warm the olive oil. Add beef cubes and cook for about 8 minutes; stirring occasionally until browned on all sides.

2 Stir in beef broth, water, onion, celery, carrot, oregano, black pepper, garlic, barley and bay leaf. Bring to a boil. Then reduce heat to low, cover and simmer for 45 minutes.

3 Stir in green beans, tomatoes and peas. Simmer, covered, until meat and vegetables are tender, about 15 more minutes. Remove bay leaf.

4 Ladle a portion (about 2 cups) of soup into each bowl. Serve and enjoy! ☺

—— Tasteful Tip ——

Barley is a very nutritious grain, which, like brown rice, is high in fiber, rich with energy and is especially flavorful in this homemade soup.

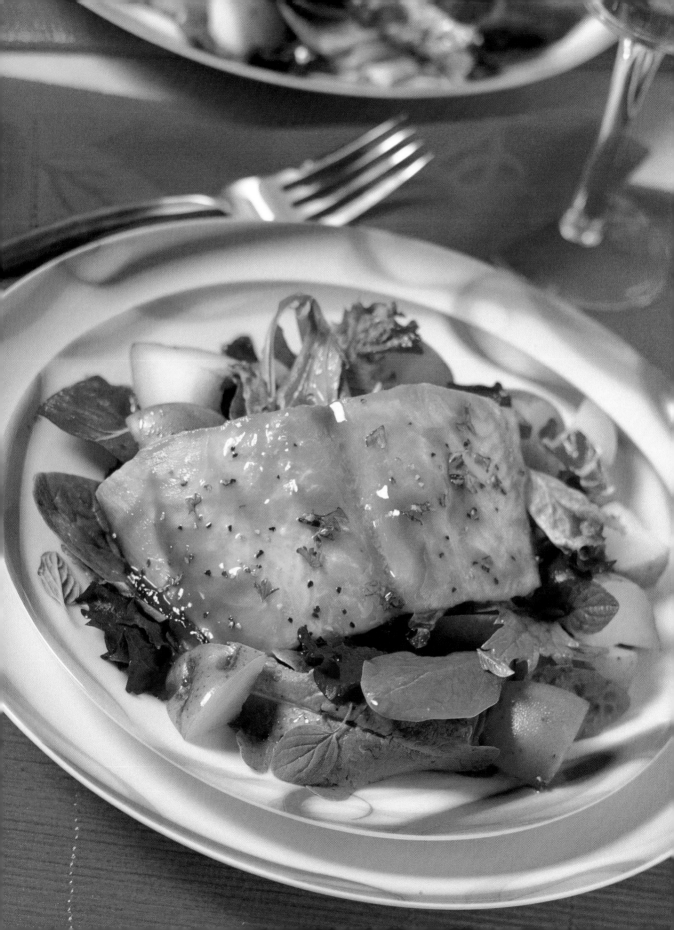

Balsamic Salmon Salad

Broiled salmon fillet glazed with teriyaki marinade
over balsamic salad and new potatoes

Servings: 2
Preparation Time: 30 minutes

INGREDIENTS

2 portions new potatoes, cubed

1 Tbsp teriyaki marinade

2 cloves garlic, minced

1 Tbsp fresh parsley, minced

2 portions salmon fillets (about 12 oz)

4 cups mixed salad greens

1 Tbsp fresh basil leaves, chopped

1 Tbsp fresh oregano leaves, chopped

1 Tbsp olive oil

2 Tbsp balsamic vinegar

1 lemon, halved

Freshly ground black pepper, to taste

DIRECTIONS

1 Steam cubed new potatoes in a covered saucepan until tender, approximately 20 minutes.

2 While potatoes are cooking, mix teriyaki marinade, garlic and parsley in a small bowl.

3 Preheat broiler. Lightly coat a broiler pan with cooking spray. Place salmon fillets on the pan, skin-side down, and brush with teriyaki marinade.

4 Broil salmon approximately 6 inches from the broiler until the fish is cooked through and flakes easily with a fork, about 8 to 10 minutes.

5 While salmon is cooking, combine salad greens, basil, oregano, olive oil and balsamic vinegar in a medium bowl and toss.

6 Divide tossed salad between two separate plates. Layer portions of potatoes and broiled salmon fillets over salad greens.

7 Top salmon and salad with a squeeze of fresh lemon and freshly ground black pepper, serve and enjoy! ☺

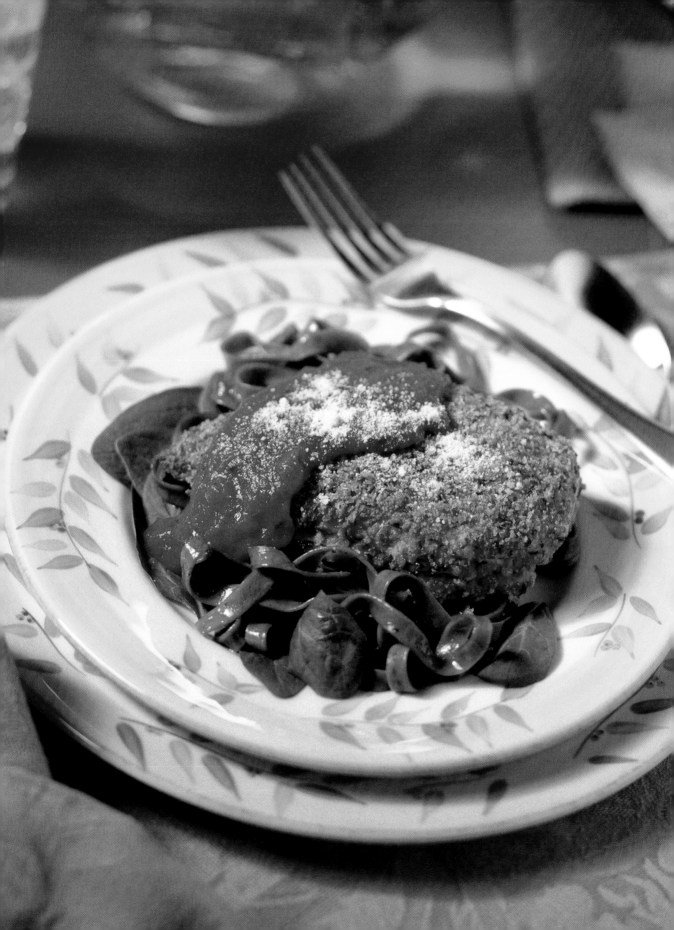

Baked Chicken Parmesan

Spinach fettuccine with breaded chicken breast,
topped with pasta sauce and Parmesan cheese

Servings: 2
Preparation Time: 40 minutes

INGREDIENTS

2 egg whites

⅓ cup Italian-seasoned breadcrumbs

4 Tbsp reduced-fat Parmesan cheese,
   grated, divided

2 portions chicken breast (about ½ lb)

2 portions spinach pasta (about 4 oz uncooked)

1 cup low-fat pasta sauce

2 cups baby spinach leaves

─────── Tasteful Tip ───────

This chicken dish is healthy and delicious! Baking the chicken, rather than frying it in fat, improves the flavor while enhancing the nutritional content.

DIRECTIONS

1 Preheat oven to 400° F.

2 In a medium mixing bowl, beat egg whites with fork until slightly frothy. Then, mix breadcrumbs and 2 tablespoons of reduced-fat Parmesan cheese in a pie plate.

3 Dip chicken breasts in egg whites and then into the breadcrumb mixture, coating both sides.

4 Lightly coat a baking sheet with cooking spray. Place chicken breasts on the baking sheet; bake for approximately 12 minutes, turn over and bake approximately 12 more minutes, until chicken is no longer pink in the center and coating is golden brown.

5 While the chicken is baking, prepare spinach pasta according to its package directions.

6 In a small saucepan, warm pasta sauce over medium heat.

7 Divide spinach leaves between two separate plates. Layer portions of warm spinach pasta and baked chicken breasts over spinach leaves. Top with pasta sauce and remaining Parmesan cheese. Serve and enjoy! ☺

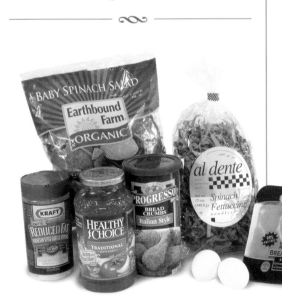

Mom's Chicken Enchiladas

Warm your heart and feed your body
with this comforting family favorite

Servings: 4
Preparation Time: 50 minutes

INGREDIENTS

4   portions chicken breast (about 1 lb)

4   green onions, sliced

2   Tbsp fresh cilantro, chopped

1   jalapeño, seeded and minced

3   cans (10 oz each) green enchilada sauce

8   corn tortillas

1   cup reduced-fat cheddar cheese, shredded

2   cups lettuce, shredded

$\frac{1}{2}$ cup salsa

$\frac{1}{2}$ cup light sour cream

1   tomato, diced

1   can (2 oz) ripe olives, sliced

———— Tasteful Tip ————

When I was growing up in Golden, Colorado, my Mom would make my brother and sister and I dinner just about every night. One meal that she loved to make and I loved to eat were these Chicken Enchiladas. By coincidence (or design), this meal fits very nicely into the Eating *for* Lifestyle as it is flavorful, nutritious and super satisfying!

———— ∞ ————

DIRECTIONS

1 Preheat oven to 350° F. Lightly coat a 9" x 13" baking dish with cooking spray.

2 Place chicken breasts in a large pot and cover with water. Bring to a boil over high heat. Reduce heat to medium and simmer until no longer pink in the center, about 15 minutes. Drain and let cool slightly. Shred cooked chicken by pulling apart with 2 forks; set aside.

3 Lightly coat a large skillet with cooking spray and place over medium-high heat. Add green onion, cilantro and jalapeño; sauté for 2 minutes. Add shredded chicken and 1 can of enchilada sauce. Cook, stirring occasionally, until heated through, about 5 minutes.

4 Pour the 2 remaining cans of enchilada sauce in a medium bowl and microwave until warm, about 2 minutes. Dip each tortilla in the heated sauce and fill with about $\frac{1}{8}$ of the chicken mixture. Roll up and place, seam-side down, in the prepared baking dish.

5 Pour remaining heated sauce over enchiladas and sprinkle with cheese. Bake until enchiladas are heated through and cheese is melted, about 15 minutes.

6 Divide lettuce onto four plates and place a portion of enchiladas on top. Top with a spoonful of salsa, a dollop of sour cream, tomatoes and olives. Serve and enjoy! 🙂

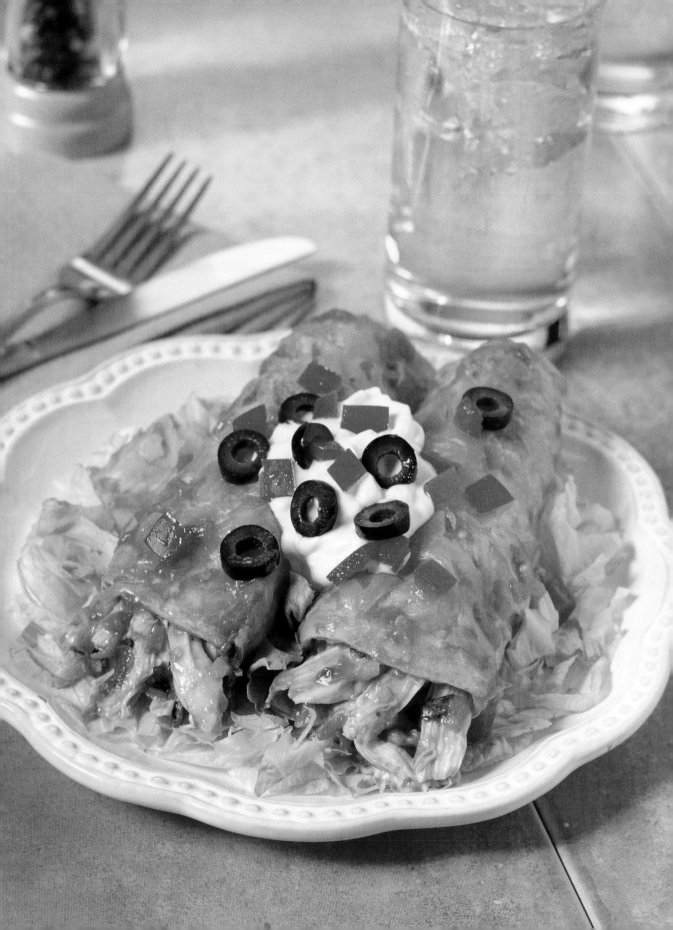

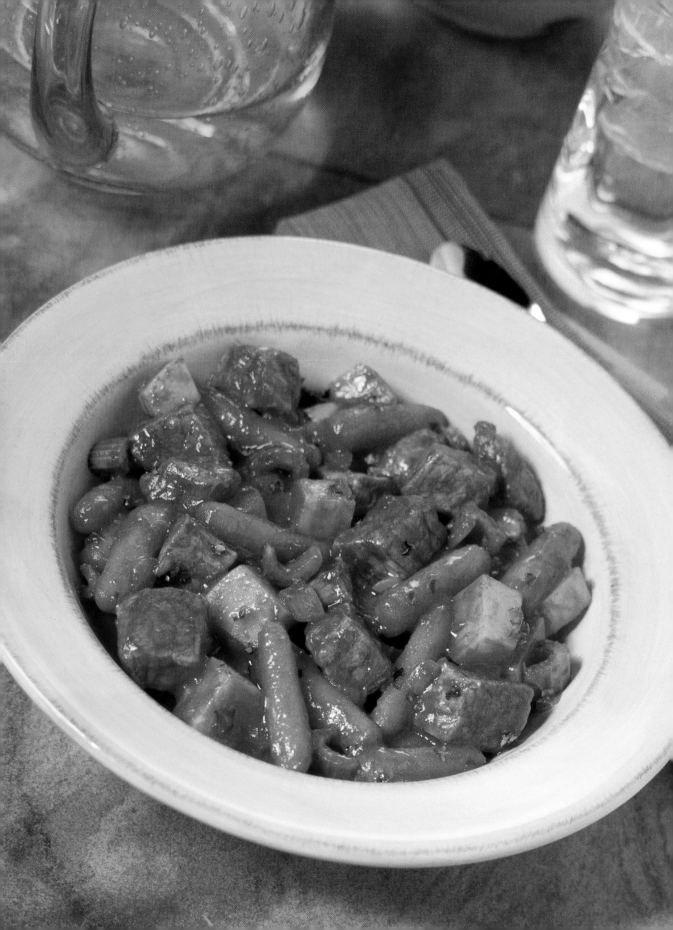

Chunky
Beef Stew

Hearty, healthy meat and potatoes with a
red-wine-accented sauce

Servings: 4
Preparation Time: 1 hour, 45 minutes

INGREDIENTS

1   onion, chopped

4   portions top round steak, cut into
    1-inch chunks (about 1 lb)

2$\frac{1}{2}$ cups low-fat, reduced-sodium beef broth

4   portions potatoes, peeled and cut into
    1-inch chunks

1   lb baby carrots

2   celery stalks, sliced

$\frac{1}{4}$ cup tomato paste

$\frac{1}{2}$ tsp ground black pepper

2   Tbsp Worcestershire sauce

1   bay leaf

$\frac{1}{4}$ cup red wine (optional)

2   Tbsp fresh parsley, chopped

—— Tasteful Tip ——

Cooking with wine (adding it to ingredients, not drinking it while you're cooking) is optional, but it does indeed help create full and satisfying flavors. Keep in mind that the alcohol content evaporates during the cooking process.

DIRECTIONS

1 Lightly coat a large pot with cooking spray and place over medium-high heat. Add onions and sauté until tender, about 5 minutes.

2 Add beef chunks and sauté until browned on all sides, about 6 minutes.

3 Add beef broth, potato chunks, carrots, celery, tomato paste, black pepper, Worcestershire sauce, bay leaf and red wine. Bring to a boil over high heat.

4 Reduce the heat to low. Cover and simmer, stirring occasionally, until the meat is tender, about 1$\frac{1}{2}$ hours. Remove bay leaf with a spoon or tongs and discard.

5 Spoon beef stew into bowls, dividing it into 4 portions. Sprinkle with parsley, serve and enjoy! ☺

Orange Roughy

Lightly breaded and seasoned baked orange roughy
with lemon parsley rice and sautéed zucchini

Servings: 4
Preparation Time: 45 minutes

INGREDIENTS

4 portions brown rice (about 1 cup uncooked)

¼ cup breadcrumbs

1 tsp Italian seasoning

¼ cup reduced-fat Parmesan cheese, grated

1 egg white

4 portions orange roughy fillets (about 1½ lbs)

3 Tbsp fresh parsley, chopped, divided

4 small zucchinis

½ red onion, chopped

1 tsp grated lemon peel

1 lemon, halved

—————— Tasteful Tip ——————

Orange roughy is a mild and delicious white fish that is high in protein and low in fat. It's not always available at your local grocery store, but when it is, consider giving it a try!

DIRECTIONS

1 Prepare brown rice according to its package directions.

2 Preheat oven to 400° F. Lightly coat a baking sheet with cooking spray.

3 In a pie plate, combine breadcrumbs, Italian seasoning and Parmesan cheese. In a small mixing bowl, whisk the egg white until slightly foamy.

4 Lightly brush both sides of the orange roughy fillets with the egg white and then coat with breadcrumbs. Arrange fillets on the prepared baking sheet and sprinkle with 1 tablespoon of parsley. Bake until the orange roughy is opaque throughout, approximately 20 minutes.

5 While the orange roughy is baking, lightly coat a large skillet with butter-flavored cooking spray and place over medium-high heat. Slice zucchini diagonally in ¼-inch slices. Add zucchini and onion to the skillet; cook for about 2 minutes. Turn zucchini slices and cook until tender, about 2 more minutes.

6 Stir the remaining fresh parsley and grated lemon peel into the cooked rice.

7 Place a portion of orange roughy onto each of 4 plates and top with a squeeze of lemon. Add a portion of rice and about one-fourth of the zucchini. Serve and enjoy! ☺

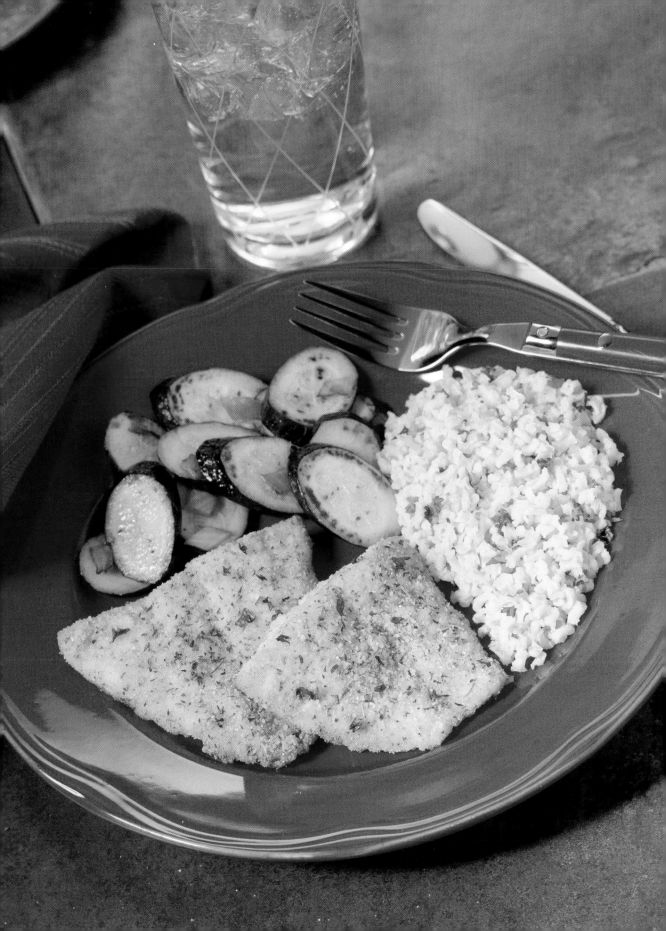

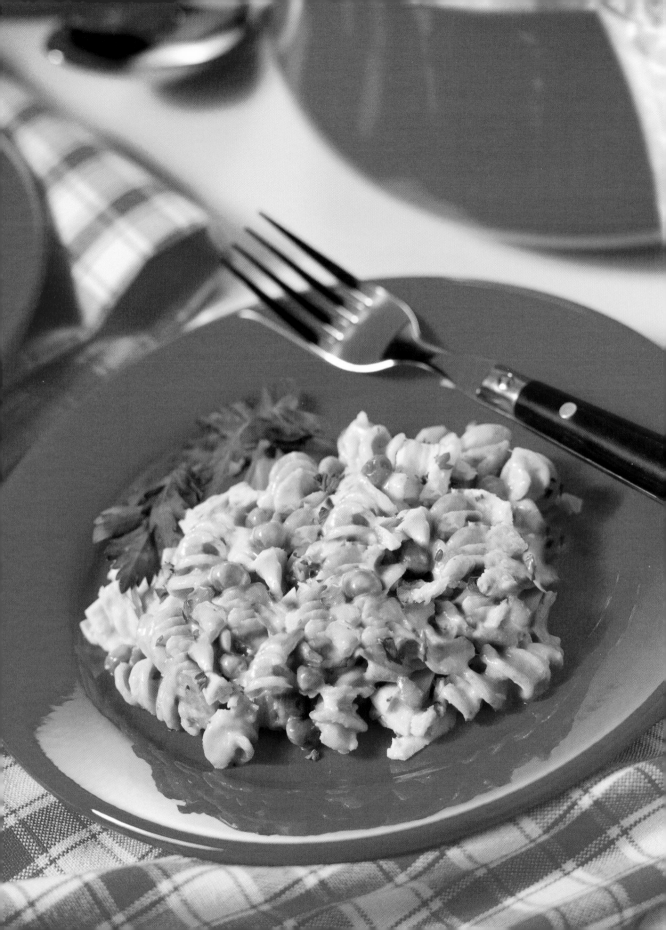

Albacore Tuna Casserole

Rotini pasta and tuna with tender green peas
in a light creamy sauce

Servings: 4
Preparation Time: 35 minutes

INGREDIENTS

4 portions rotini pasta (about 8 oz uncooked)

2 cans (6 oz) albacore tuna, water packed, drained

1 can (10 oz) low-fat, reduced-sodium cream of mushroom soup, condensed

½ cup skim milk

1 cup frozen peas

— Tasteful Tip —

Extra servings or "planned-overs" of Albacore Tuna Casserole can be stored in small Tupperware® containers in the refrigerator. It makes an excellent "ready-made" lunch for the following day. Just reheat in the microwave for approximately 3 to 6 minutes (until warm in the center), and you're all set!

DIRECTIONS

1 Preheat oven to 350° F.

2 Prepare rotini pasta according to its package directions.

3 Lightly coat an 8" x 8" baking dish with cooking spray.

4 Place cooked pasta in baking dish and add tuna, soup, skim milk and peas; mix well.

5 Bake uncovered until the casserole begins to bubble, about 20 minutes.

6 Remove casserole from oven and let stand for 5 minutes. Then divide into 4 portions, serve and enjoy! ☺

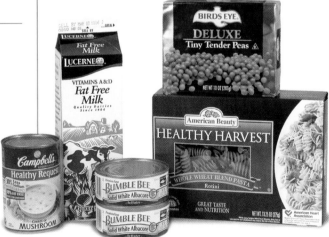

Tangy BBQ Chicken

*Tender chicken topped with homemade
 barbecue sauce served with brown rice*

Servings: 2
Preparation Time: 45 minutes

INGREDIENTS

2 portions brown rice (about $^1/_2$ cup uncooked)

3 tsp olive oil, divided

2 portions chicken breast (about $^1/_2$ lb)

$^1/_2$ onion, diced

1 cup tomato juice

$^1/_3$ cup vinegar

Hot pepper sauce, to taste

2 cloves garlic, minced

$^1/_4$ tsp ground black pepper

1 tsp Worcestershire sauce

$^1/_2$ red bell pepper, diced

1 Tbsp chives, sliced

DIRECTIONS

1 Prepare brown rice according to its package directions.

2 While the rice is cooking, heat 2 teaspoons of olive oil in a medium skillet over medium heat. Add chicken breasts, cover and cook the chicken for 6 minutes, turn over and cook approximately 6 more minutes, until no longer pink in the center.

3 While the chicken is cooking, heat the remaining olive oil in a medium saucepan over medium heat. Add onion and sauté until it is golden brown, about 4 minutes. Add tomato juice, vinegar, hot pepper sauce, garlic, black pepper and Worcestershire sauce; stir well. Simmer sauce over low heat for 10 minutes.

4 When the chicken is done, add it to the sauce and simmer for 3 more minutes.

5 Stir the diced bell pepper and chives into the cooked rice.

6 Place a portion of chicken breast and sauce with a portion of rice on two separate plates. Serve and enjoy! ☺

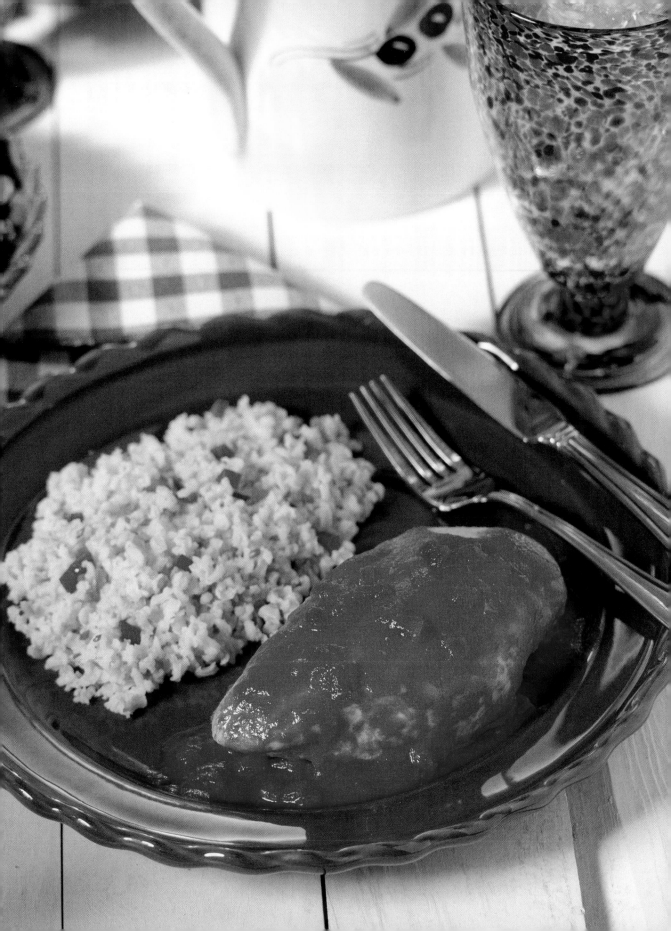

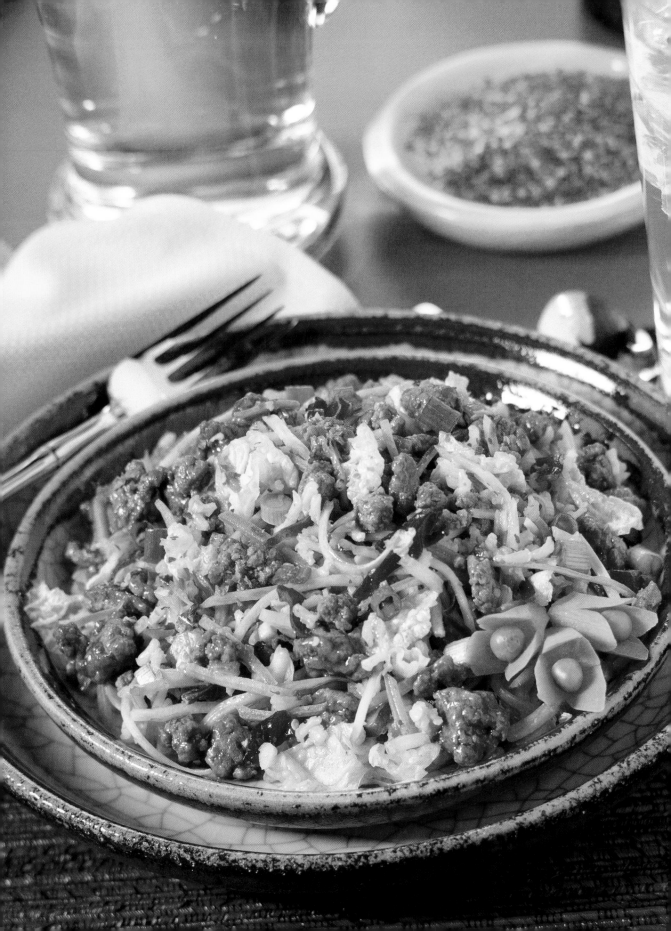

Sesame Beef Stir-Fry

Lean ground beef, brown rice, broccoli and napa cabbage stir-fried in sesame-soy sauce

Servings: 2
Preparation Time: 45 minutes

INGREDIENTS

2 portions brown rice (about ½ cup uncooked)

2 portions lean ground beef (about ½ lb)

1 Tbsp toasted sesame oil

2 cloves garlic, minced

3 green onions, sliced

1 cup broccoli slaw (found near bagged salads in produce department)

1 cup napa cabbage, shredded

1 Tbsp lite soy sauce

Crushed red pepper flakes, to taste

DIRECTIONS

1 Prepare brown rice according to its package directions.

2 While the rice is cooking, in a medium skillet or wok, brown the ground beef over medium heat until no longer pink. Remove the beef from the skillet, drain and set aside.

3 Heat sesame oil in the skillet over medium-high heat. Add garlic and green onions; stir-fry for 2 minutes. Add the broccoli slaw and cabbage; stir-fry for 2 minutes. Add rice and soy sauce; stir-fry for 2 more minutes.

4 Return the cooked ground beef to the skillet with the rice and vegetable mixture and season with red pepper flakes, to taste. Stir until ingredients are well combined and heated through, about 2 minutes.

5 Divide into 2 portions, serve and enjoy! ☺

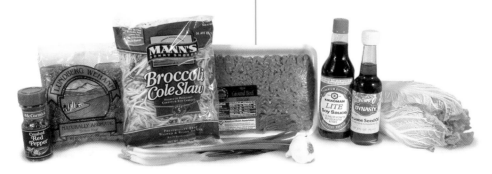

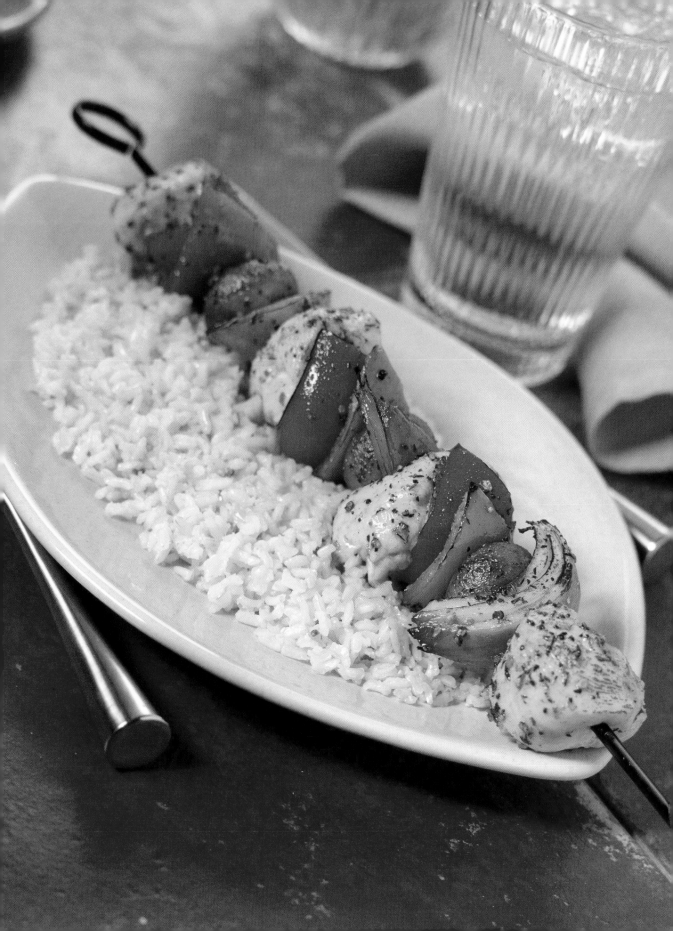

Chicken Kabobs

Skewered chicken and fresh vegetables
cooked over an open-flame grill

Servings: 4
Preparation Time: 45 minutes

INGREDIENTS

4 portions brown rice (about 1 cup uncooked)

4 portions chicken breast (about 1 lb), cut into 1 1/2-inch squares

2 green bell peppers, cut into 1 1/2-inch pieces

2 red bell peppers, cut into 1 1/2-inch pieces

12 fresh mushrooms, whole

1 onion, cut into wedges

1 Tbsp olive oil

2 tsp McCormick® Montreal Chicken seasoning

—— Tasteful Tip ——

*Cooking with an open-flame grill is a great way to bring out the best flavors in foods. However, when grilling is not a feasible option, remember that oven-broiling is the next best thing. For example, these kabobs can be cooked by placing them on a broiler pan, about 6 inches below the heat source. Cook for about 5 minutes, turn and cook for another 5 minutes. And, always be sure chicken is no longer pink in center before you serve it up.

DIRECTIONS

1 Prepare the rice according to its package directions.

2 Preheat grill.*

3 On four skewers, alternately thread a piece of chicken, then green pepper, red pepper, mushroom and onion. Repeat until all ingredients are used.

4 Lightly brush the olive oil over kabobs and sprinkle with Montreal chicken seasoning.

5 Grill kabobs for 5 minutes; turn and grill until the chicken is no longer pink in the center, about 5 more minutes.

6 Place a portion of rice and one kabob on each plate. Serve and enjoy! ☺

Indian
Chicken

Spiced grilled chicken with Tabbouleh-stuffed tomato

Servings: 4
Preparation Time: 50 minutes

INGREDIENTS

1 cup water

2/3 cup bulgur wheat (found in rice section)

2 lemons, halved

1 cup fresh parsley, chopped

1/2 cup fresh mint leaves, chopped

4 green onions, sliced

1 Roma tomato, diced

2 Tbsp olive oil, divided

1/2 tsp ground black pepper

1/4 tsp salt

1 Tbsp Hungarian paprika

1 Tbsp cumin

1/2 tsp dried oregano

1 tsp dried coriander

1/2 tsp crushed red pepper flakes

4 portions chicken breast (about 1 lb)

4 large tomatoes

DIRECTIONS

1 In a small saucepan, boil one cup of water. Then remove from heat and pour boiling water into a medium mixing bowl. Add bulgur wheat, cover and let stand for 20 minutes to soften. (You don't cook the bulgur wheat over heat.)

2 Add lemon juice, parsley, mint, green onion, diced Roma tomato, 1 tablespoon olive oil, black pepper and salt to bulgur wheat; stir to combine. Cover and refrigerate for at least 20 minutes. (The combination of these ingredients is called Tabbouleh, pronounced "ta-bū-lee.")

3 Preheat grill to high. In a pie plate, combine paprika, cumin, oregano, coriander and red pepper flakes. Lightly coat the chicken breasts with remaining olive oil and rub with spice mixture, making sure they are well coated on each side.

4 Place chicken on hot grill and cook for approximately 6 minutes; turn and grill for approximately 6 more minutes until no longer pink in the center.

5 While chicken is grilling, cut tomatoes into quarters, but do *not* cut all the way through. Gently open tomatoes and fill with a portion of Tabbouleh.

6 Place a portion of Indian chicken and a Tabbouleh-filled tomato on each plate. Serve and enjoy! ☺

 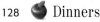

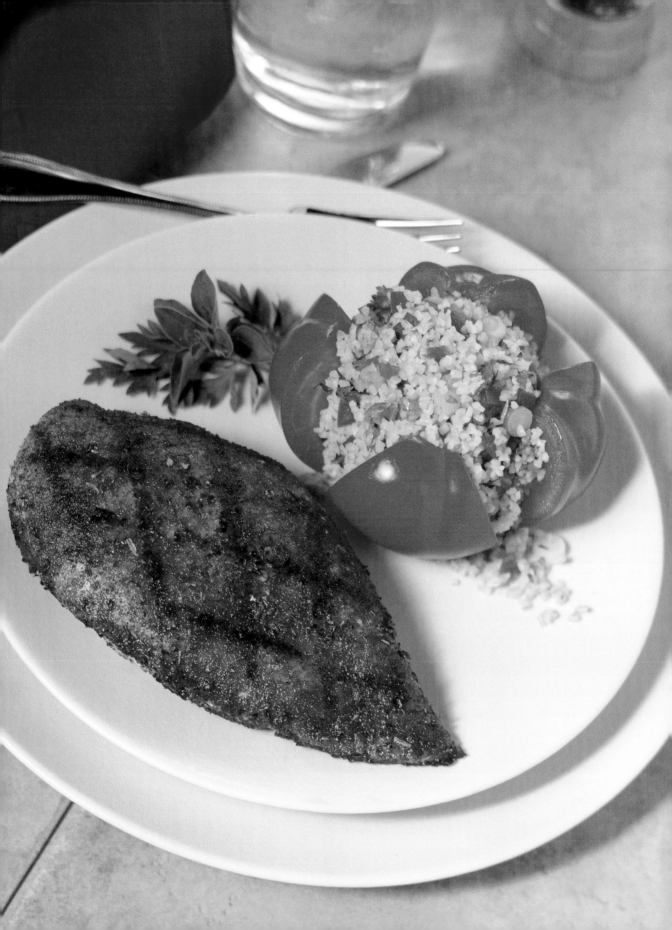

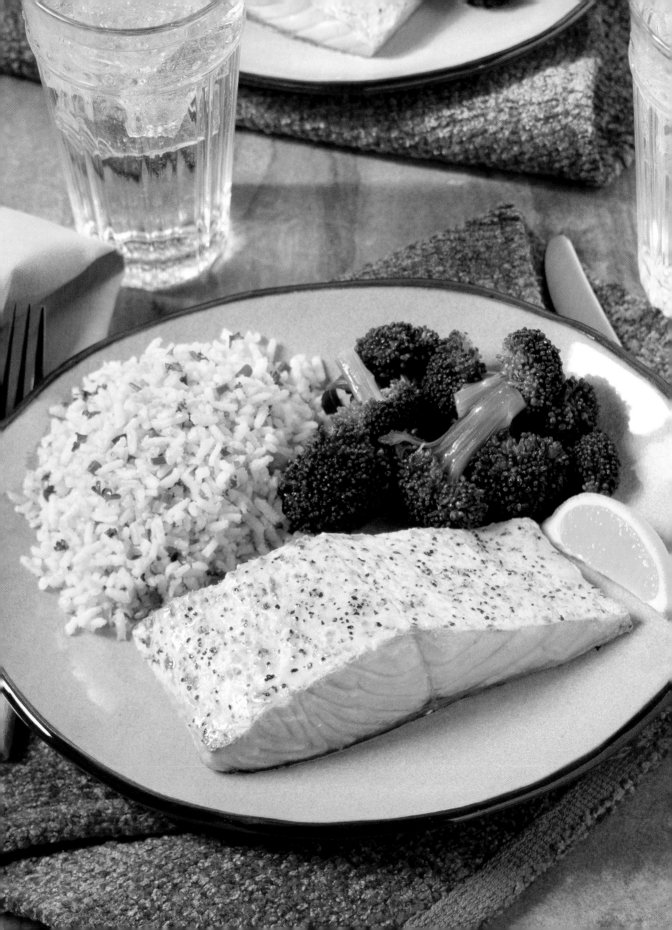

Lemon-Peppered Salmon Fillet

Eating for Life 101: A delicious broiled salmon fillet, a portion of brown rice and a serving of steamed broccoli

Servings: 2
Preparation Time: 45 minutes

INGREDIENTS

2 portions brown rice (about $\frac{1}{2}$ cup uncooked)

2 Tbsp fat-free mayonnaise

1 tsp lemon-pepper seasoning

2 lemons, halved, divided

2 portions salmon fillet (about 12 oz)

$\frac{1}{2}$ lb broccoli florets

3 green onions, minced

2 Tbsp fresh parsley, minced

——— Tasteful Tip ———

Well-done, medium or a little on the "rare" side, how you like your salmon doesn't really affect the quality of essential fatty acids (EFAs) which are abundantly supplied in this especially nutritious fish. EFAs are so important because they play a vital role in maintaining the proper biological functioning of everything from muscles to memory. One of the reasons salmon tastes so good is because our bodies are craving these essential fats!

DIRECTIONS

1 Prepare brown rice according to its package directions.

2 While the rice is cooking, preheat broiler.

3 In a small mixing bowl, combine fat-free mayonnaise, lemon-pepper seasoning and the juice of one lemon.

4 Lightly coat a broiler pan with cooking spray. Place salmon fillets on the broiler pan (skin-side down) and brush lemon-pepper sauce over the top. Broil salmon approximately 6 inches from the broiler until the fillets are cooked through and flake easily with a fork, about 12 to 15 minutes.

5 While the salmon is broiling, steam the broccoli in a covered pan for 6 to 8 minutes or until crisp-tender.

6 Stir the green onion and parsley into the cooked rice.

7 Place portions of salmon and rice on two separate plates along with a serving of broccoli. Top salmon and broccoli with a squeeze of fresh lemon. Serve and enjoy! ☺

Enchilada Soup with Avocado

Tender chunks of chicken in a flavorful soup, topped with cheddar cheese, avocado and crisp tortilla strips

Servings: 8

Preparation Time: 55 minutes

INGREDIENTS

1 Tbsp olive oil

6 cloves garlic, minced

1 Tbsp cilantro, chopped

8 corn tortillas, divided

8 portions chicken breast (about 2 lbs)

1 can (15 oz) puréed tomatoes

2 onions, finely chopped

6 cups fat-free, reduced-sodium chicken broth

2 cups water

1 can (6 oz) tomato paste

1 Tbsp ground cumin

2 tsp chili powder

2 bay leaves

Ground red pepper, to taste

3/4 cup reduced-fat cheddar cheese, shredded

1 avocado, peeled, pitted and diced

——— Tasteful Tip ———

You'll notice that this recipe makes eight servings. That's because it is such a great "planned-over." Extra servings of this Enchilada Soup can be frozen and stored for up to two months.

DIRECTIONS

1 Warm olive oil in a large pot over medium-low heat. Add garlic and cilantro; sauté for 3 minutes. Chop 4 of the tortillas into approximately 1-inch squares and add to pot; sauté until softened, about 5 minutes.

2 While tortillas are cooking, slice chicken into bite-size pieces. Add chicken, puréed tomatoes, onions, chicken broth, water, tomato paste, cumin, chili powder and bay leaves; bring to a boil over high heat.

3 Reduce heat to low, add ground red pepper and simmer for 30 minutes, stirring occasionally.

4 While the soup is simmering, preheat your oven to 400° F. Using scissors, cut the remaining tortillas into approximately 1/4-inch-wide strips, and place on baking sheet in a single layer. Bake until lightly browned, about 7 minutes. (They will crisp as they cool.)

5 After the soup has simmered for 30 minutes, remove the bay leaves. Then ladle a portion (about 1 1/2 cups) of soup into each bowl and top with the shredded cheese, diced avocado and tortilla strips. Serve and enjoy! ☺

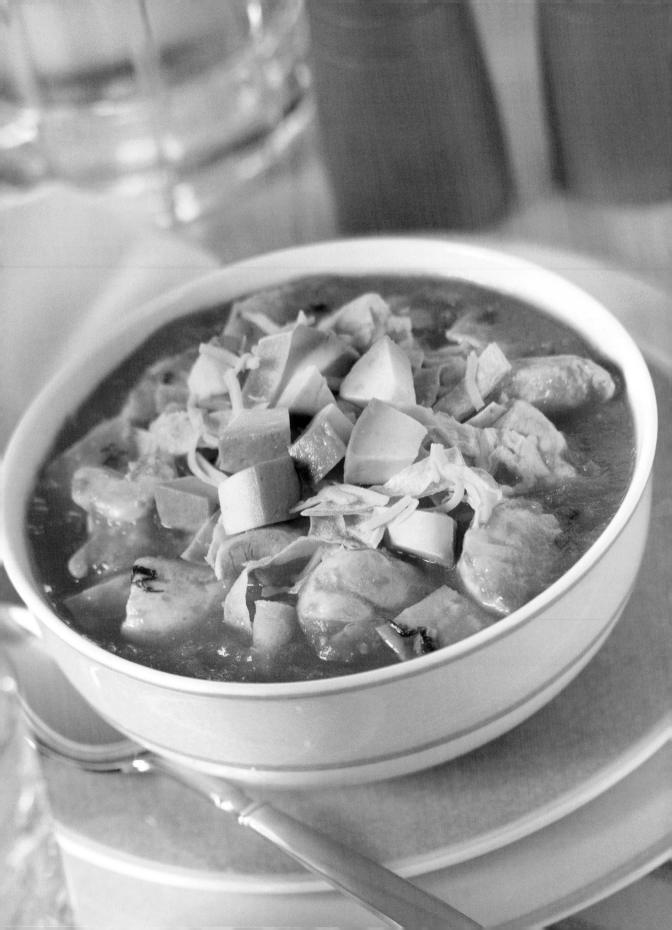

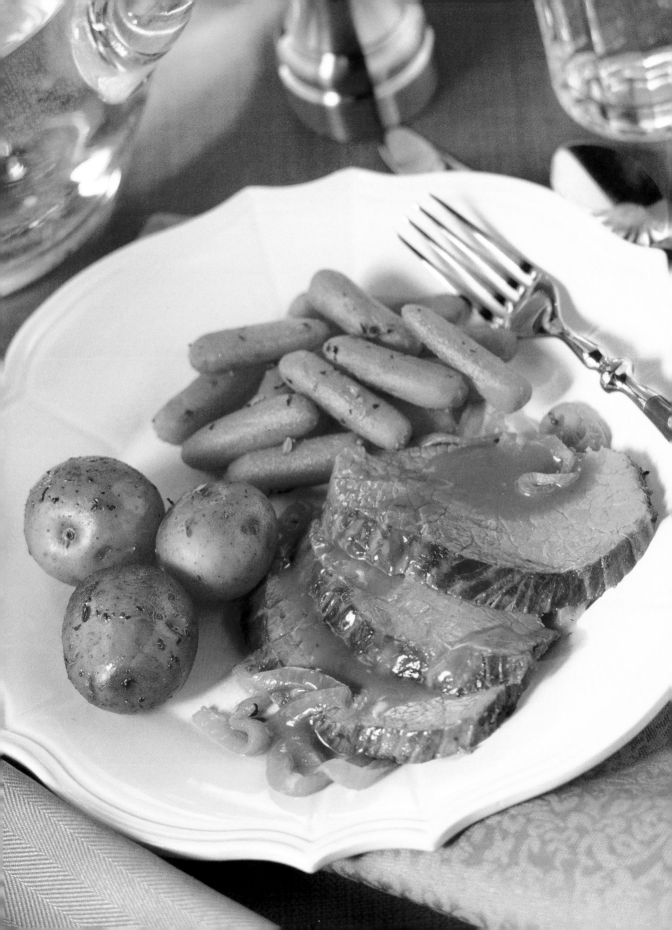

Pot Roast

Tender slow-cooked beef roast with
new potatoes and baby carrots

Servings: 8
Preparation Time: up to 10 hours*

INGREDIENTS

3-lb boneless beef bottom round roast,
    trimmed of all visible fat

2 onions, sliced

2 Tbsp Hungarian paprika

$\frac{1}{2}$ tsp dried basil

$\frac{1}{2}$ tsp dried oregano

$\frac{1}{2}$ tsp dried thyme

3 cloves garlic, minced

$\frac{1}{2}$ cup water

$\frac{1}{2}$ cup red wine (optional)

1 can (15 oz) low-fat, reduced-sodium beef broth

$\frac{1}{4}$ tsp ground black pepper

1$\frac{1}{2}$ lbs baby carrots

2 lbs small new potatoes

DIRECTIONS

1 Lightly coat a large skillet with cooking
spray and place over medium-high heat.
Add roast and brown on all sides, about
3 to 5 minutes per side. Place browned
roast in Crockpot.

2 Add onion slices to skillet and cook, stirring occasionally, until golden, about 5 minutes. Add paprika, basil, oregano, thyme
and garlic; cook 2 more minutes. Place
onion mixture over roast in Crockpot.

3 Add water, wine, broth, black pepper,
carrots and potatoes to Crockpot. Cover
and cook until tender, about 10 hours on
low heat or 5 hours on high heat.

4 Remove roast from the Crockpot and
set on cutting board. Use a large spoon to
skim fat off cooking broth.

5 Slice roast and place a portion on each
plate along with a portion of potatoes and a
serving of carrots. Top sliced roast with a
couple spoonfuls of broth. Serve and enjoy! ☺

Tasteful Tip

*It only takes about 20 minutes to prepare this meal, but the cooking time can be up to 10 hours. What you do is place the ingredients in a Crockpot and set it to slow cook on the low setting and leave it for the day. For example, if you're going to be at work all day, you can put it in the Crockpot in the morning and take it out in the evening when you get home. If you're not going to be out all day, you can set the Crockpot to the high setting and cook for approximately five hours. By making eight servings at once, you will be able to save extra servings in the refrigerator or by freezing them for future nutritious, delicious meals that can be prepared in minutes.

Caribbean Pork Tenderloin

*Succulent mango salsa over broiled pork tenderloin
with spinach and pearl barley*

Servings: 4
Preparation Time: 40 minutes

INGREDIENTS

¾ cup pearl barley

1½ cups reduced-sodium vegetable broth

¾ cup water

1 ripe mango, peeled and pitted, diced

1 red bell pepper, seeded and chopped

1 jalapeño, seeded and chopped

½ red onion, chopped

½ tsp lime peel, grated

1 lime, juiced

¼ cup fresh cilantro, chopped

¼ tsp salt

4 portions pork tenderloin (about 1 lb),
trimmed of fat

¼ tsp ground black pepper

1 tsp five-spice powder (found in
Asian food section)

3 Tbsp hoisin sauce (found in Asian
food section)

1 tsp toasted sesame oil

2 cups baby spinach

DIRECTIONS

1 Preheat oven to 450° F.

2 Place a large saucepan over medium heat.
Add barley and stir constantly until barley
is toasted (pale golden), about 5 minutes.

3 Add low-sodium vegetable broth and
water to toasted barley; bring to a boil
over high heat. Reduce heat to medium-
low, cover and simmer until barley is tender
and liquid is absorbed, about 35 minutes.

4 While barley is cooking, combine mango,
bell pepper, jalapeño, onion, lime peel,
lime juice, cilantro and salt in a medium
mixing bowl. Cover and refrigerate to let
the flavors blend.

5 Lightly coat a broiler pan with cooking
spray. Season pork tenderloin with black
pepper and five-spice powder. Place pork
in oven and bake 10 minutes. In a small
mixing bowl, combine hoisin sauce and
sesame oil. Coat tenderloin with sauce
and bake until juices run clear, about 15
more minutes. Remove tenderloin from
oven, let sit for 5 minutes and then cut
into ¼-inch slices.

6 Divide the spinach between 4 plates.
Top each with a portion of sliced tenderloin
and a spoonful of salsa. Add a portion of
barley, serve and enjoy! ☺

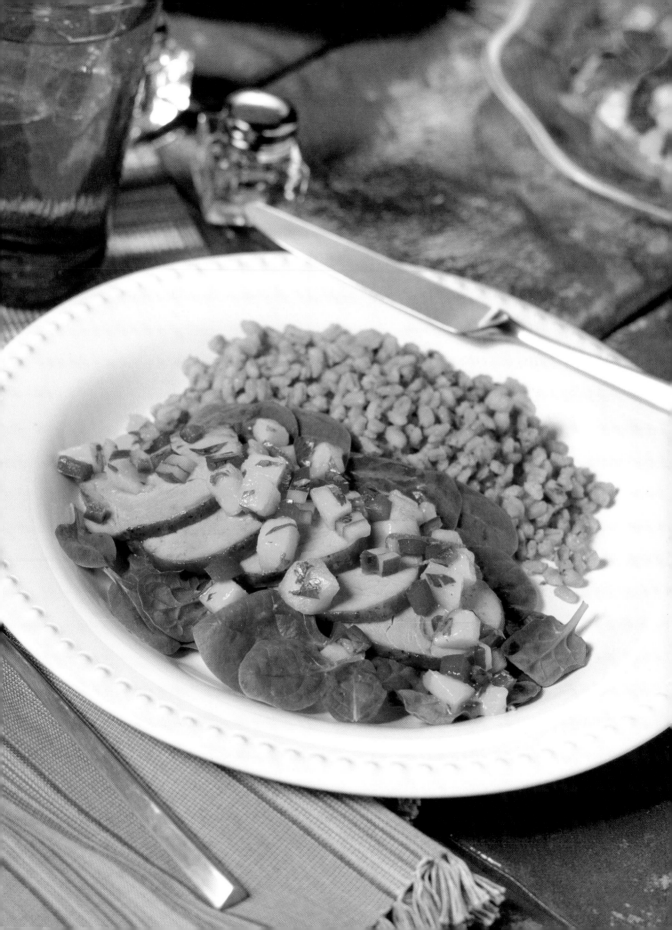

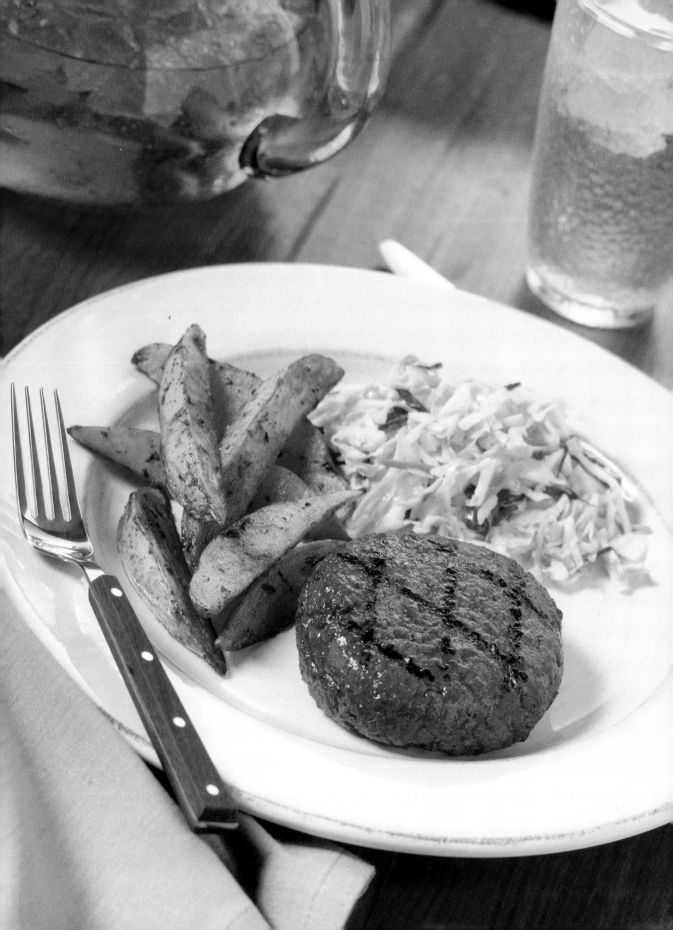

Colorado Buffalo Burger

Seasoned baked fries, cool coleslaw and a lean ground buffalo patty

Servings: 4

Preparation Time: 40 minutes

INGREDIENTS

2   Tbsp olive oil

2   Tbsp hot pepper sauce

1   tsp ground thyme

1   tsp Hungarian paprika

1   tsp ground cumin

4   portion-size white potatoes, cut into wedges

1/4   tsp black pepper

4   cups packaged coleslaw mix

1/4   onion, chopped

1/2   cup fat-free mayonnaise

2   Tbsp vinegar

2   tsp sugar substitute

4   portions lean ground buffalo (about 1 lb)

Tasteful Tip

*Buffalo, or bison, is very similar to beef. The meat has a wonderful, slightly sweet taste, is 98 percent fat free and contains high levels of minerals and vitamins. The key to cooking buffalo is not to over-cook it. For the best-tasting burgers, cook them rare to medium.

DIRECTIONS

1 Preheat oven to 450° F. Lightly coat a baking sheet with cooking spray.

2 In a large mixing bowl, combine olive oil, hot pepper sauce, thyme, paprika and cumin. Add potato wedges and toss to coat.

3 Spread coated potatoes in a single layer on baking sheet. Season with black pepper. Place in oven and bake for 15 minutes; turn and bake until golden brown, about 15 more minutes.

4 In a medium mixing bowl, combine coleslaw mix, onion, mayonnaise, vinegar and sugar substitute. Cover with plastic wrap and place in refrigerator.

5 Preheat grill to high. Then form ground buffalo into 4 portion-size patties. Place on hot grill, close lid and turn down to medium heat. Cook for 5 minutes; turn and cook to desired doneness*, about 5 more minutes.

6 Place a portion-size buffalo burger, a portion of fries and about one-fourth of the coleslaw on each plate. Serve and enjoy! ☺

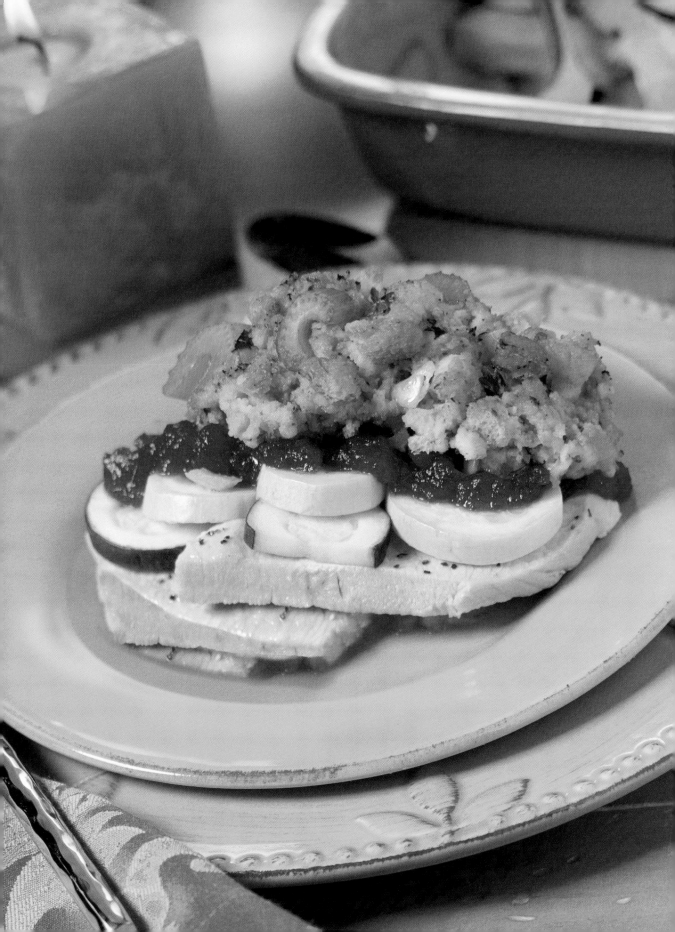

Deluxe
Turkey Dinner

Tender turkey breast, layered with steamed squash,
cranberry sauce and herb-seasoned dressing

Servings: 4
Preparation Time: 55 minutes

INGREDIENTS

1 cup herb-seasoned stuffing mix

1 cup fat-free, reduced-sodium chicken broth

2 stalks celery, chopped

½ onion, chopped

4 portions turkey breast slices (about 1 lb)

Freshly ground black pepper, to taste

1 zucchini, sliced

1 yellow squash, sliced

1 cup whole-berry cranberry sauce

DIRECTIONS

1 Preheat oven to 350° F.

2 Prepare stuffing according to its package directions, substituting fat-free chicken broth in place of butter. Add celery and onion to stuffing, and mix thoroughly.

3 Lightly coat an 8"x 8" baking dish with cooking spray. Layer turkey breast slices evenly into the bottom of the baking dish and season with freshly ground black pepper.

4 Evenly layer sliced squash on turkey, and top with a layer of cranberry sauce. Spoon prepared stuffing on top of cranberry sauce.

5 Cover with foil and bake until the turkey is cooked through, approximately 40 minutes.

6 Turn oven to broil setting. Remove foil and place under broiler for 5 minutes to brown the dressing.

7 Divide into 4 portions, serve and enjoy! ☺

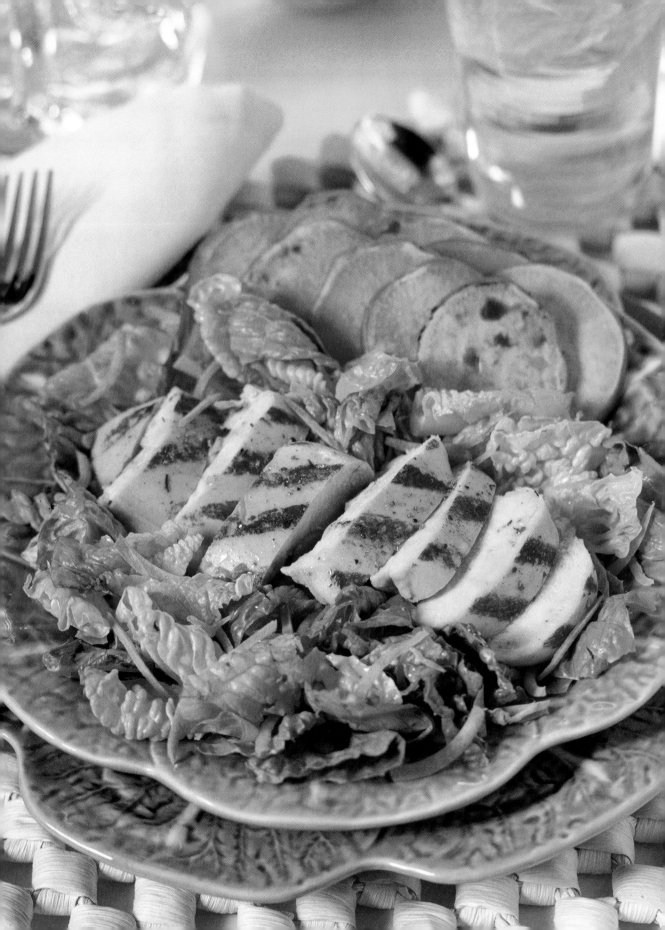

Grilled
Chicken Salad

Tender chicken strips on a bed of romaine lettuce
with lemon dressing and yam slices

Servings: 2
Preparation Time: 20 minutes

INGREDIENTS

2 portions yam, peeled, sliced

2 portions chicken breast (about 8 oz)

1 Tbsp olive oil

1 lemon, halved

$1/4$ tsp Spike® seasoning

4 cups romaine lettuce, cut into bite-size pieces

1 carrot, shredded

Freshly ground black pepper, to taste

DIRECTIONS

1 Preheat grill to high.

2 Lightly coat a small skillet with cooking spray and place over low heat. Place yam slices in the skillet and cook 8 minutes, turn and cook another 8 minutes, or until fork tender.

3 While the yams are cooking, place the chicken on a hot grill and cook for about 6 minutes on each side, until no longer pink in the center. Let the chicken cool slightly, then slice into $1/2$-inch strips and set aside.

4 In a small mixing bowl, combine the oil, lemon juice and Spike seasoning; mix well and set aside.

5 Divide romaine lettuce and place on two separate plates. Sprinkle with shredded carrot. Top with a portion of sliced chicken.

6 Pour lemon dressing over salads and top with freshly ground black pepper. Place a portion of cooked yam slices on each plate. Serve and enjoy! ☺

Baked Halibut

*Lemon Parmesan rice, steamed asparagus spears
and fresh baked halibut steak*

Servings: 4
Preparation Time: 45 minutes

INGREDIENTS

4 portions brown rice (about 1 cup uncooked)

4 portion-size halibut steaks (about 1 1/2 lbs)

1/4 tsp ground black pepper

3/4 cup fat-free plain yogurt

1/4 cup breadcrumbs

1 clove garlic, minced

1 1/2 tsp chives, chopped

3 Tbsp reduced-fat Parmesan cheese,
   grated, divided

1 tsp paprika

1 1/2 lbs asparagus spears, trimmed

1 tsp grated lemon peel

1 lemon, halved

DIRECTIONS

1 Prepare brown rice according to package directions.

2 Preheat oven to 400° F.

3 While rice is cooking, lightly coat a broiler pan with cooking spray. Arrange halibut steaks on the broiler pan and season with black pepper.

4 In a medium mixing bowl, combine yogurt, breadcrumbs, garlic and chives. Spread the yogurt mixture evenly over halibut steaks. Sprinkle 2 tablespoons Parmesan cheese over the yogurt mixture, and top with paprika.

5 Bake, uncovered, until the halibut is opaque throughout, approximately 15 to 20 minutes.

6 Place asparagus spears in an 8"x 8" baking dish; add 2 tablespoons of water. Cover with plastic wrap and pierce with a fork several times to vent. Microwave on high until crisp tender, about 4 to 6 minutes. Remove from microwave and let stand 2 minutes.

7 Mix grated lemon peel and remaining tablespoon of Parmesan into cooked rice.

8 Place portions of halibut and rice on each of 4 plates along with about one-fourth of the asparagus. Top baked halibut with a squeeze of lemon. Serve and enjoy! ☺

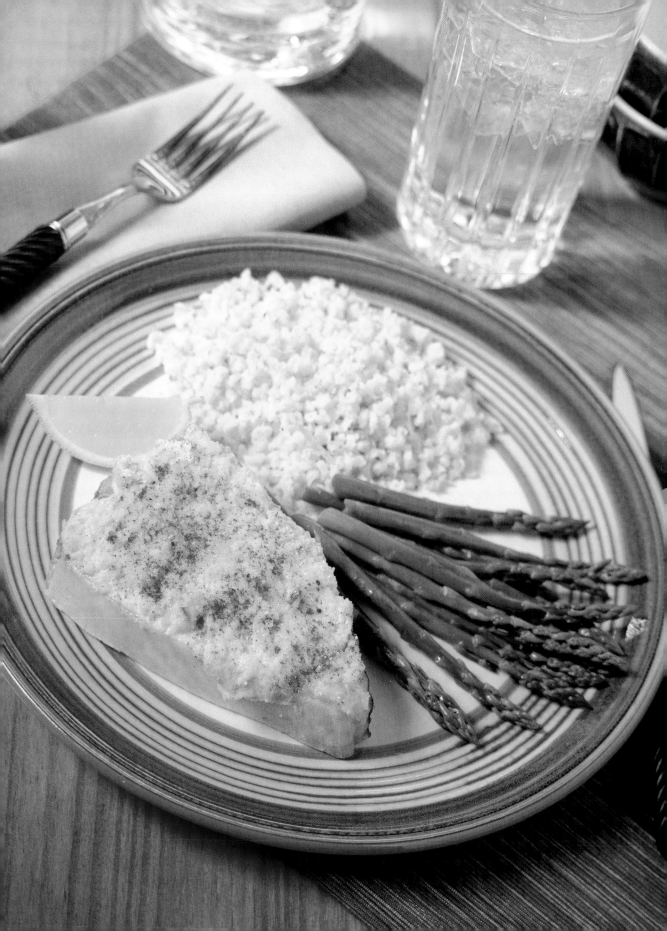

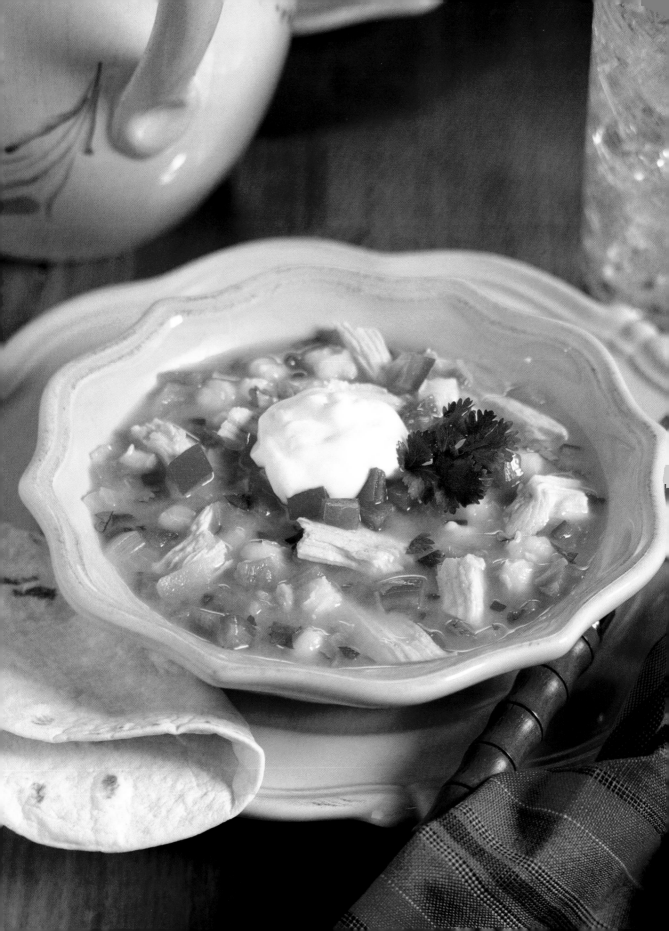

Dad's Great Green Chili

Flavorful green chili with shredded chicken,
fresh tomato and BP's* special spices

Servings: 8
Preparation Time: 1 hour, 15 minutes

INGREDIENTS

8   cups fat-free, reduced-sodium chicken broth

1   onion, finely chopped

8   portions chicken breast (about 2 lbs)

2   packages Knorr® Roasted Chicken Gravy Mix

3   cans (7 oz each) mild diced green chilies

6   cloves garlic, minced

$\frac{1}{2}$ cup fresh cilantro, chopped

$\frac{1}{2}$ tsp ground cumin

2   jalapeños, seeded and chopped

1   can (28 oz) white hominy, drained

8   (6-inch) flour tortillas

1   tomato, diced

$\frac{1}{2}$ cup fat-free sour cream

—— Tasteful Tip ——

This recipe makes eight servings of delicious green chili, which is great for "planned-overs." Store extra servings in single-portion Tupperware® containers and freeze for up to two months. Microwave to reheat for quick, great-tasting meals!

❧

*BP is my father's nickname. His full name is William *James* Phillips, and my middle name is *Nathaniel*. So, technically, he is not a "senior," and I am not a "junior." Anyway... his Green Chili *really* is great!

DIRECTIONS

1 In a large pot, combine chicken broth, onion and chicken breasts. Heat to boiling over high heat. Then reduce heat to low and simmer until the chicken is no longer pink in the center, about 20 minutes. Remove chicken from the broth and set aside to cool.

2 Use a whisk to blend gravy mix into the broth. Then add chilies, garlic, cilantro, cumin, jalapeños and hominy. Bring to a boil over medium-high heat; then reduce heat to low.

3 Shred the cooked chicken by pulling it apart with two forks, and add it back into the broth. Cover and simmer for 40 minutes.

4 Warm flour tortillas by placing them between two damp paper towels and microwaving on high for 45 seconds.

5 Spoon a portion of the green chili (about 1$\frac{1}{2}$ cups) into each bowl, top with a spoonful of diced tomato and a tablespoon of sour cream.

6 Fold a warmed tortilla, and place it beside the bowl of chili for dipping. Serve and enjoy! ☺

Marinated Flank Steak

*Mushroom gravy over flavorfully marinated steak slices,
with Italian green beans and baked potato*

Servings: 4
Preparation Time: 1 hour, 20 minutes

INGREDIENTS

$^1\!/_3$ cup lite soy sauce

1 Tbsp balsamic vinegar

1 Tbsp olive oil

4 cloves garlic, crushed

1 tsp ground ginger

$^1\!/_2$ tsp ground black pepper

1 flank steak (about 1 $^1\!/_2$ lbs)

4 portion-size potatoes

1 bag (14 oz) frozen cut Italian green beans

8 oz fresh mushrooms, sliced

1 $^1\!/_4$ cups water

1 pkg Knorr® Hunter mushroom gravy mix

2 Tbsp Butter Buds®

1 green onion, sliced

——— Tasteful Tip ———

Flank steak is a lean and flavorful cut of beef. Try slicing it across the grain (the grain in beef is akin to the grain in wood) into very thin pieces to make it tender.

DIRECTIONS

1 In a large Ziploc® bag, combine soy sauce, vinegar, olive oil, garlic, ginger and black pepper. Using a fork, pierce flank steak several times on both sides and place in Ziploc® bag with marinade. Seal bag and refrigerate for at least an hour.

2 Preheat oven to 450° F. Wash and dry potatoes and pierce several times with a fork. Bake directly on the oven rack until tender, about 45 minutes.

3 After potatoes have baked for about 30 minutes, prepare Italian green beans according to package directions.

4 Move potatoes to bottom rack of oven and preheat broiler. Remove steak from marinade and place on a broiler pan. Broil 3 inches from heat source for about 6 minutes on each side.

5 Lightly coat a medium skillet with cooking spray and place over medium-high heat. Sauté mushrooms for about 2 minutes. Add water and gravy mix. Bring to a boil, stirring constantly. Reduce heat to low, simmer until thickened, about 5 minutes.

6 Slice steak across the grain into $^1\!/_8$-inch slices. Place a portion of steak and a portion of baked potato with a serving of Italian green beans on each plate. Slice potato open and top with Butter Buds and green onion. Top steak with gravy. Serve and enjoy! ☺

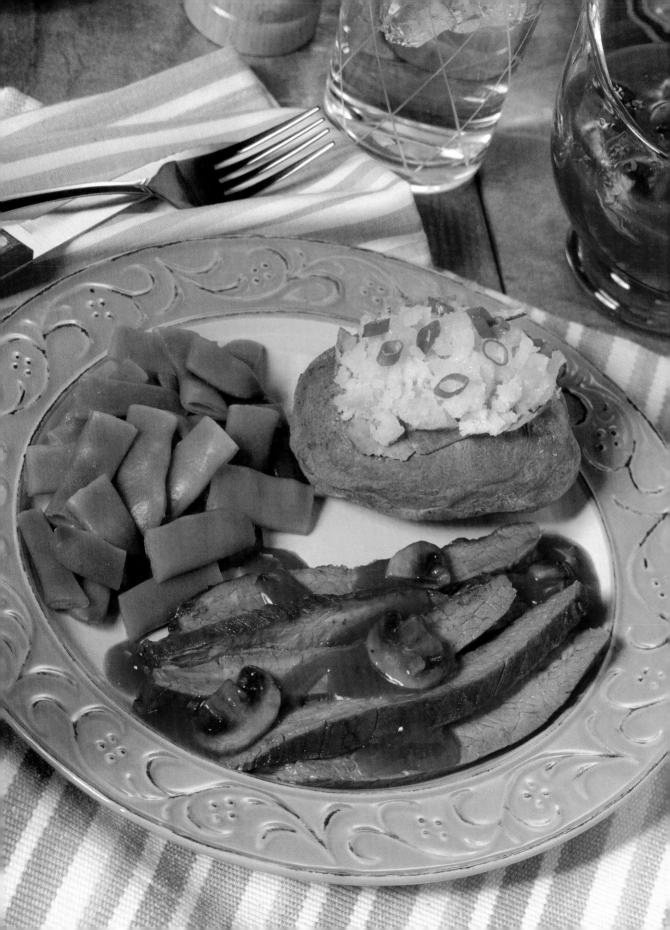

Spicy Buffalo Chicken Sandwich

*Hot wings-style chicken breast on a whole-grain bun,
blue cheese dip, carrots and celery sticks*

Servings: 4
Preparation Time: 22 minutes

INGREDIENTS

- 2 tsp Hungarian paprika
- 2 tsp chili powder
- 4 portions chicken breast (about 1 lb)
- 1 Tbsp olive oil
- 1/2 cup hot pepper sauce
- 3/4 cup fat-free sour cream
- 2 green onions, sliced
- 1 oz blue cheese, crumbled
- 4 whole-grain buns, split
- 4 lettuce leaves
- 8 celery stalks, cut into sticks
- 6 large carrots, peeled and cut into sticks

DIRECTIONS

1 In a small bowl, combine paprika and chili powder. Then sprinkle spice blend over chicken breasts.

2 Lightly coat a large skillet with cooking spray and place over medium-low heat. Place chicken breasts in skillet; cook for 6 minutes. Turn and cook until no longer pink in the center, about 6 more minutes.

3 Place a large saucepan over low heat. Add olive oil and heat for 1 minute. Stir in hot pepper sauce.

4 When the chicken breasts are done, remove from skillet, place in saucepan and coat evenly with hot pepper sauce mixture.

5 In a small mixing bowl, combine sour cream, green onion and blue cheese.

6 Place a whole-grain bun on each of four plates, top with lettuce leaf and a portion-size chicken breast. Arrange about one-fourth of the blue cheese dip, celery and carrot sticks on each plate. Serve and enjoy! ☺

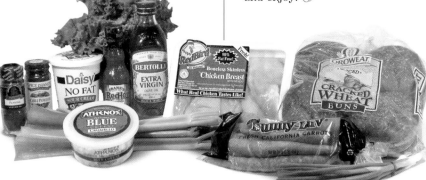

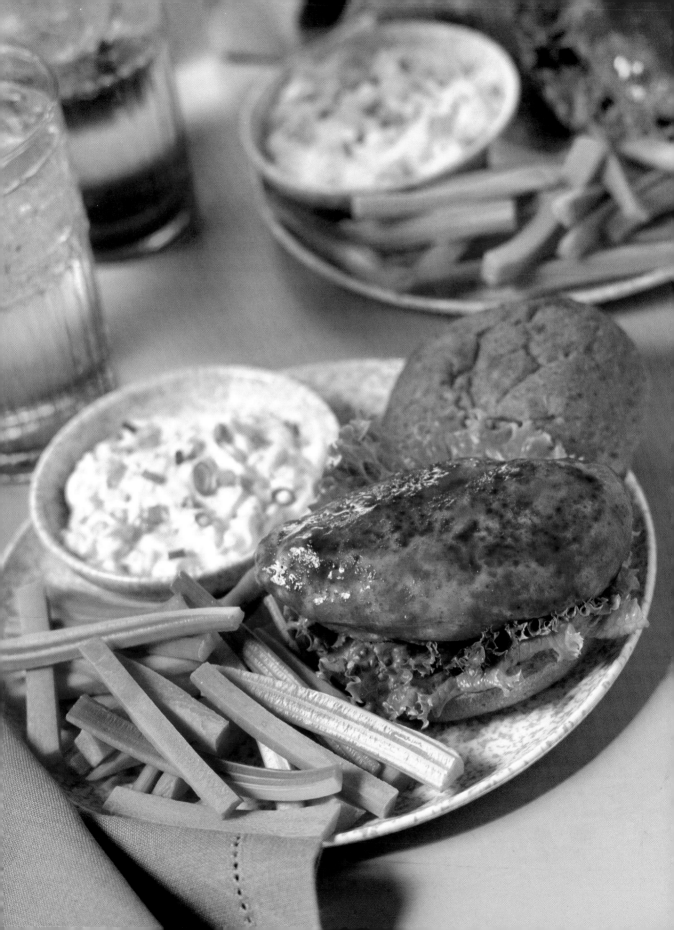

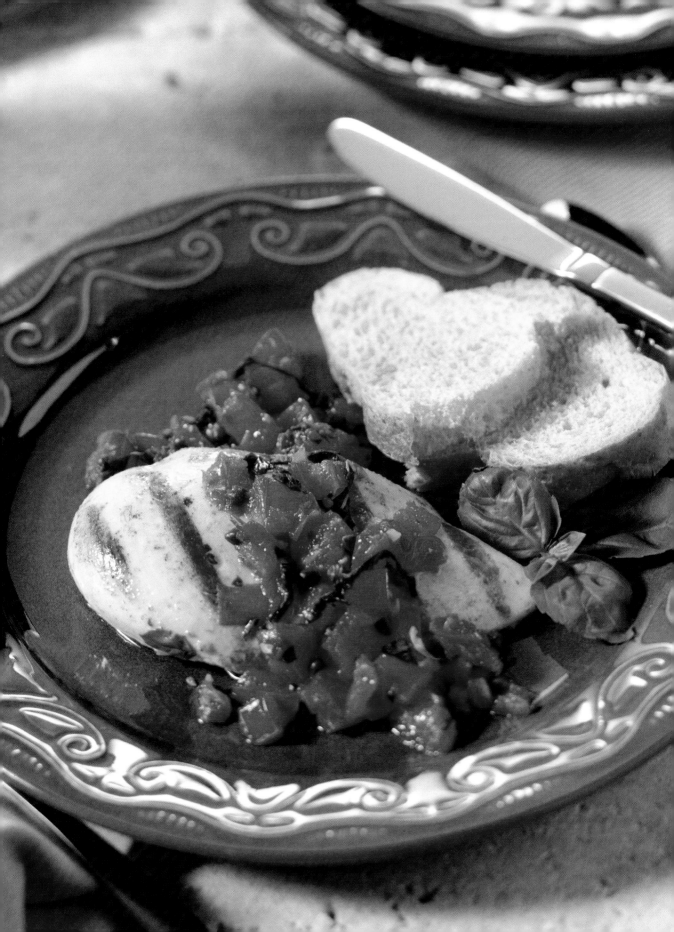

Grilled Chicken Tuscan Style

Sautéed tomatoes, basil and capers
over grilled chicken breast with whole-wheat bread

Servings: 2
Preparation Time: 20 minutes

INGREDIENTS

2 portions chicken breast (about $^1/_2$ lb)

1 Tbsp olive oil

2 tomatoes, diced

2 Tbsp capers, drained and rinsed

$^1/_2$ tsp Mrs. Dash® Tomato-Basil-Garlic seasoning

$^1/_4$ cup fresh basil, sliced, divided

2 portions whole-wheat bread

DIRECTIONS

1 Preheat grill to high.

2 Place chicken on hot grill and cook for about 6 minutes; turn and grill for about 6 more minutes, until no longer pink in the center.

3 While the chicken is cooking, heat olive oil in a large skillet over medium-low heat. Add tomatoes and capers; sauté until soft, about 10 minutes.

4 Stir in Mrs. Dash seasoning and half of the sliced basil; sauté for 2 more minutes.

5 Place a portion of chicken on two separate plates and top each with half the tomato and caper mixture; sprinkle with the remaining fresh basil.

6 Place a portion of whole-wheat bread on each plate. Serve and enjoy! ☺

French Dip Sandwich

*Tender roast beef, double dipped in homemade au jus
on a whole-grain roll with crisp green salad*

Servings: 4
Preparation Time: 20 minutes

INGREDIENTS

- 1 Tbsp olive oil
- 1 shallot, chopped
- 1 Tbsp all-purpose flour
- 3 Tbsp dry sherry (optional)
- 2 cans (10$\frac{1}{2}$ oz each) beef consommé
- 1 bag (10 oz) romaine salad blend
- $\frac{1}{3}$ cup Newman's Own® Light Balsamic Vinaigrette
- Freshly ground black pepper, to taste
- 4 whole-grain rolls, split
- 4 portions lean roast beef, thinly sliced (about 1 lb)
- 1 tsp McCormick® Montreal Steak Seasoning
- 8 cherry peppers

DIRECTIONS

1 Place a large skillet over medium heat, add olive oil and heat for 1 minute. Add shallots and sauté 2 minutes. Add flour and sauté 2 more minutes. Whisk in sherry and cook for 3 minutes.

2 While whisking, slowly pour in beef consommé. Bring to a boil over high heat. Then reduce heat to low and simmer.

3 Place salad greens in a large mixing bowl. Drizzle with vinaigrette, toss to coat and season with black pepper. Divide into 4 salad bowls.

4 Set out 4 dinner plates. Place a roll and a ramekin (or small cup) on each plate.

5 Divide roast beef into 4 portions. Use tongs to dip a portion of roast beef into warm au jus sauce, place inside roll and sprinkle with steak seasoning.

6 Fill ramekins with extra au jus sauce for dipping. Place 2 cherry peppers on each plate. Serve and enjoy! 😊

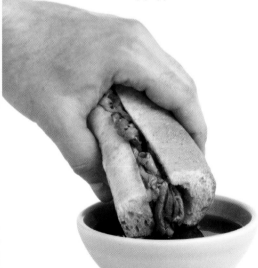

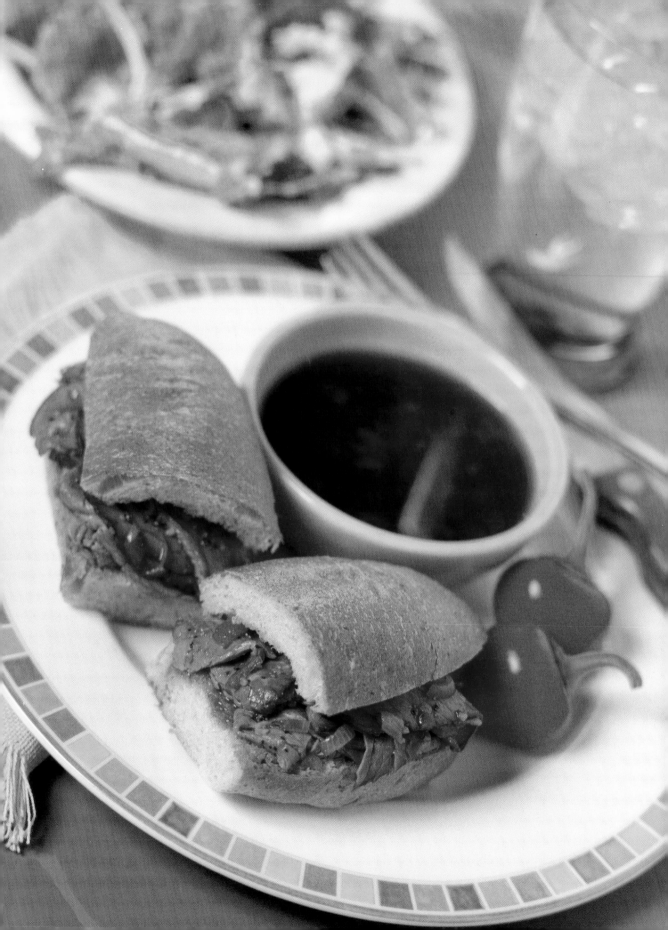

Chicken Minestrone

Italian-inspired soup with chicken, fresh vegetables,
beans and pasta topped with Parmesan cheese

Servings: 6
Preparation Time: 35 minutes

INGREDIENTS

2 Tbsp olive oil

2 slices Canadian bacon, chopped

1 onion, chopped

2 celery stalks, sliced

4 cloves garlic, crushed

1 medium zucchini, diced

1 bay leaf

1 can (15 oz) cannellini beans, drained and rinsed

1 can (15 oz) red kidney beans, drained and rinsed

6 cups fat-free, reduced-sodium chicken broth

2 cups water

6 portions chicken breast, cut into ½-inch chunks (about 1½ lbs)

¾ cup Ditalini pasta

1 box (10 oz) frozen green beans

1 bag (5 oz) baby spinach

3 Tbsp fresh basil, sliced

2 Tbsp fresh Parmesan, grated

DIRECTIONS

1 Place a large pot over medium-high heat. Add oil and heat for 1 minute. Add Canadian bacon and sauté for 4 minutes. Add onions, celery, garlic, zucchini and bay leaf, sauté for another 5 minutes.

2 Add cannellini beans, red kidney beans, chicken broth and water to the pot. Bring to a boil over high heat. Then add chicken and cook for 10 more minutes.

3 Reduce heat to medium high; add pasta and green beans. Cook until pasta is tender, about 8 minutes.

4 Remove bay leaf from soup with tongs or a spoon. Stir in spinach and cook until slightly wilted, about 1 minute.

5 Ladle a portion (about 2 cups) of minestrone into each bowl. Top with fresh basil and Parmesan. Serve and enjoy! ☺

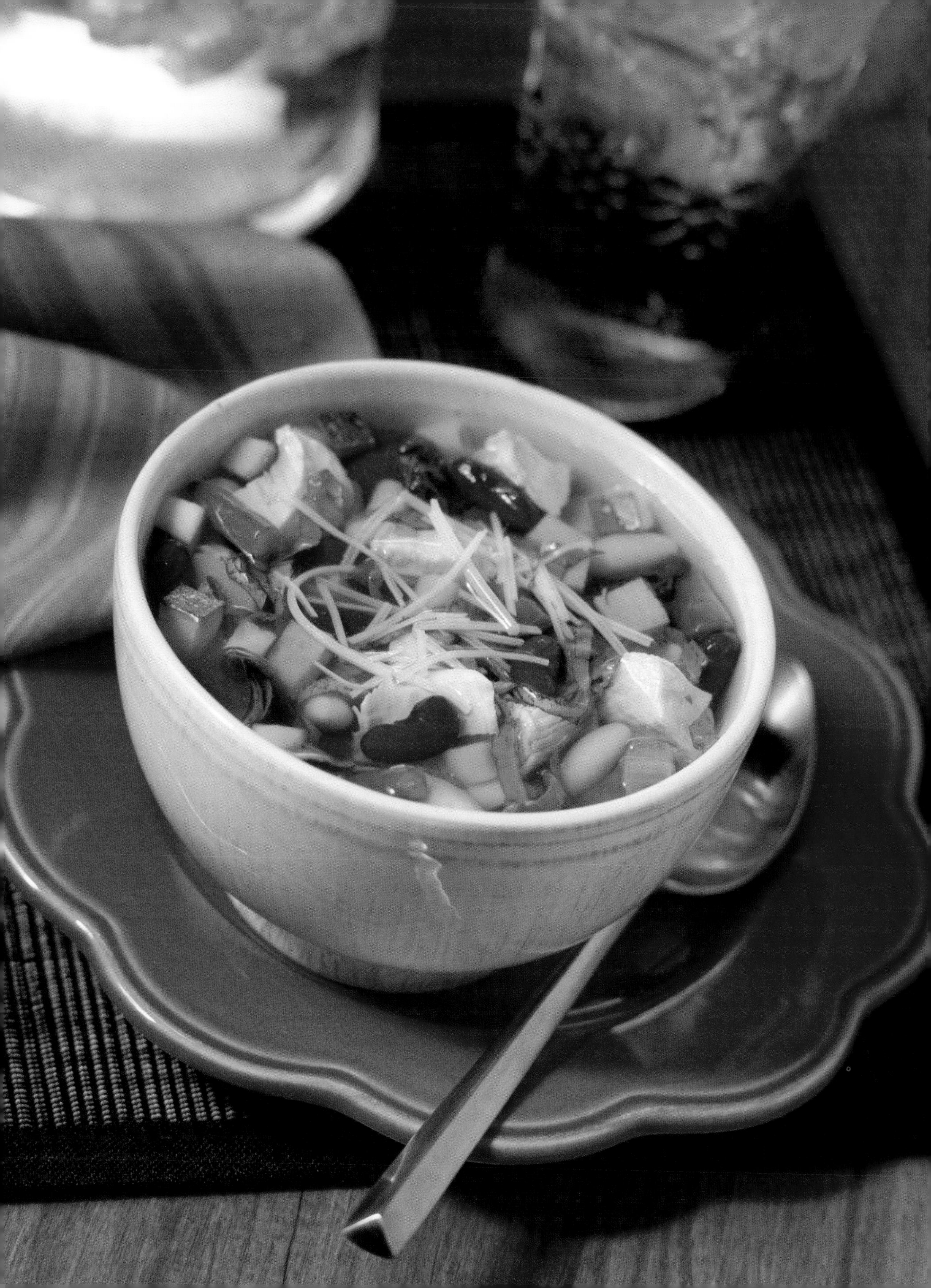

Greek Chicken Pitas

Mediterranean-style chicken, fresh tomato and lettuce
with cucumber-dill sauce in a pita

Servings: 2
Preparation Time: 35 minutes

INGREDIENTS

1 lemon, halved

½ cup water

2 portions chicken breast (about ½ lb)

2 Tbsp Greek seasoning

½ tsp lemon-pepper seasoning

⅓ cup fat-free plain yogurt

½ small cucumber, peeled, seeded and chopped

1 clove garlic, minced

1 Tbsp fresh chives, chopped

1 Tbsp fresh dill, chopped

2 pitas

2 lettuce leaves

2 tomato slices

DIRECTIONS

1 In a large Ziploc® bag, combine lemon juice and water; set aside. Coat the chicken breasts with Greek seasoning and lemon-pepper seasoning, then place in Ziploc bag with lemon juice mixture. Close the bag and gently squeeze to make sure chicken is coated. Set in refrigerator to marinate for at least 15 minutes.

2 While chicken is marinating, preheat the grill to high. Then combine the yogurt, cucumber, garlic, chives and dill in a small mixing bowl; cover and refrigerate.

3 Place marinated chicken on hot grill and cook for approximately 6 minutes, turn and grill 6 more minutes until no longer pink in the center. Let the chicken cool slightly, then cut into strips.

4 Slice top off pitas, open and fill with a lettuce leaf, tomato slice and a portion of sliced chicken. Top each with half the cucumber-dill sauce. Serve and enjoy! ☺

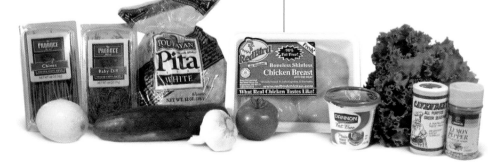

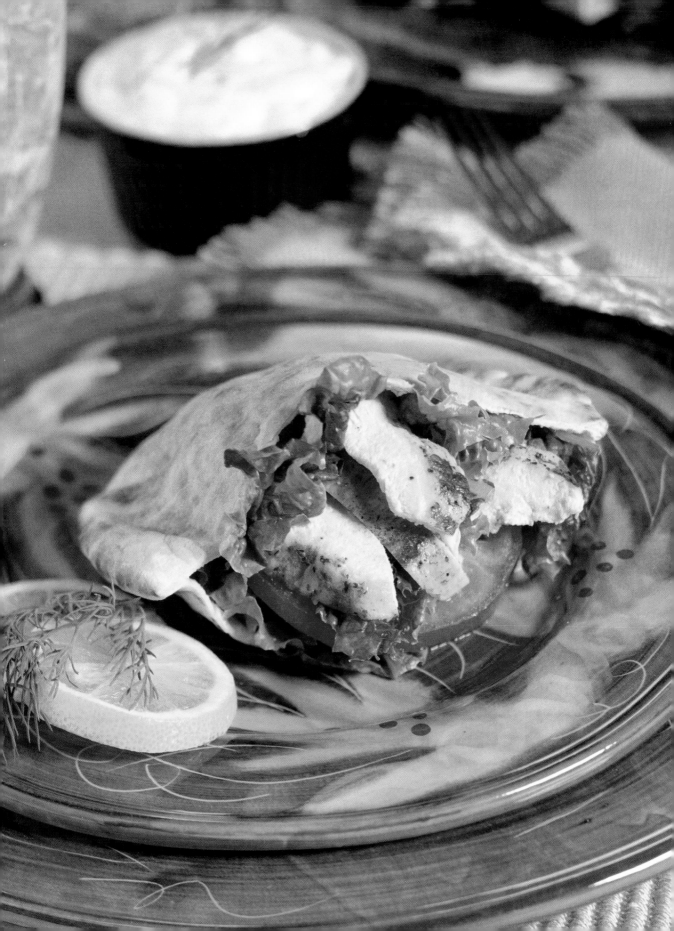

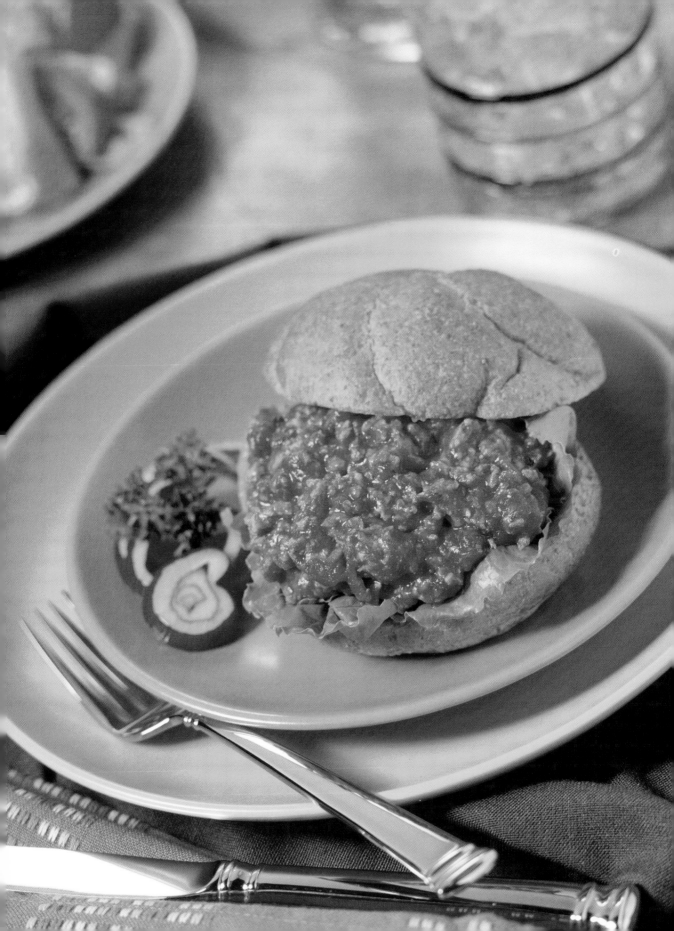

Sloppy Joes

Ground turkey and savory tomato sauce on a soft wheat roll

Servings: 4
Preparation Time: 25 minutes

INGREDIENTS

4 portions lean ground turkey (about 1 lb)

1/4 tsp ground black pepper

1/2 red onion, chopped

1 can (8 oz) no-salt-added tomato sauce

1/2 cup ketchup

1/4 cup barbecue sauce

1 tsp chili powder

Dash of hot pepper sauce

4 wheat buns or rolls, split

4 lettuce leaves

Tasteful Tip

For convenience, the ground turkey mixture can be prepared in advance and refrigerated for up to three days or frozen in portion-size servings for up to two months. These Sloppy Joes are great for lunches or quick dinners!

DIRECTIONS

1 In a large skillet, combine ground turkey, black pepper and onion. Cook over medium heat, stirring occasionally, until the turkey is no longer pink.

2 Stir in tomato sauce, ketchup, barbecue sauce, chili powder and hot pepper sauce. Simmer for about 10 minutes over low heat, stirring occasionally, until mixture has thickened.

3 Place a wheat bun on each plate. Top each with a lettuce leaf and a portion of turkey mixture. Serve and enjoy! ☺

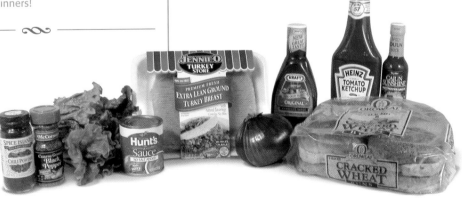

Herbed Chicken

Rosemary red potatoes and steamed baby carrots
with herb-marinated broiled chicken

Servings: 4
Preparation Time: 55 minutes

INGREDIENTS

1 cup fat-free plain yogurt, divided

2 tsp Italian seasoning, divided

2 cloves garlic, minced, divided

$\frac{1}{4}$ tsp ground black pepper, divided

1 Tbsp fresh basil, chopped

1 lemon, halved

4 portions chicken breast (about 1 lb)

4 portions new red potatoes (about 1$\frac{1}{2}$ lbs)

2 Tbsp reduced-fat Parmesan cheese, grated

1 lb baby carrots, trimmed

1 tsp fresh rosemary, chopped

1 Tbsp Butter Buds®

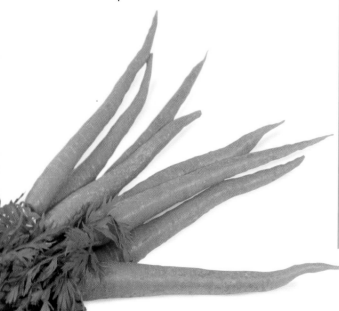

DIRECTIONS

1 In a large mixing bowl, combine $\frac{3}{4}$ cup yogurt, 1 tsp Italian seasoning, 1 clove minced garlic, $\frac{1}{8}$ tsp black pepper, fresh basil and lemon juice. Add chicken to yogurt marinade. Cover and refrigerate for at least 30 minutes.

2 While chicken is marinating, cut potatoes into quarters and place them in a large saucepan. Cover with water, bring to a boil over high heat, then reduce heat to low. Cover and simmer until tender, about 20 minutes.

3 Preheat broiler and lightly coat a broiler pan with cooking spray. Place marinated chicken on the pan and broil 6 inches from the heat source for about 15 minutes. Top chicken with Parmesan cheese and broil until lightly browned, about 2 more minutes.

4 Place baby carrots in a medium saucepan with about 1 inch of water. Bring to a boil over high heat, then cover and reduce heat to low. Steam until tender, about 9 minutes.

5 In a small bowl, combine remaining $\frac{1}{4}$ cup yogurt, 1 tsp Italian seasoning, 1 clove minced garlic, $\frac{1}{8}$ tsp black pepper, rosemary and Butter Buds. Drain potatoes and return to saucepan. Stir in yogurt mixture to coat.

6 Place a portion of chicken and a portion of potatoes with about one-fourth of the carrots on each plate. Serve and enjoy! ☺

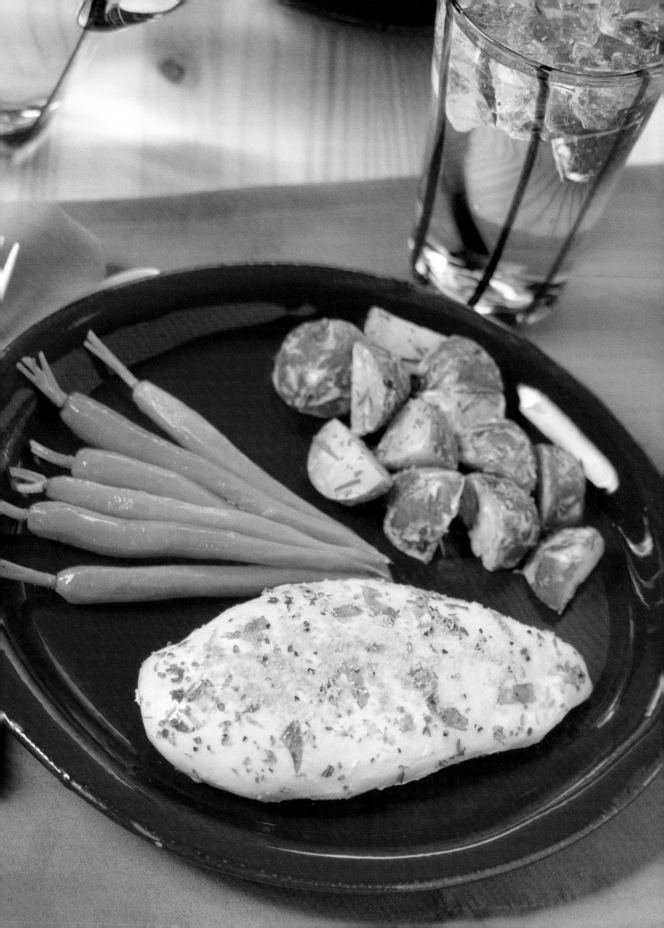

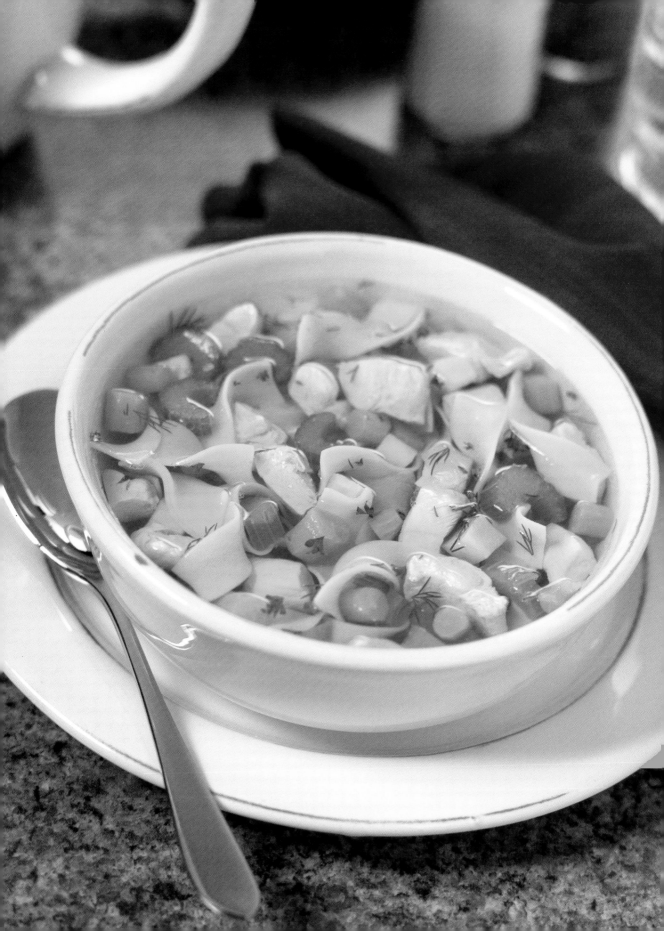

Chicken Noodle Soup

Wholesome, healthy, homemade,
good ol' fashioned chicken soup

Servings: 8
Preparation Time: 30 minutes

INGREDIENTS

2 Tbsp olive oil

1 onion, chopped

4 carrots, peeled and chopped

2 parsnips, peeled and chopped

4 celery stalks, chopped

4 bay leaves

$\frac{1}{2}$ tsp ground black pepper

12 cups fat-free, reduced-sodium chicken broth

2 cups water

8 portions chicken breast (about 2 lbs),
   cut into bite-size pieces

8 portions wide egg noodles (about 1 lb)

$\frac{1}{4}$ cup fresh parsley, chopped

2 Tbsp fresh dill, chopped

DIRECTIONS

1 Heat olive oil in a large pot over medium heat. Add chopped onion and sauté for about 4 minutes.

2 Add carrots, parsnips, celery, bay leaves, black pepper, chicken broth and water. Bring to a boil over high heat.

3 Add uncooked chicken pieces to broth and bring back up to a boil.

4 Add noodles and simmer until tender, about 8 minutes. Reduce heat to low.

5 Remove bay leaves, then stir in parsley and dill.

6 Ladle a portion (about 2 cups) of soup into each bowl. Serve and enjoy! ☺

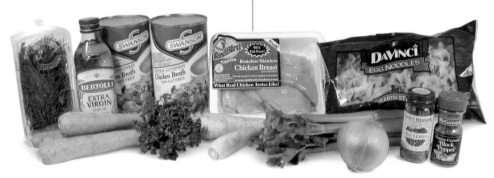

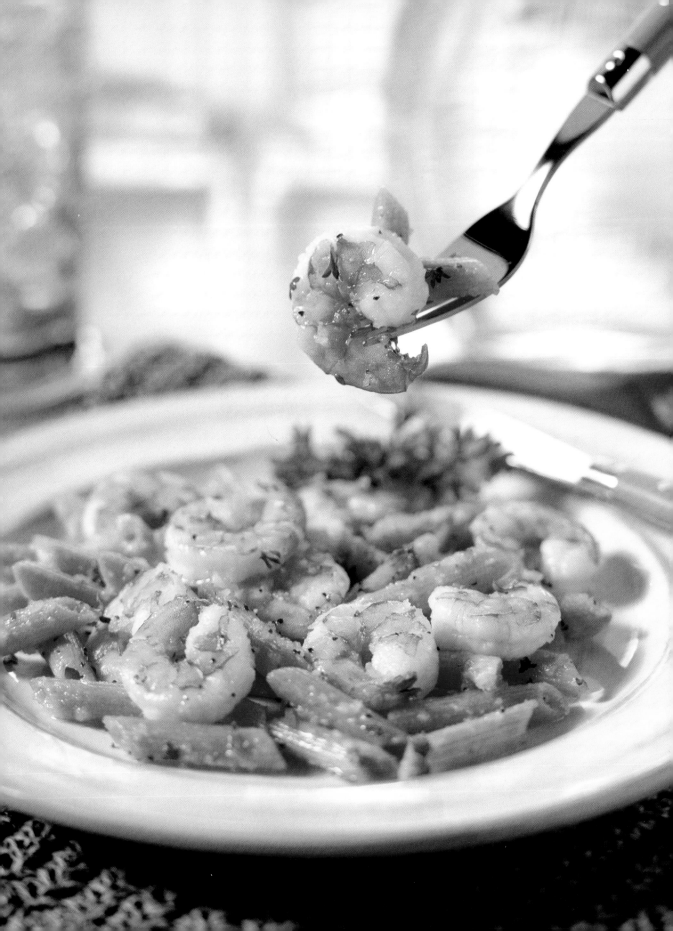

Shrimp Scampi

Shrimp sautéed in a white wine and garlic sauce with penne pasta

Servings: 2
Preparation Time: 25 minutes

INGREDIENTS

2 portions whole-wheat penne pasta (about 4 oz uncooked)

1 Tbsp olive oil

3 cloves garlic, minced

2 portions raw shrimp, peeled and deveined (about 1/2 lb)

3 Tbsp Butter Buds®, divided

3 Tbsp white wine (or chicken broth)

1/4 tsp ground black pepper

1 lemon, halved

3 Tbsp reduced-fat Parmesan cheese, grated

2 Tbsp fresh parsley, chopped

——— Tasteful Tip ———

The Eating *for* Life version of this traditionally rich-tasting dish uses olive oil and Butter Buds® instead of butter. You'll enjoy the rich taste without the saturated fat!

DIRECTIONS

1 Prepare penne pasta according to its package directions.

2 While the pasta is cooking, heat olive oil and garlic in a wok or large skillet over medium heat.

3 Add shrimp to the skillet and cook, stirring frequently, until it's almost pink (three-quarters done), about 2 minutes.

4 Add 1 Tbsp of Butter Buds and white wine to shrimp; sauté about 2 more minutes.

5 Place cooked pasta in a large mixing bowl and combine it with remainder of the Butter Buds and black pepper; mix gently.

6 Add cooked shrimp to pasta and gently mix it all together.

7 Divide into two portions and spoon onto plates. Top with a squeeze of lemon, Parmesan cheese and fresh parsley. Serve and enjoy! ☺

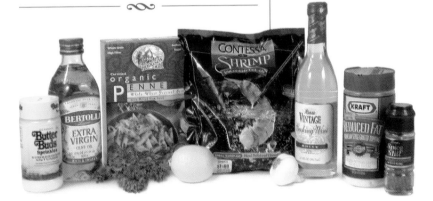

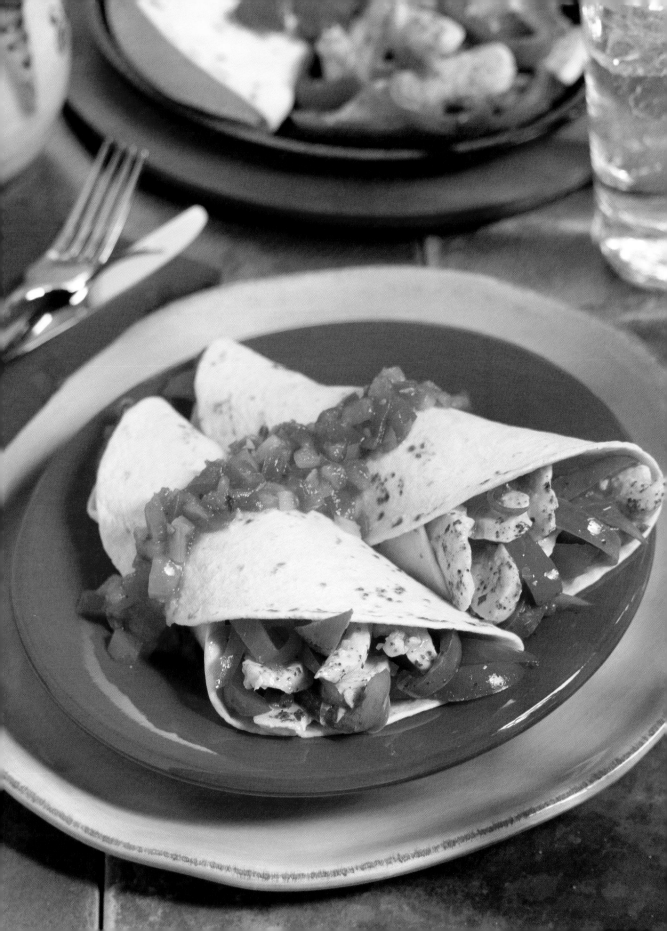

Chicken Fajitas

*Marinated chicken, sautéed bell pepper and onion
with spicy salsa in a hot flour tortilla*

Servings: 2
Preparation Time: 55 minutes

INGREDIENTS

2   portions chicken breast (about $^1/_2$ lb),
    cut into $^1/_2$-inch strips

2   Tbsp fat-free Italian salad dressing

1   tsp chili powder

1   onion, sliced

1   green bell pepper, cut into $^1/_4$-inch strips

1   red bell pepper, cut into $^1/_4$-inch strips

4   (6-inch) flour tortillas

$^1/_4$ cup salsa

DIRECTIONS

1 In a large Ziploc® bag, combine sliced chicken and Italian dressing. Make sure chicken is coated, and seal the bag. Place in refrigerator to marinate at least 30 minutes. (Marinate longer, perhaps overnight, to enhance flavor even more.)

2 Lightly coat a large skillet with cooking spray and place over medium-high heat. Add the chicken, marinade and chili powder; sauté until chicken is no longer pink in the center, about 7 minutes. Transfer chicken to a plate and cover with foil to keep warm.

3 Lightly coat the same skillet with cooking spray; add onions and sauté until soft, about 5 minutes. Add green and red bell peppers and sauté until tender, about 7 more minutes.

4 Add cooked chicken back to the skillet, combine with the onion and peppers and sauté until heated through, about 2 more minutes.

5 Warm tortillas in the microwave between 2 dampened paper towels for about 45 seconds. Place 2 tortillas on each plate and fill each with about one-fourth of the chicken mixture. Top with salsa, serve and enjoy! ☺

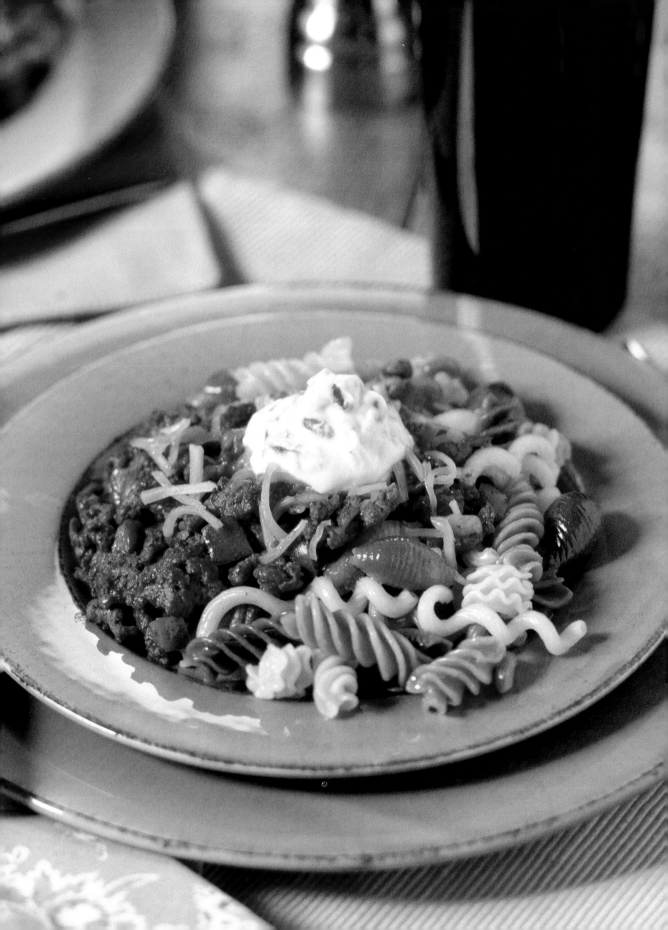

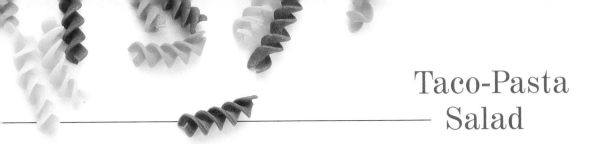

Taco-Pasta Salad

Spicy ground beef served with
pasta, bell pepper, salsa and sour cream

Servings: 2
Preparation Time: 20 minutes

INGREDIENTS

2 portions rotini pasta (about 4 oz uncooked)

2 portions lean ground beef (about ½ lb)

¼ cup water

1 Tbsp taco seasoning mix

1 green bell pepper, diced

2 Tbsp salsa

2 Tbsp fat-free sour cream

2 Tbsp reduced-fat cheddar cheese, shredded

——— Tasteful Tip ———

This simple and easy-to-prepare Taco-Pasta Salad is great for quick dinners! Extra servings or "planned-overs" can be stored in airtight Tupperware® containers and refrigerated for tomorrow's lunch. It's even good served cold. So simple!

DIRECTIONS

1 Prepare rotini pasta according to its package directions.

2 While the pasta is cooking, brown ground beef in a medium skillet over medium heat until no longer pink. Drain the beef of any excess fat and return it to the skillet.

3 Add water, taco seasoning and bell pepper to cooked ground beef; simmer until the sauce thickens, stirring occasionally.

4 While the beef is simmering, combine salsa and sour cream in a small bowl.

5 Place a portion of pasta on two separate plates. Top with a portion of ground beef mixture. Sprinkle each with half of the cheese and a dollop of salsa-sour cream sauce. Serve and enjoy! ☺

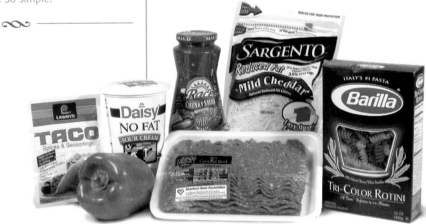

Chili Rellenos Casserole

Green chilies filled with melted Monterey Jack cheese
baked in a light egg soufflé

Servings: 4
Preparation Time: 45 minutes

INGREDIENTS

3 cans (4 oz) whole green chilies, drained

4 oz reduced-fat Monterey Jack cheese

1 1/4 cup egg substitute

1/2 cup flour

1/2 cup skim milk

1/2 cup reduced-fat cheddar cheese, shredded

1 tsp chili powder

2 green onions, sliced

1/2 cup salsa

DIRECTIONS

1 Preheat oven to 350° F.

2 Lightly coat an 11" x 7" baking dish with cooking spray.

3 Lay whole green chilies out on paper towels. Slice Monterey Jack cheese into the same number of pieces as there are chilies. Insert a slice of cheese inside each chili and arrange evenly in baking dish.

4 In a medium mixing bowl, whisk together egg substitute, flour and milk. Pour egg mixture over chilies in baking dish.

5 Layer shredded cheddar cheese on top of casserole, then sprinkle with chili powder and green onion.

6 Bake for 35 minutes or until top is golden brown and toothpick inserted in center comes out "clean." (If the toothpick does not come out clean, that means the casserole is not yet cooked through. Give it a few more minutes, and test it again.)

7 Cut into 4 portions and top with salsa. Serve and enjoy! ☺

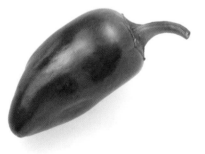

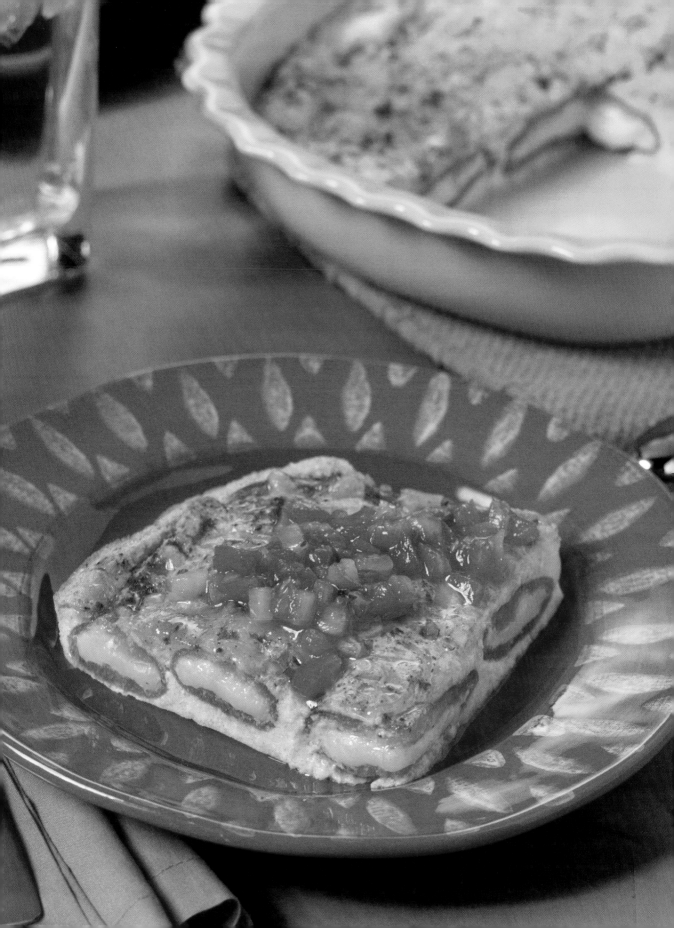

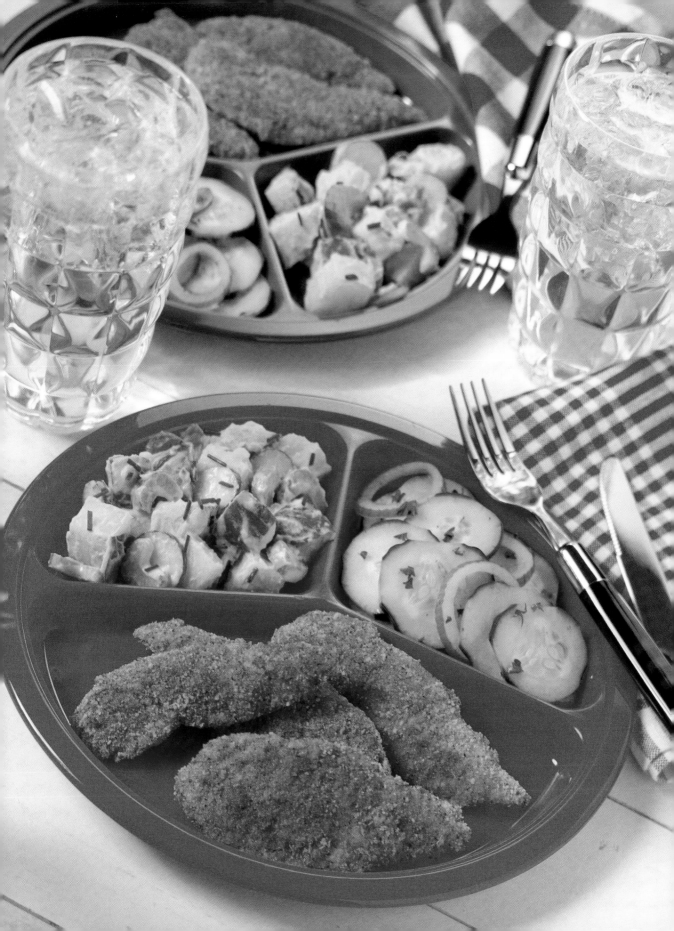

Chicken
Tenders

Buttermilk baked chicken strips with
potato salad and crisp cucumbers

Servings: 4
Preparation Time: 50 minutes

INGREDIENTS

4 portions red potatoes, diced

1 red onion, thinly sliced

2 cucumbers, thinly sliced

$1/3$ cup cider vinegar

$1/3$ cup water

1 Tbsp sugar substitute

$3/4$ tsp ground black pepper, divided

1 Tbsp fresh parsley, chopped

1 Tbsp white vinegar

1 cup low-fat buttermilk

1 cup breadcrumbs

1 tsp paprika

1 tsp poultry seasoning

$1/4$ tsp ground red pepper

$1/4$ tsp allspice

4 portions chicken breast tenders (about 1 lb)

$1/2$ white onion, peeled

1 Tbsp yellow mustard

$1/2$ cup fat-free mayonnaise

$1/3$ cup radishes, sliced

1 stalk celery, sliced

DIRECTIONS

1 Place potatoes in a large saucepan and cover with water. Boil over high heat until "fork tender," about 15 minutes.

2 In a medium glass bowl, combine red onion, cucumber, cider vinegar, water, sugar substitute, $1/4$ teaspoon black pepper and fresh parsley. Cover and refrigerate.

3 Drain potatoes and return to hot saucepan. Sprinkle with white vinegar, then place in a large glass bowl; set aside to cool.

4 Preheat oven to 400° F. Lightly coat a broiler pan with cooking spray.

5 Pour buttermilk into a pie plate. In another pie plate, combine breadcrumbs, paprika, poultry seasoning, red pepper, allspice and $1/4$ teaspoon black pepper.

6 Dip chicken in buttermilk, then coat with breadcrumbs on both sides and place on broiler pan. Bake for 6 minutes, turn and bake 6 more minutes, until no longer pink in the center.

7 Grate a tablespoon of white onion over the cooked potatoes. Stir in mustard, mayonnaise, $1/4$ teaspoon black pepper, radishes and celery.

8 Place a portion of chicken tenders and a portion of potato salad with a serving of cucumbers on each plate. Serve and enjoy! ☺

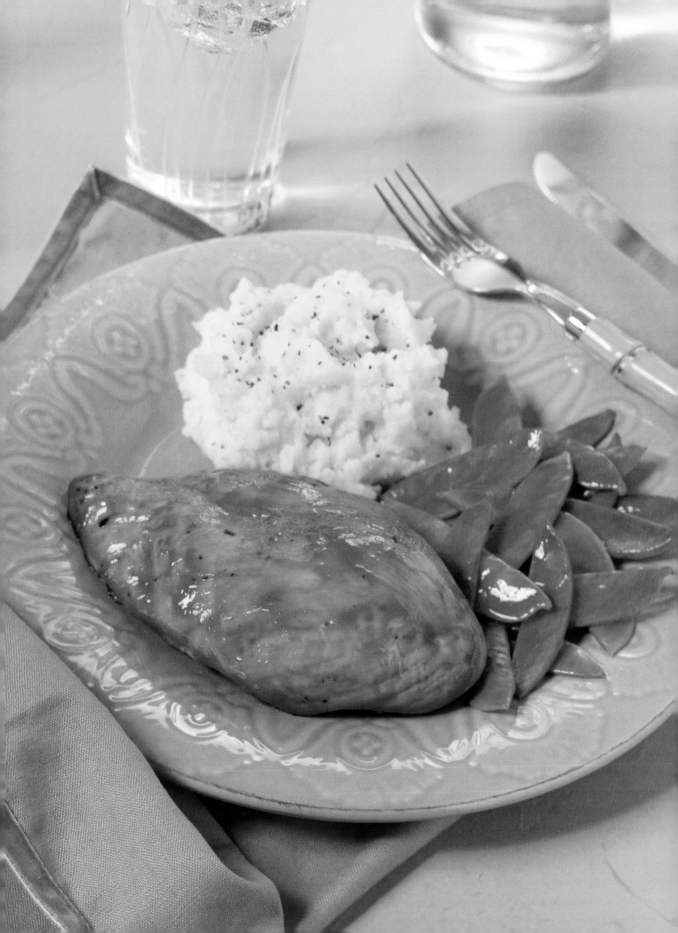

Teriyaki Chicken

Broiled breast of chicken, steamed snow peas
and wasabi mashed potatoes

Servings: 4
Preparation Time: 55 minutes

INGREDIENTS

4 portions chicken breast (about 1 lb)

¼ cup teriyaki marinade

4 portion-size potatoes

1 lb snow peas, trimmed (stem end and string removed)

1 tsp powdered wasabi

¼ tsp ground black pepper

¼ cup skim milk

¼ cup fat-free sour cream

—— Tasteful Tip ——

Chicken breast, potatoes and a steamed vegetable... this is basic and in some ways best when it comes to the Eating *for* Lifestyle. Be sure to keep an eye on your portion sizes and be conscious of when you feel *your* satisfaction level.

DIRECTIONS

1 In a large Ziploc® bag, combine chicken breasts and teriyaki marinade. Make sure chicken is coated and seal the bag. Place in refrigerator to marinate for at least 30 minutes.

2 While the chicken is marinating, peel potatoes and then cut into 1-inch chunks. Place potatoes in a large saucepan and cover with water. Bring to a boil over high heat. Then, reduce heat to low, cover and simmer until tender, about 20 minutes.

3 Preheat broiler. Lightly coat a broiler pan with cooking spray. Remove chicken from the marinade and place it on the pan. Broil chicken 6 inches from heat source, without turning, until no longer pink in the center, about 15 minutes.

4 Place snow peas in a medium saucepan with about 1 inch of water. Bring to a boil over high heat, then cover and reduce heat to low. Steam until crisp-tender, about 3 minutes.

5 Drain potatoes. Then mash with wasabi and black pepper. Add skim milk and sour cream and continue to mash until light and fluffy.

6 Place a portion of chicken and a portion of mashed potatoes with about one-fourth of the snow peas on each plate. Serve and enjoy! ☺

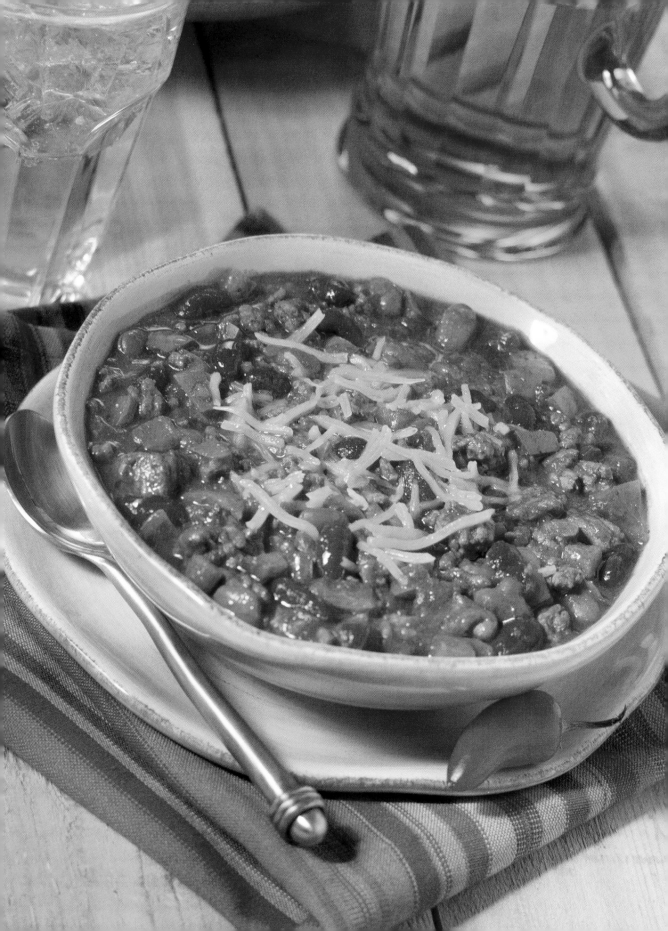

Hot Stuff Chili!

Four-alarm chili con carne; high in nutrition and even higher in flavor

Servings: 8
Preparation Time: 1 hour, 45 minutes

INGREDIENTS

8 portions lean ground beef (about 2 lbs)

1 white onion, chopped

8 cloves garlic, minced

1 green bell pepper, diced

$\frac{1}{4}$ cup fresh Italian parsley, chopped

3 jalapeños, seeded and chopped

$\frac{1}{3}$ cup fresh red chili powder*

1$\frac{1}{2}$ tsp ground cumin

3 cans (15 oz) low-fat, reduced-sodium beef broth

$\frac{1}{3}$ cup dry vermouth (optional)

1 can (28 oz) crushed tomatoes

1 can (15 oz) kidney beans, drained and rinsed

1 can (15 oz) chili beans

$\frac{1}{2}$ cup sharp reduced-fat cheddar cheese, shredded

—— Tasteful Tip ——

*For "powerful flavor," try the chili powder often found in cellophane packages in the Mexican food section (not the spice section) of your grocery store. Choose mild, medium or **HOT** (if you dare!), depending on how you like it.

DIRECTIONS

1 Place a large pot over medium heat. Add ground beef, onion, garlic, bell pepper, parsley and jalapeños. Cook, stirring occasionally, until ground beef is no longer pink, about 8 minutes.

2 Stir in chili powder and cumin; cook for another 2 minutes.

3 Add beef broth, dry vermouth, tomatoes and beans; bring to a boil over high heat.

4 Reduce heat; cover and simmer for 90 minutes.

5 Ladle a portion of chili (about 1$\frac{1}{2}$ cups) into each bowl and top with about a tablespoon of cheese. Serve and enjoy! ☺

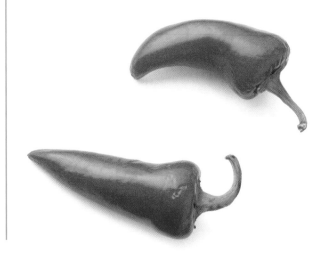

Tuna Steak Sandwich

*Pan-seared, peppered tuna fillet with
lettuce and tomato on a whole-wheat bun*

Servings: 2
Preparation Time: 30 minutes

INGREDIENTS

1   lemon, halved

2   Tbsp white wine (optional)

2   portions tuna steak (about 12 oz)

1   tsp blackened redfish seasoning

2   whole-wheat buns, split

2   lettuce leaves

2   tomato slices

——————— Tasteful Tip ———————

*Searing is simple. You just preheat the skillet over
high heat until you can drop a bead of water on it
and it immediately boils and evaporates. When it is
that hot, it's ready. All you do then is put the meat
(in this case, the tuna) on the skillet and let it cook!

DIRECTIONS

1 In a large Ziploc® bag, combine lemon
juice and white wine. Add tuna to the
lemon juice mixture and make sure it is
coated; place in refrigerator to marinate
for at least 15 minutes.

2 Remove the tuna from the marinade and
sprinkle both sides with blackened redfish
seasoning.

3 Lightly coat a skillet with cooking spray
and place over high heat. When skillet is
really hot, add the tuna steaks and sear for
2 minutes.* Then turn steaks and reduce
the heat to low, cover with foil and cook
approximately 5 minutes for rare or
7 minutes for medium.

4 Place tuna steaks on whole-wheat rolls
with lettuce and tomato. Serve and enjoy! ☺

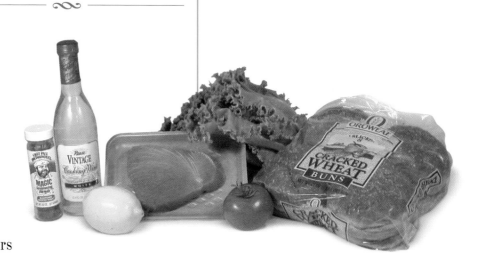

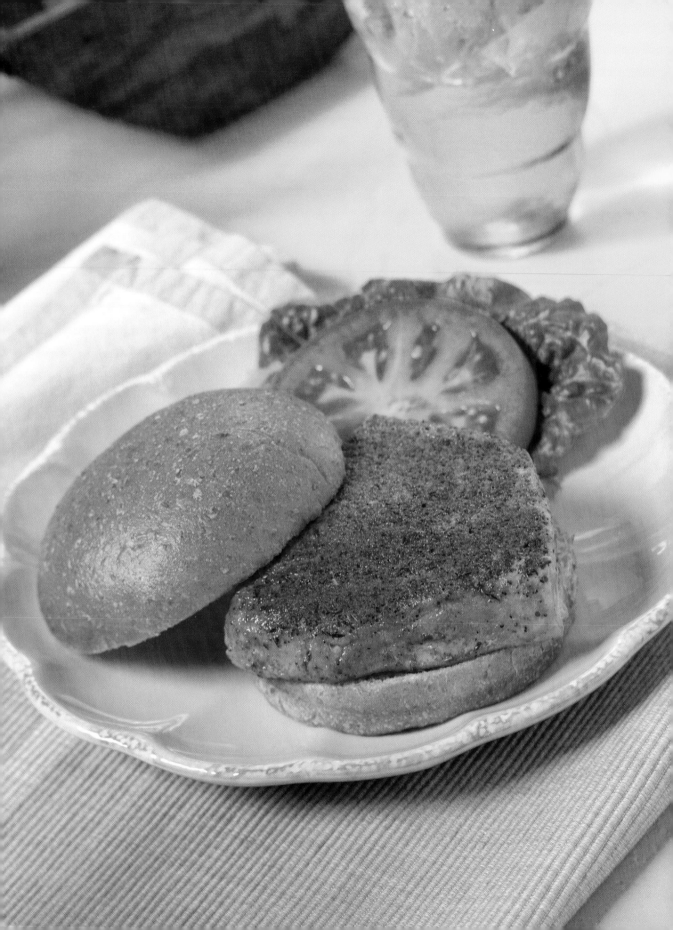

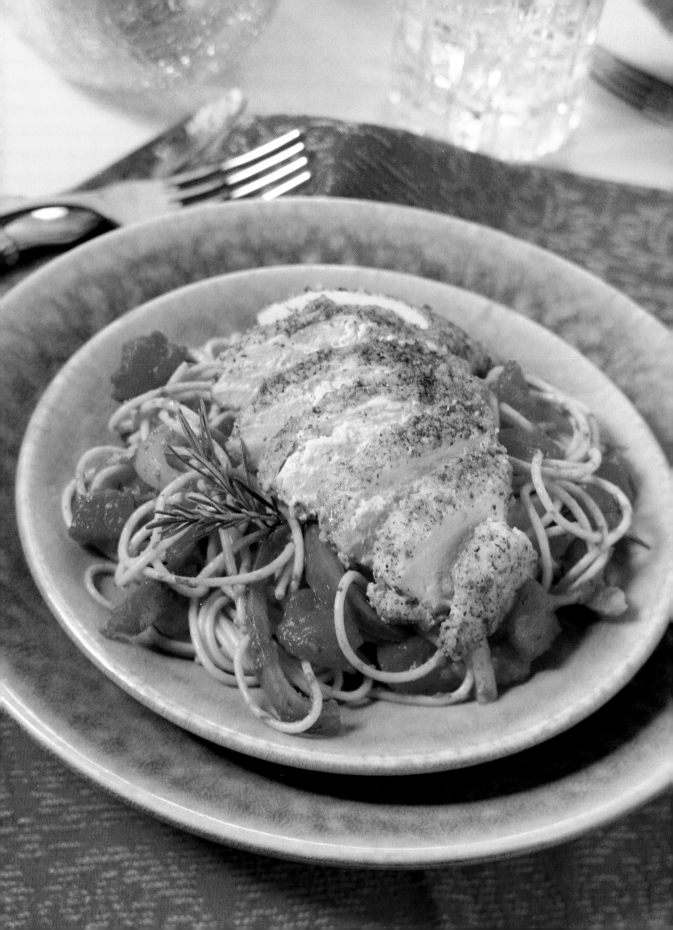

Chicken Pomodoro

Succulent sautéed tomatoes with
Italian-seasoned chicken and pasta

Servings: 4
Preparation Time: 30 minutes

INGREDIENTS

4   portions spaghetti (about 8 oz uncooked)

2   egg whites

4   tsp Mrs. Dash® Tomato-Basil-Garlic seasoning

¼   cup reduced-fat Parmesan cheese, grated

4   portions chicken breast (about 1 lb)

2   Tbsp olive oil

3   tomatoes, diced (or one 15-oz can)

1   green bell pepper, sliced

1   yellow bell pepper, sliced

¾   tsp Italian seasoning

4   Tbsp red wine (or chicken broth)

DIRECTIONS

1 Prepare spaghetti according to its package directions.

2 In a medium mixing bowl, lightly beat the egg whites. In a pie plate, combine the Mrs. Dash seasoning and Parmesan cheese.

3 Dip chicken breasts in egg whites then into the seasoned Parmesan, coating both sides.

4 Heat olive oil in a large nonstick skillet over medium heat. Place chicken breasts in skillet; cover and cook for approximately 6 minutes; turn and cook for 6 more minutes until no longer pink in the center. Transfer the cooked chicken breasts to a plate; cover with foil to keep warm.

5 Add tomatoes and bell peppers to skillet and sauté over medium heat until the peppers begin to soften, approximately 3 minutes. Stir in Italian seasoning and red wine, continue to cook for 2 minutes.

6 Add pasta to the skillet with sautéed tomatoes and peppers; mix gently.

7 Slice cooked chicken. Divide pasta mixture into four portions, top with a portion of sliced chicken, serve and enjoy! ☺

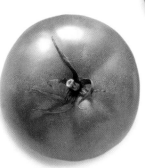
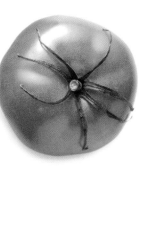

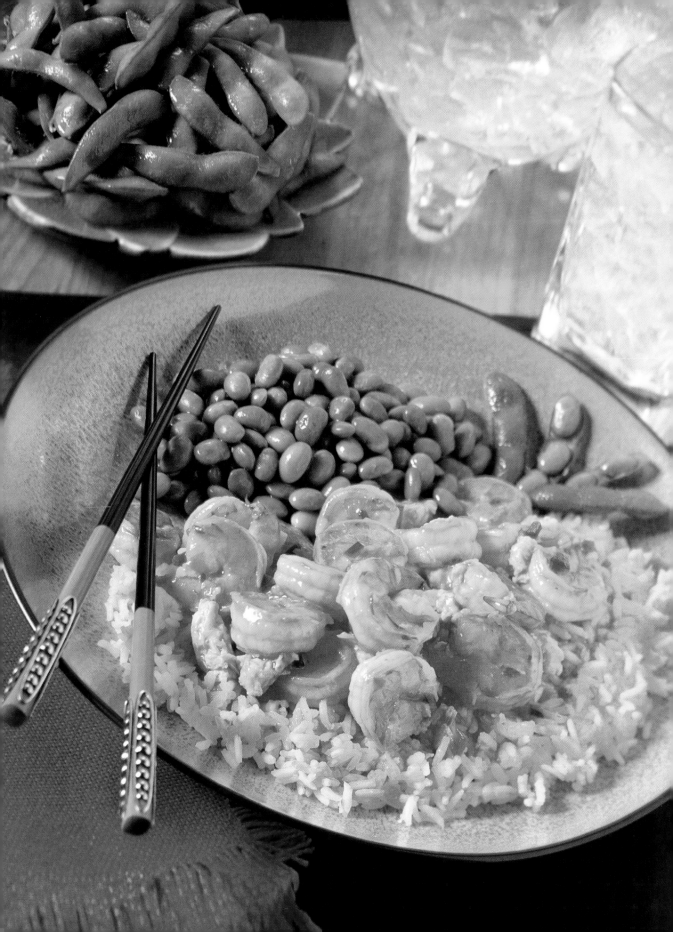

Singapore Shrimp

Stir-fried sweet and spicy shrimp
over steamed rice with soybeans

Servings: 4
Preparation Time: 25 minutes

INGREDIENTS

4   portions jasmine rice (about 1 cup uncooked)

1   package (12 oz) soybeans in the pod

4   portions raw shrimp, peeled and deveined
    (about 1 pound)

1$\frac{1}{2}$ tsp cornstarch

$\frac{1}{8}$ tsp white pepper

$\frac{1}{4}$ cup fat-free, reduced-sodium chicken broth

$\frac{1}{4}$ cup ketchup

2   Tbsp lite soy sauce

2   Tbsp rice vinegar

2   Tbsp chili garlic sauce (found in the Asian
    foods section)

2   tsp olive oil

6   cloves garlic, minced

1   tsp fresh ginger, grated

1   shallot, minced

1   jalapeño, seeded and minced

$\frac{1}{4}$ cup egg substitute

—— Tasteful Tip ——

*Soybeans in the pod are commonly referred to by
their Japanese name edamame [eh-dah-MAH-meh].
They are a delicious and nutritious, protein-rich
vegetable! To eat, simply use your fingers to push
the seeds from the pod.

DIRECTIONS

1 Prepare jasmine rice according to its
package directions; keep warm.

2 While the rice is cooking, prepare
soybeans (edamame*) according to its
package directions.

3 Then, in a medium mixing bowl, stir
together shrimp, cornstarch and white
pepper; set aside.

4 In a small mixing bowl, combine chicken
broth, ketchup, soy sauce, rice vinegar and
chili garlic sauce; set aside.

5 Heat oil in a wok or large skillet over
high heat. Add garlic, ginger, shallot and
jalapeño; stir-fry for 30 seconds. Add shrimp
mixture to the wok or skillet and stir-fry for
2 minutes. Then add the chicken broth mixture and stir-fry for 1 more minute.

6 While stirring, slowly pour the egg
substitute into the shrimp mixture.
Continue to cook, stirring constantly, for
another 30 seconds.

7 Divide the rice into four portions. Spoon
a portion of shrimp over each serving of
rice. Place a fourth of the soybeans on
each plate, serve and enjoy! ☺

Italian-Style Turkey Burger

Melted provolone and marinara over grilled portabella,
seasoned turkey patty and toasted Italian bread

Servings: 4
Preparation Time: 25 minutes

INGREDIENTS

4 portions lean ground turkey breast
(about 1 lb)

$^1/_2$ cup tomato sauce

$^1/_2$ cup reduced-fat Parmesan cheese,
grated, divided

1 Tbsp Italian seasoning

2 tsp Dijon mustard

4 portabella mushrooms

2 tsp olive oil

4 slices Italian bread

2 cups marinara sauce

4 slices reduced-fat provolone cheese

——— Tasteful Tip ———

This Eating *for* Life meal is a fun and flavorful alternative to the traditional American cheeseburger.
It's easy to make and may very well become one of
your favorites!

DIRECTIONS

1 Preheat broiler. Also, preheat grill.

2 In a medium mixing bowl, combine
ground turkey, tomato sauce, $^1/_4$ cup
Parmesan cheese, Italian seasoning
and Dijon mustard. Form mixture into
4 portion-size patties.

3 Place turkey patties on hot grill and
cook for about 6 minutes. Turn and cook
until no longer pink in the center, about
6 more minutes.

4 Clean mushrooms by wiping them with
a damp cloth. Remove and discard stems.
Brush mushroom caps with olive oil. Place
on hot grill and cook for 2 minutes, turn
and cook 2 more minutes; set aside.

5 Place Italian bread slices on a baking
sheet and place under broiler until lightly
toasted, about 3 minutes.

6 Top each toasted bread slice with a
cooked turkey burger, a portabella mushroom, $^1/_2$ cup marinara sauce and a slice
of provolone. Place under broiler until
cheese melts and sauce is warmed
through, about 3 minutes.

7 Top each with about a tablespoon of
Parmesan cheese. Serve and enjoy! ☺

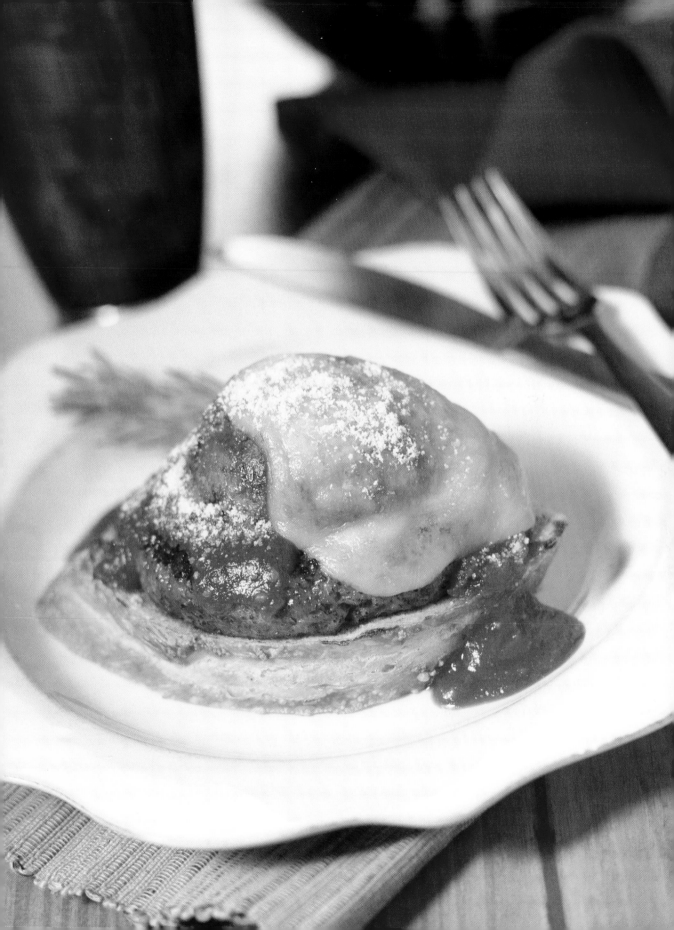

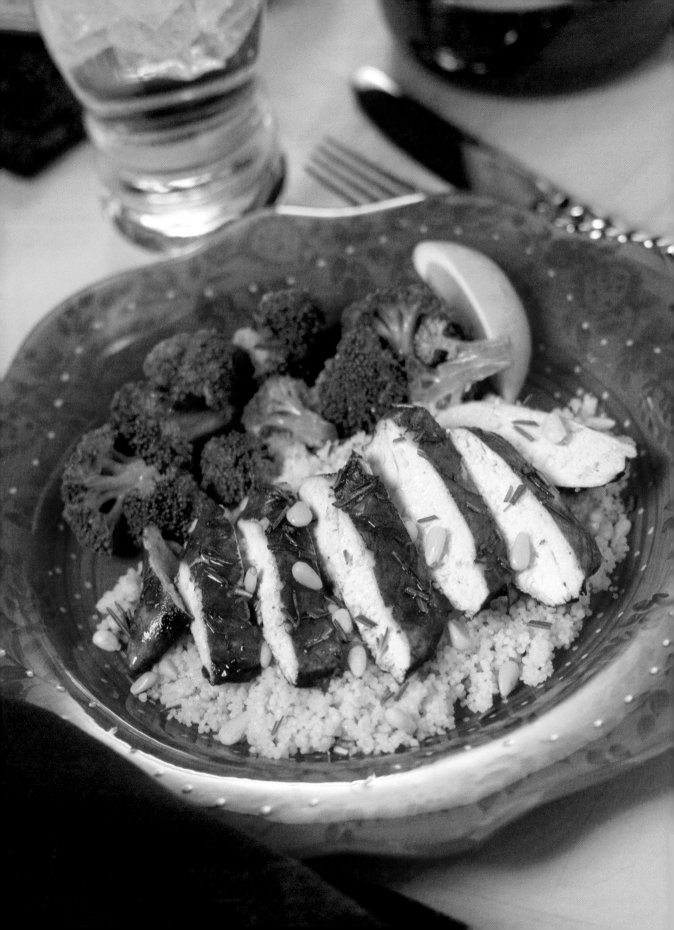

Rosemary Chicken

Balsamic glazed chicken breast topped with fresh rosemary
and pine nuts with couscous and steamed broccoli

Servings: 4
Preparation Time: 25 minutes

INGREDIENTS

3   Tbsp balsamic vinegar

2   Tbsp olive oil, divided

3   Tbsp fresh rosemary, chopped, divided

¼   tsp ground black pepper

3   cloves garlic, minced

4   portions chicken breast (about 1 pound)

1½   cups water

1   cup plain couscous

1   lb broccoli florets

2   Tbsp pine nuts

1   lemon, halved

DIRECTIONS

1 In a pie plate, mix balsamic vinegar, 1 Tbsp olive oil, 2 Tbsp fresh rosemary, black pepper and garlic. Add chicken and turn to coat.

2 Lightly coat a large skillet with cooking spray and place over medium-high heat. Place chicken in skillet and cook for 6 minutes. Turn and cook until no longer pink in the center, about 6 more minutes.

3 In a medium saucepan, combine water and remaining 1 Tbsp olive oil and bring to a boil over high heat. Stir in couscous, cover, remove from heat and allow to stand for 5 minutes. Fluff with a fork before serving.

4 While the couscous is cooking, place the broccoli in a baking dish with 2 Tbsp of water. Cover and microwave on high for 4 minutes. Stir broccoli and return to microwave until crisp-tender, about 4 more minutes.

5 Slice cooked chicken. Place a portion of couscous on each of 4 plates and top with a portion of chicken along with a serving of broccoli.

6 Top each with about a fourth of the pine nuts, remaining fresh rosemary and a squeeze of lemon. Serve and enjoy! ☺

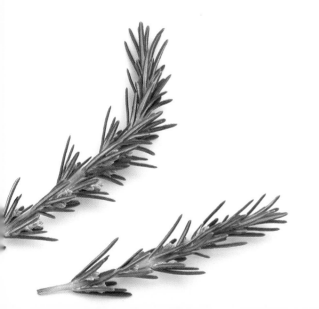

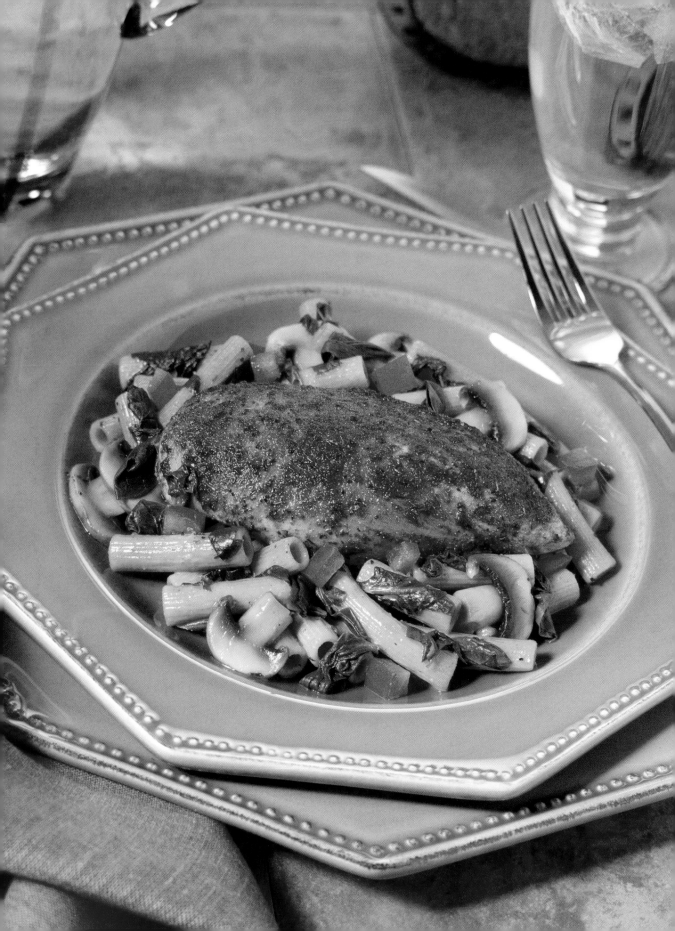

Cajun
Chicken

Spicy blackened chicken breast over pasta mixed with spinach and tomato in a buttery cream sauce

Servings: 2
Preparation Time: 25 minutes

INGREDIENTS

2 portions whole-wheat rigatoni (about 4 oz uncooked)

2 portions chicken breast (about $^1/_2$ lb)

2 Tbsp Cajun seasoning

$^1/_2$ cup skim milk

1 bag (5 oz) baby spinach leaves

8 oz fresh mushrooms, sliced

1 Tbsp Butter Buds

1 tomato, chopped

DIRECTIONS

1 Prepare rigatoni according to its package directions.

2 Lightly coat a large skillet with cooking spray and place over medium heat. Coat chicken breasts with Cajun seasoning.

3 Place chicken breasts in skillet; cook for approximately 6 minutes; turn and cook for 6 more minutes until no longer pink in the center. Transfer the cooked chicken breasts to a plate; cover with foil to keep warm.

4 Add milk, cooked pasta, spinach, mushrooms and Butter Buds to skillet; mix well.

5 Cover and simmer over low heat, stirring occasionally, until heated through, approximately 5 minutes.

6 Divide pasta mixture into two portions and top with a portion of Cajun chicken. Garnish with tomatoes, serve and enjoy! ☺

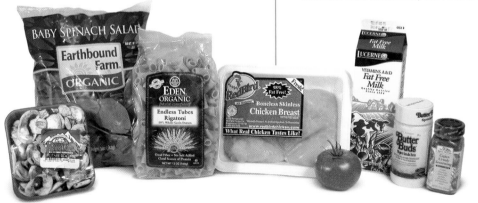

Desserts

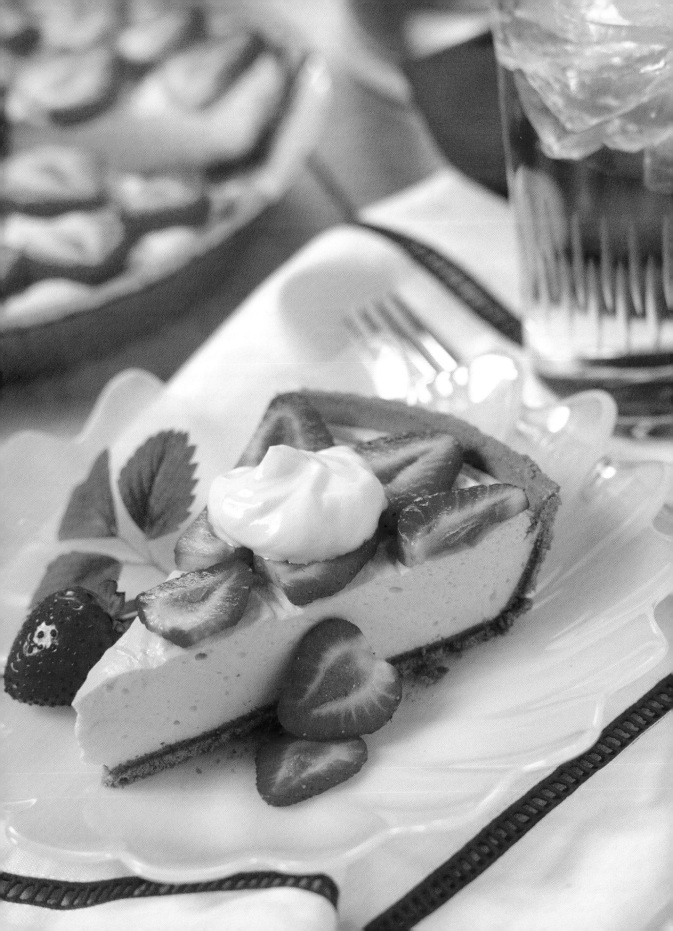

Strawberry Cheesecake

Sliced strawberries over protein-enriched
cheesecake in a graham cracker crust

Servings: 8
Preparation Time: 3 hours

INGREDIENTS

1 cup low-fat cottage cheese

1 Tbsp vanilla extract

3 Tbsp Splenda® granular

12 oz fat-free cream cheese, softened at
   room temperature

1 cup egg substitute

1 Ready Crust® reduced-fat graham cracker crust

$\frac{1}{2}$ cup fat-free sour cream

2 tsp sugar substitute

1 cup fresh strawberries, sliced

Tasteful Tip

Adding low-fat cottage cheese to "dessert-like" recipes, such as this Strawberry Cheesecake, is a new technique for many people. But it's actually a really nice way to fortify the protein content, and it produces a smooth texture and rich flavor as well!

∽

DIRECTIONS

1 Preheat oven to 350° F.

2 Spoon cottage cheese into blender and blend until smooth, about 30 seconds. Add vanilla extract and Splenda; blend for about 15 more seconds.

3 Add the softened cream cheese and blend for about 30 seconds, scraping down the sides as needed. While blending, gradually add the egg substitute and continue to blend until smooth, about 45 seconds.

4 Pour cheese filling into Ready Crust and bake until set, about 35 minutes.

5 Remove cheesecake from oven and cool for about 15 minutes. Then cover and refrigerate for at least 2 hours.

6 Prior to serving, in a small mixing bowl, combine sour cream and sugar substitute.

7 Slice cheesecake into 8 portions, top with sliced strawberries and sour cream. Serve and enjoy! ☺

Peaches 'n' Cream

Fresh sliced peaches and whipped topping
over creamy vanilla pudding

Servings: 4
Preparation Time: 25 minutes

INGREDIENTS

1 cup cold skim milk

6 oz light fat-free vanilla yogurt

2 scoops (about 48 grams of protein)
   vanilla protein powder (whey or soy)

1 package (4-serving size) vanilla fat-free,
   sugar-free instant pudding mix

2 peaches, sliced

1 cup Cool Whip® Free

DIRECTIONS

1 In a large mixing bowl, whisk together milk and yogurt until smooth. Stir in protein powder. Add pudding mix and whisk until well blended, about 2 minutes.

2 Spoon a portion of pudding mixture into each of 4 dessert bowls. Chill in refrigerator for at least 20 minutes.

3 Top with sliced peaches and a dollop of Cool Whip. Serve and enjoy! ☺

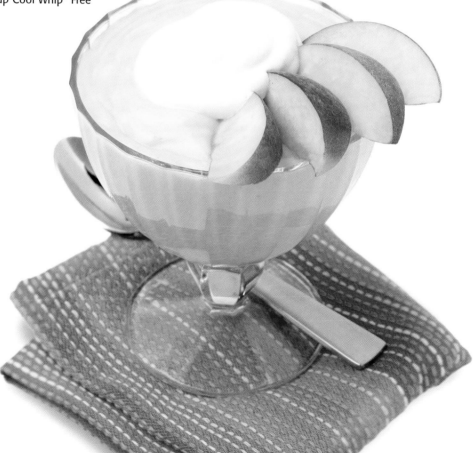

Anyday Sundae

Believe it... this sundae is actually nutritious!

Servings: 2
Preparation Time: 10 minutes

INGREDIENTS

½ cup skim milk

1 scoop (about 24 grams of protein)
vanilla protein powder (whey or soy)

2 cups frozen banana slices*
(about 2 medium bananas)

4 tsp chocolate syrup

4 Tbsp Fat Free Reddi-wip®

2 tsp chopped nuts

2 maraschino cherries

DIRECTIONS

1 Pour skim milk into blender. Add protein powder and blend on high speed for about 15 seconds.

2 Add frozen banana slices and blend on high speed for 45 seconds or until smooth (stopping blender to stir with spoon and scrape down sides as needed).

3 Spoon into 2 dessert bowls. Top each sundae with 2 teaspoons of chocolate syrup, 2 tablespoons of Reddi-wip, a teaspoon of chopped nuts and a maraschino cherry. Serve and enjoy! ☺

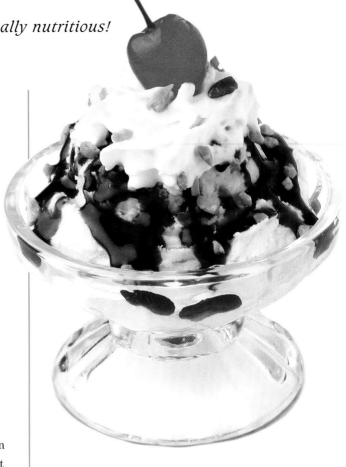

—— Tasteful Tip ——

*It's the frozen banana slices in this recipe that give it that rich, wonderful "ice cream-like" consistency. If you've never frozen a banana, here's how: Simply peel a slightly overripe banana and slice it into 1-inch chunks. Place the slices in a Ziploc® freezer bag overnight or longer. Before making this sundae, place banana slices in a measuring cup and let them thaw at room temperature for about 20 minutes, or just microwave them for about 20 seconds. Toss 'em in the blender after that! Yum!

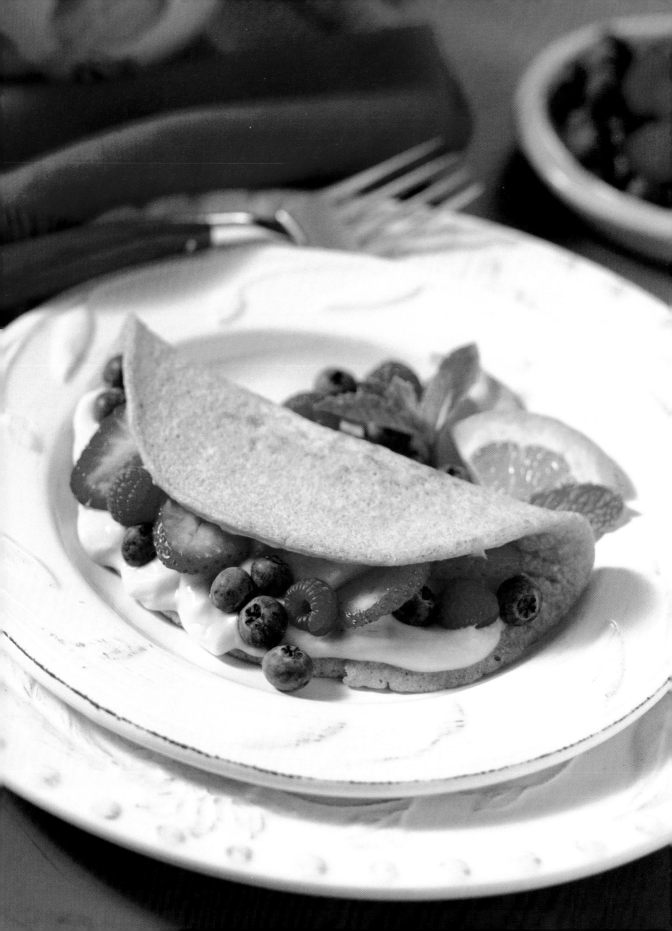

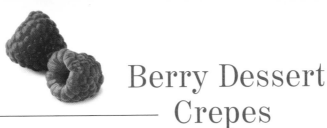

Berry Dessert
Crepes

Crepes with fresh berries and raspberry yogurt filling

Servings: 2
Preparation Time: 15 minutes

INGREDIENTS

¼ cup egg substitute

¼ cup skim milk

⅓ cup whole-wheat flour

½ tsp sugar substitute

6 oz light, fat-free raspberry yogurt

3 Tbsp vanilla protein powder (whey or soy)

1 cup fresh berries of your choice

——— Tasteful Tip ———

Crepes can be made ahead of time and stacked (unfilled) placing wax paper between them. Unfilled crepes can be sealed in Ziploc® bags and refrigerated for several days or frozen for up to two months. Thaw frozen crepes in the refrigerator or at room temperature. Then carefully peel them apart and fill.

DIRECTIONS

1 In a medium mixing bowl, whisk the egg substitute, milk, flour and sugar substitute until well blended.

2 Lightly coat a small nonstick skillet with butter-flavored cooking spray and place over medium heat.

3 Pour half of the crepe batter into the heated skillet, then quickly lift and tilt the skillet to spread the batter. Return to heat. When the edges of the crepe are dry, carefully flip it over and cook until lightly browned, about 2 minutes.

4 Place crepe on a small plate and repeat with remaining batter.

5 In a small mixing bowl, combine yogurt and protein powder; mix well. Divide filling into two portions and spoon into crepes. Top each with half of the berries. Fold the crepe over the filling, serve and enjoy! ☺

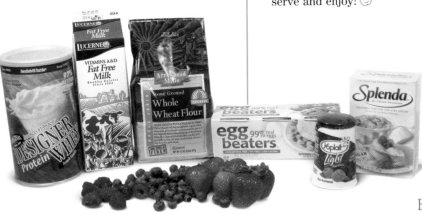

Bananas Foster Style

Maple-glazed fried bananas with cottage cheese

Servings: 1
Preparation Time: 5 minutes

INGREDIENTS

1 banana, sliced

2 Tbsp sugar-free maple syrup

1 portion low-fat cottage cheese (about $^1/_2$ cup)

DIRECTIONS

1 Lightly coat a small nonstick skillet with butter-flavored cooking spray and place over medium heat. Add sliced bananas and fry for about 1 minute.

2 Add maple syrup to the skillet and gently stir to coat the banana slices; continue to cook for another minute.

3 Place cottage cheese on a small serving plate and microwave on high until heated through, about 20 seconds.

4 Top cottage cheese with maple-glazed banana slices. Serve and enjoy!

Enriched Double Chocolate Pudding

Exceptionally nutritious, rich and satisfying chocolate dessert

Servings: 2
Preparation Time: 25 minutes

INGREDIENTS

- 1 cup cold skim milk
- 1 packet chocolate Myoplex® Lite
- 2 Tbsp fat-free, sugar-free chocolate instant pudding mix

Tasteful Tip

This nutritious pudding is made with Myoplex Lite nutrition shake mix, which contains a very high-quality blend of protein, vitamins and minerals. If you prefer a different brand of nutrition shake mix, it's a-okay to use that, too!

DIRECTIONS

1 Pour skim milk in blender. Then add Myoplex powder and blend on medium speed for 15 seconds.

2 Add the pudding mix and blend on high speed until thick and creamy, about 45 more seconds (stopping blender to stir with spoon and scrape down sides as needed).

3 Spoon into 2 dessert bowls and chill in refrigerator for at least 20 minutes, then serve and enjoy! ☺

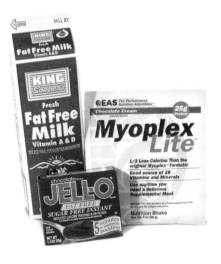

Walnut Brownies

Rich cocoa brownies with walnuts and warmth!

Servings: 12
Preparation Time: 25 minutes

INGREDIENTS

$^1\!/_2$ cup soy flour

$^1\!/_4$ cup whole-wheat flour

$^1\!/_2$ cup Splenda® granular

$^1\!/_4$ cup unsweetened cocoa powder

$^1\!/_2$ tsp baking powder

$^1\!/_4$ tsp salt

$^1\!/_4$ cup canola oil

2 tsp vanilla extract

6 egg whites, beaten

$^1\!/_4$ cup unsweetened applesauce

$^1\!/_4$ cup water

$^1\!/_3$ cup walnut pieces

DIRECTIONS

1 Preheat oven to 350° F. Lightly coat an 8" x 8" baking dish with butter-flavored cooking spray.

2 In a large mixing bowl, sift together soy flour, whole-wheat flour, Splenda, cocoa powder, baking powder and salt.

3 In a medium mixing bowl, combine canola oil, vanilla extract, egg whites, applesauce and water. Pour applesauce mixture into flour mixture and stir just until well combined.

4 Pour brownie batter into baking dish and sprinkle with walnuts. Bake until edges spring back when you touch them gently (center will be soft), about 15 minutes.

5 Allow brownies to cool and then cut into 12 pieces.

6 Serve one brownie with a glass of your favorite vanilla protein powder mixed with water or skim milk and enjoy! ☺

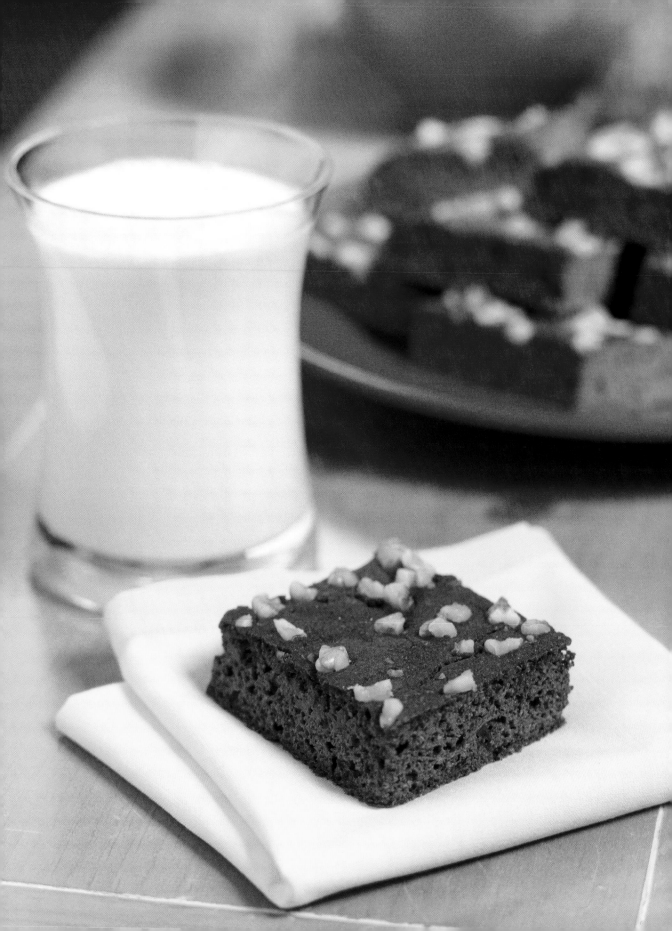

Chocolate Mousse

Light pudding texture and wonderful chocolate taste!

Servings: 2
Preparation Time: 25 minutes

INGREDIENTS

1   cup cold skim milk

1   packet chocolate Myoplex® Lite

2   Tbsp fat-free, sugar-free chocolate instant
    pudding mix

3/4 cup Cool Whip® Lite

DIRECTIONS

1 Pour skim milk in blender. Then add
Myoplex powder and blend on medium
speed for 15 seconds.

2 Add pudding and blend on high speed
until smooth, about 45 more seconds (stopping blender to stir with spoon and scrape
down sides as needed).

3 Pour chocolate mixture into a medium
mixing bowl and gently fold in the
Cool Whip.

4 Spoon into 2 dessert
glasses and chill in
refrigerator for at
least 20 minutes.
Serve and enjoy! ☺

Berry
Parfait

Strawberries and blueberries layered with cool almond yogurt and cottage cheese

Servings: 2
Preparation Time: 10 minutes

INGREDIENTS

$\frac{1}{2}$ cup strawberries, sliced, fresh or frozen, thawed and drained

$\frac{1}{2}$ cup blueberries, fresh or frozen, thawed and drained

2 packets sugar substitute (Splenda® or Equal®)

2 portions low-fat cottage cheese (about 1 cup)

6 oz light, fat-free vanilla yogurt

$\frac{1}{4}$ tsp vanilla extract

$\frac{1}{4}$ tsp almond extract

DIRECTIONS

1 Place strawberries in a small bowl and sprinkle with a packet of sugar substitute.

2 Place blueberries in a separate small bowl and sprinkle with the second packet of sugar substitute.

3 In a medium mixing bowl, combine cottage cheese, vanilla yogurt, vanilla extract and almond extract; mix well.

4 Layer blueberries, then yogurt mixture and strawberries in two parfait glasses (or other tall glasses). Serve and enjoy! ☺

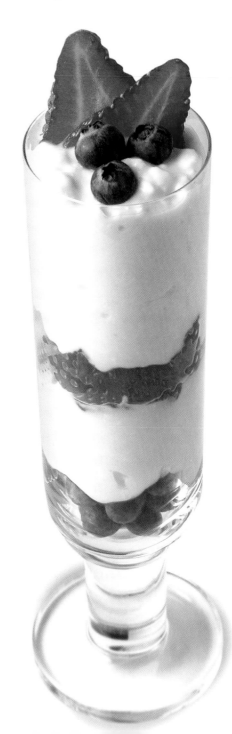

Banana Cream Pudding

Protein- and vitamin-enriched banana cream pie filling

Servings: 2
Preparation Time: 25 minutes

Ingredients

1 cup cold skim milk

1 packet vanilla Myoplex® Lite

2 Tbsp fat-free, sugar-free banana
   instant pudding mix

1 banana, sliced

½ cup Cool Whip® Free

--------- Tasteful Tip ---------

This pudding recipe is a great dessert dish for your
Eating *for* Lifestyle! It's made with Myoplex Lite nutrition shake mix, which is very nutrient rich and
healthy. Remember, if you have a nutrition shake
mix or protein powder you prefer other than
Myoplex, please use that instead.

Directions

1 Pour skim milk in blender. Then add
   Myoplex powder and blend on medium
   speed for 15 seconds.

2 Add pudding mix and blend on high
   speed until thick and creamy, about 45
   more seconds (stopping blender to stir with
   spoon and scrape down sides as needed).

3 Spoon into 2 dessert glasses and chill
   in refrigerator for at least 20 minutes.

4 Top each serving with half the banana
   slices and a dollop of Cool Whip. Serve
   and enjoy! ☺

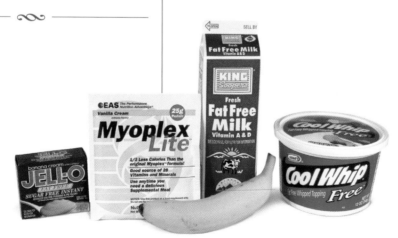

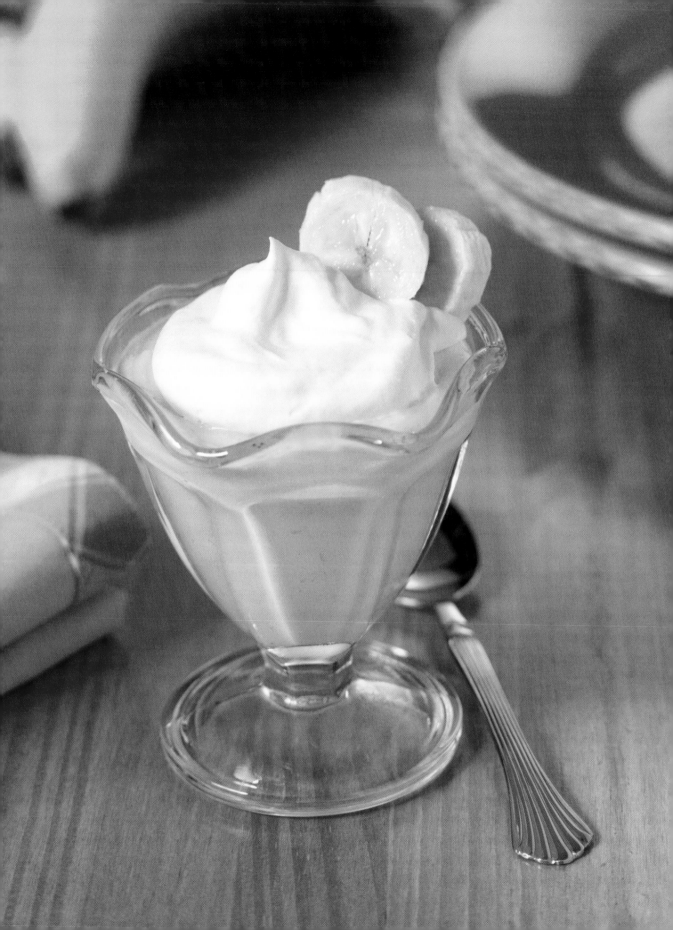

Pistachio Pudding

Smooth, satisfying and simply dessert delicious!

Servings: 2
Preparation Time: 25 minutes

INGREDIENTS

1 cup cold skim milk

1 packet vanilla Myoplex® Lite

2 Tbsp fat-free, sugar-free pistachio instant pudding mix

1 Tbsp chopped pistachios

DIRECTIONS

1 Pour skim milk into blender. Add Myoplex powder and blend on medium speed for about 15 seconds.

2 Add pudding mix and blend on high speed until pudding becomes thick and creamy, about 45 more seconds (stopping blender to stir with spoon and scrape down sides as needed).

3 Spoon into 2 dessert glasses and chill in refrigerator for at least 20 minutes.

4 Top each serving with half the chopped pistachios. Serve and enjoy! 🍎

Fortified
Fudgesicle

Rich chocolate-flavored protein pudding pop

Servings: 6
Preparation Time: 3 hours

INGREDIENTS

¹/₂ cup fat-free evaporated milk

1¹/₂ cup low-fat cottage cheese

1 package (4-serving size) fat-free, sugar-free
   chocolate instant pudding mix

DIRECTIONS

1 Pour fat-free evaporated milk in blender.
Add cottage cheese and blend at medium
speed until smooth, about 45 seconds.

2 Add the pudding mix and blend on high
speed until thick and creamy, about 45 more
seconds (stopping blender to stir with spoon
and scrape down sides as needed).

3 Spoon pudding mixture into 6 popsicle
molds or paper cups. Insert wooden sticks
and place in freezer for about 3 hours.
Serve and enjoy! 🍎

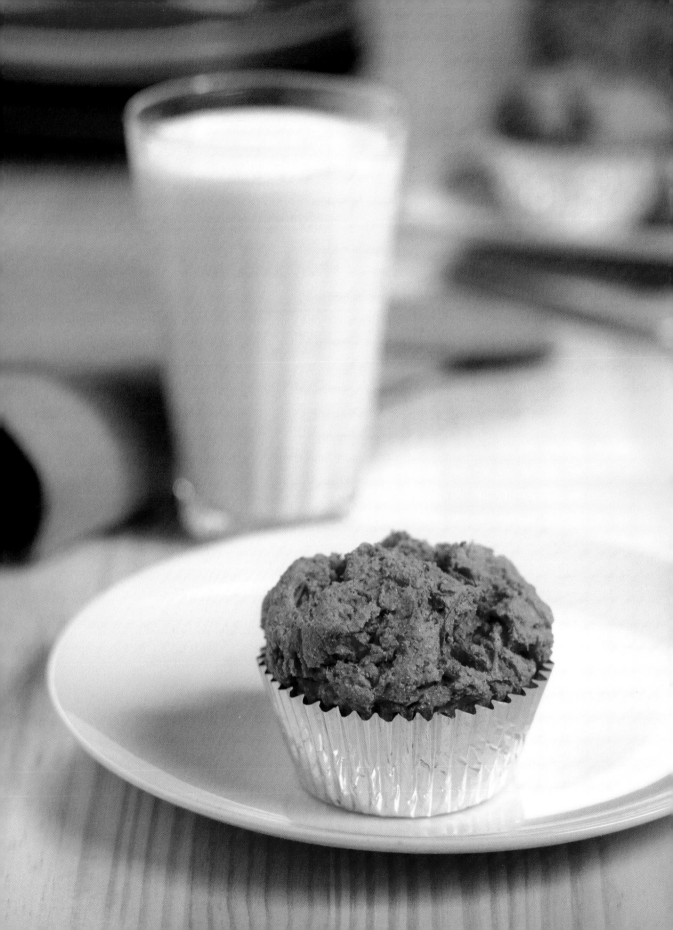

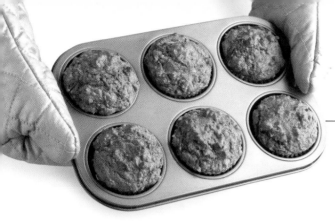

Carrot Cake Muffins

Completely dessert delicious!

Servings: 12
Preparation Time: 30 minutes

INGREDIENTS

12 foil muffin liners

1 cup whole-wheat flour

1 cup oat flour

2 tsp baking soda

1 1/2 tsp cinnamon

3/4 cup wheat germ

1/2 cup brown sugar substitute

9 Tbsp vanilla protein powder (soy or whey)

3/4 tsp salt

3/4 cup unsweetened applesauce

3/4 cup skim milk

4 large egg whites, beaten

2 cups carrots, shredded

——— Tasteful Tip ———

This recipe makes 12 delicious muffins, and they can easily be stored in the refrigerator in an airtight container for two days or frozen individually in Ziploc® freezer bags for up to two months.

DIRECTIONS

1 Preheat oven to 375° F.

2 Line 12 muffin cups with foil liners. Lightly coat the liners with butter-flavored cooking spray.

3 In a large mixing bowl, sift together wheat flour, oat flour, baking soda and cinnamon. Then add the wheat germ, brown sugar substitute, protein powder and salt. Stir to combine.

4 In another bowl, combine applesauce, skim milk and egg whites. Pour applesauce mixture into flour mixture. Stir just until all ingredients are moistened (batter will be lumpy). Then, gently fold in the carrots until evenly combined.

5 Spoon the batter into the foil-lined muffin cups until each is almost full. Bake until golden and a wooden toothpick inserted in the center of muffin comes out "clean," about 18 minutes.

6 Serve one carrot cake muffin with a glass of your favorite vanilla protein powder mixed with cold water or skim milk and enjoy! ☺

Butterscotch Bliss

*A cloud of Cool Whip® with nutritious,
creamy butterscotch pudding*

Servings: 2
Preparation Time: 25 minutes

INGREDIENTS

1   cup cold skim milk

1   packet vanilla Myoplex® Lite

2   Tbsp fat-free, sugar-free butterscotch
    instant pudding mix

2/3 cup Cool Whip® Lite

DIRECTIONS

1 Pour skim milk in blender. Then add
Myoplex powder and blend on medium
speed for 15 seconds.

2 Add pudding mix and blend on high
speed until thick and creamy, about 45
more seconds (stopping blender to stir with
spoon and scrape down sides as needed).

3 Line 2 dessert bowls with Cool Whip
and fill the center of each with
half the pudding. Chill in refrigerator for at least 20 minutes.
Serve and enjoy! ☺

Black Forest Pudding

*Layers of nutrient-enriched chocolate
pudding, cherries and whipped topping*

Servings: 2
Preparation Time: 25 minutes

INGREDIENTS

1 cup cold skim milk

1 packet chocolate Myoplex® Lite

2 Tbsp fat-free, sugar-free chocolate
instant pudding mix

$\frac{1}{2}$ cup sugar-free cherry pie filling

$\frac{1}{2}$ cup Cool Whip® Free

DIRECTIONS

1 Pour skim milk in blender. Then add
Myoplex powder and blend on medium
speed for 15 seconds.

2 Add pudding mix and blend on high speed
until thick and creamy, about 45 more seconds (stopping blender to stir with spoon
and scrape down sides as needed).

3 Spoon layers of pudding and cherry pie
filling in 2 dessert glasses. Chill in refrigerator for at least 20 minutes.

4 Top each with a dollop of Cool Whip.
Serve and enjoy! 😊

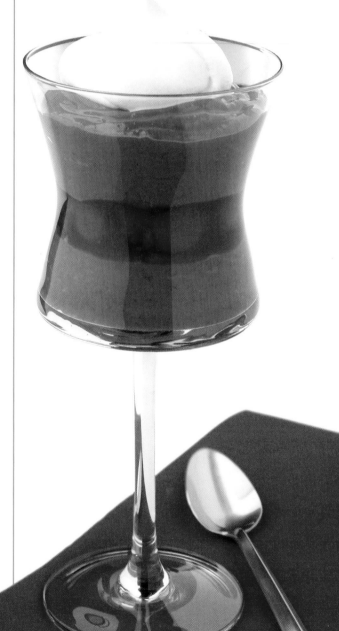

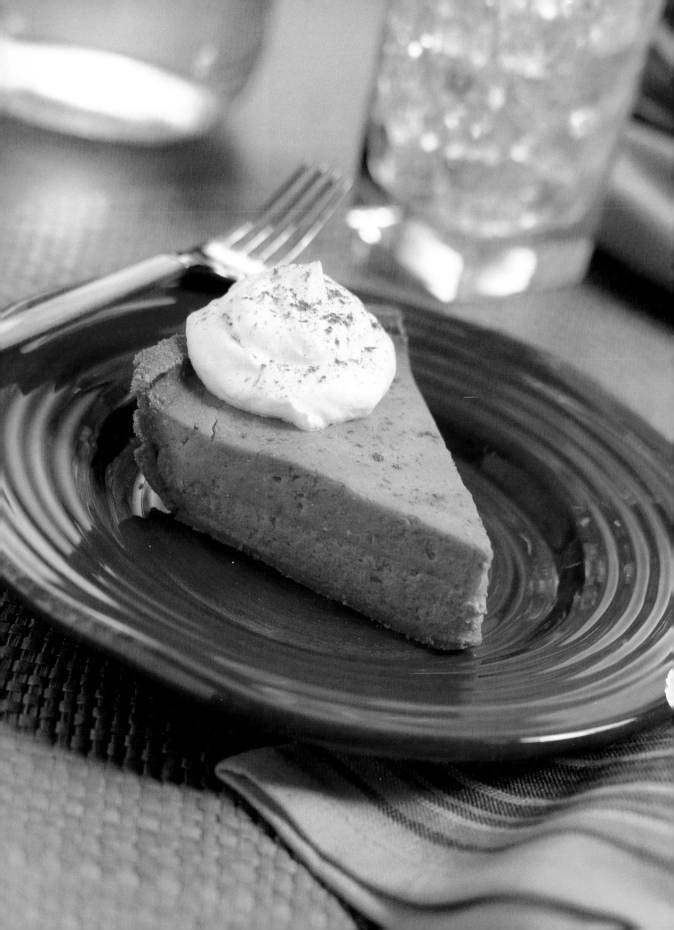

Pumpkin
Cheesecake

Protein-enhanced pumpkin pie filling
in a light graham cracker crust

Servings: 8
Preparation Time: 3 hours

INGREDIENTS

2 cups low-fat ricotta cheese

1 can (15 oz) pumpkin puree*

½ cup sugar-free maple syrup

5 Tbsp sugar substitute

1 tsp pumpkin pie spice

1 tsp vanilla extract

¾ cup vanilla protein powder (whey or soy)

1 Ready Crust® reduced-fat graham cracker crust

1 cup Cool Whip Free*

——— Tasteful Tip ———

*In order to achieve the nutritional balance as well as the delicious dessert taste of this dish, it's important to use pumpkin *puree* rather than traditional pumpkin pie filling.

DIRECTIONS

1 Preheat oven to 400° F.

2 In a large mixing bowl, combine ricotta cheese, pumpkin puree, maple syrup, sugar substitute, pumpkin pie spice, vanilla extract and protein powder; mix well.

3 Pour the filling mixture into the crust and smooth it with the back of a spoon to even out. Bake until the filling is set, about 40 minutes. (You'll know it's done when you can stick a wooden toothpick into the center and it comes out "clean.")

4 Remove pie from the oven and let it cool for 15 minutes. Then refrigerate for at least 2 hours.

5 Slice into 8 portions and place each on a small plate. Top with a dollop of Cool Whip and a dash of pumpkin pie spice. Serve and enjoy! ☺

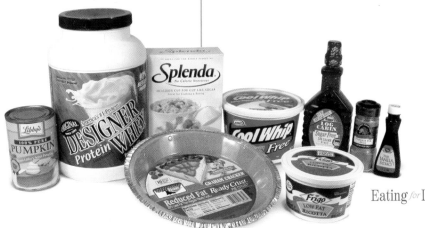

Breakfasts

Spanish Omelet

Flavorful omelet with salsa, melted cheese and golden brown Potatoes O'Brien

Servings: 1
Preparation Time: 15 minutes

INGREDIENTS

1   portion Potatoes O'Brien, frozen (about ⅔ cup)

1   whole egg

3   egg whites

1   Tbsp skim milk

¼   tsp chili powder

⅛   tsp ground cumin

⅛   tsp freshly ground black pepper

1   slice reduced-fat cheese

¼   cup salsa

DIRECTIONS

1 Lightly coat a small nonstick skillet with cooking spray and cook potatoes over medium-high heat until golden brown, about 10 minutes.

2 While potatoes are cooking, in a small mixing bowl, whisk together egg, egg whites and skim milk. Add chili powder, cumin and black pepper; blend well.

3 Lightly coat a medium nonstick skillet with cooking spray and place over medium heat. Add egg mixture to skillet. As eggs begin to set, run a spatula around the edge of the skillet, lifting set eggs so uncooked eggs flow underneath.

4 When the eggs are set but still moist, add the slice of cheese to one side of the omelet and top with salsa. Fold omelet over filling. Cook until cheese starts to melt, about 1 minute.

5 Place the omelet and potatoes on a warmed plate. Serve and enjoy! 😊

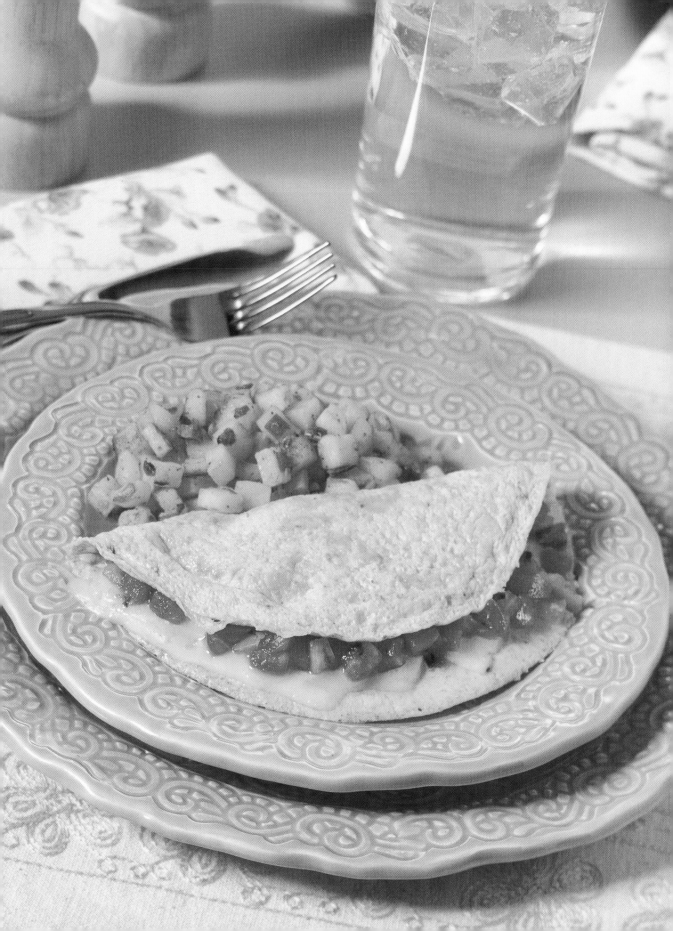

Golden Pancakes

Protein pancakes make breakfast a dessert!

Servings: 2
Preparation Time: 15 minutes

Ingredients

1 cup uncooked whole-grain oats (non-instant)

6 egg whites

1 cup fat-free cottage cheese

¼ tsp vanilla extract

¼ tsp ground cinnamon

2 packets sugar substitute

½ cup sugar-free maple syrup

¼ cup mixed berries

Directions

1 Lightly coat a nonstick skillet or griddle with cooking spray; place over medium heat.

2 In a blender, combine oats, egg whites, cottage cheese, vanilla, cinnamon and sugar substitute. Blend on medium speed until smooth, about 1 minute.

3 Pour batter, about ¼ cup at a time, onto hot skillet. Cook pancake until bubbly on top and dry around edges, about 3 minutes. Turn and cook other side until golden brown, about 2 more minutes.

4 While pancakes are cooking, microwave maple syrup until warm, about 20 seconds.

5 Place a portion of pancakes on 2 separate plates. Top with warm maple syrup and mixed berries. Serve and enjoy! ☺

Breakfast
Du Jour

Whole-grain cereal and scrambled eggs are a good beginning!

Servings: 1
Preparation Time: 10 minutes

INGREDIENTS

$^{1}/_{2}$ cup egg substitute

1 portion Kellogg's® Complete Oat Bran Flakes

$^{1}/_{2}$ cup skim milk

sugar substitute, to taste

DIRECTIONS

1 Lightly coat a small nonstick skillet with cooking spray and place over medium heat.

2 Pour egg substitute into skillet. As eggs begin to set, use a spatula to lift cooked portion. Cook until eggs are set, about 4 minutes.

3 Place scrambled eggs on a small plate. Put cereal in a bowl, pour in milk and sprinkle with sugar substitute.

4 Serve and enjoy! ☺

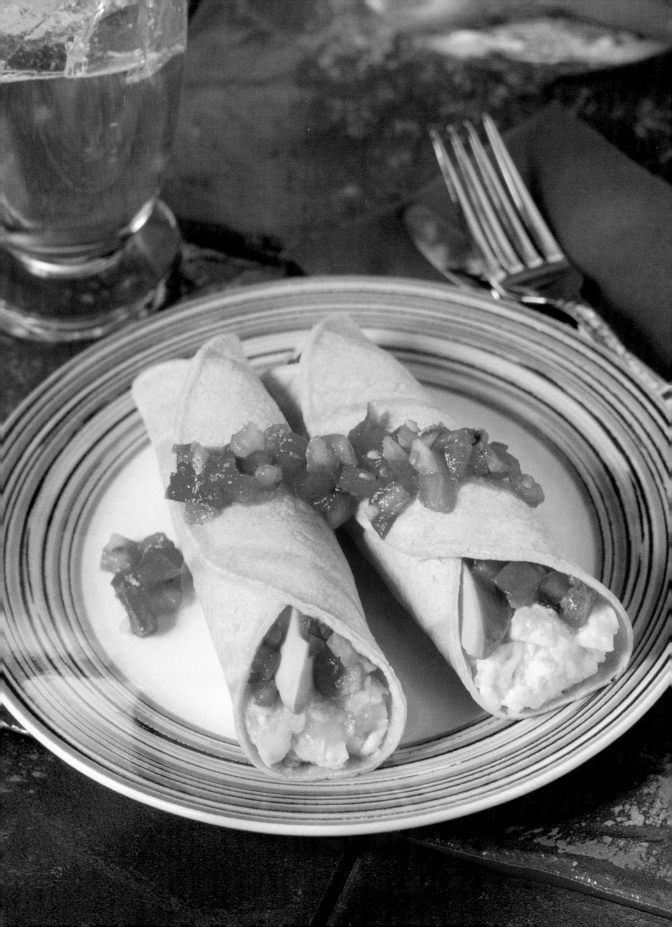

Egg-Cellent Enchiladas

Quick, delicious, nutritious Eating for Lifestyle breakfast!

Servings: 1

Preparation Time: 8 minutes

INGREDIENTS

1   whole egg

3   egg whites

2   Tbsp reduced-fat cheddar cheese, shredded

2   corn tortillas

¼   avocado, sliced

¼   cup salsa, divided

DIRECTIONS

1 Lightly coat a small nonstick skillet with cooking spray and place over medium heat.

2 Whisk egg and egg whites until blended; pour into skillet and scramble for about 2 minutes. Add cheddar cheese and stir until eggs are set and cheese is melted, about 2 more minutes.

3 Lightly dampen two paper towels and place the corn tortillas between them. Microwave on high for 30 seconds.

4 Fill each tortilla with half the scrambled eggs and cheese, sliced avocado and a spoonful of salsa.

5 Roll up, top with remaining salsa, serve and enjoy! ☺

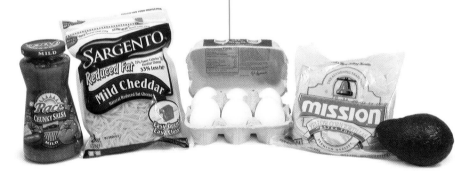

Ham and
Egg Sandwich

Lean ham, scrambled eggs and melted cheddar cheese
on grilled whole-wheat bread

Servings: 1
Preparation Time: 10 minutes

INGREDIENTS

1 whole egg

3 egg whites

2 Tbsp skim milk

1/8 tsp ground black pepper

2 slices whole-wheat bread

1 slice lean ham

1 slice reduced-fat cheddar cheese

DIRECTIONS

1 Lightly coat a small nonstick skillet with butter-flavored cooking spray and place over medium heat.

2 In a small mixing bowl, whisk together egg, egg whites, skim milk and black pepper. Pour egg mixture into skillet and stir until set. Remove from skillet and set aside.

3 Lightly respray the skillet and add one slice of bread. Layer with ham, cooked eggs and cheese. Top with remaining bread slice.

4 Cook over medium heat until bottom is golden brown, about 3 minutes. Turn and cook for another 2 minutes or until the cheese is melted and the bread is golden brown. Serve and enjoy! ☺

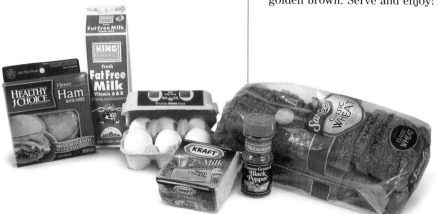

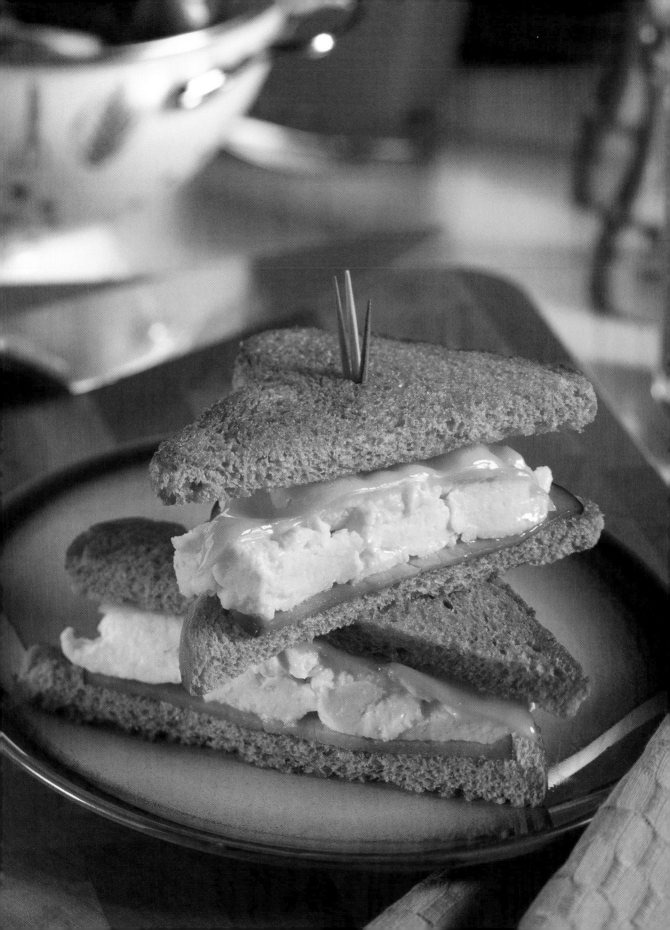

Eggs and Oats

Simple and nutritious way to start your day

Servings: 1
Preparation Time: 10 minutes

INGREDIENTS

½ cup whole-grain oats (non-instant)

1 whole egg

3 egg whites

ground black pepper, to taste

½ cup skim milk

sugar substitute, to taste

DIRECTIONS

1 Cook whole-grain oats according to package directions.

2 Lightly coat a small nonstick skillet with cooking spray and place over medium heat.

3 In a small mixing bowl, whisk the egg and egg whites until slightly frothy. Pour into skillet. As eggs begin to set, use a spatula to lift cooked portion. Cook until eggs are set, about 4 minutes.

4 Place scrambled eggs on a small plate and top with pepper. Spoon cooked oats into a serving bowl, pour in milk and sprinkle with sugar substitute.

5 Add a cup of coffee if you'd like. Serve and enjoy! ☺

Denver Omelet

*Delicious omelet filled with diced ham, bell pepper
and onion with whole-wheat toast*

Servings: 1
Preparation Time: 15 minutes

INGREDIENTS

1 whole egg

3 egg whites

1 Tbsp skim milk

¼ tsp ground black pepper

¼ green bell pepper, diced

¼ red bell pepper, diced

1 slice onion, chopped

¼ cup lean ham, diced

2 Tbsp reduced-fat cheddar cheese, shredded

1 slice whole-wheat bread

DIRECTIONS

1 Lightly coat a small nonstick skillet with cooking spray; place over medium-low heat.

2 In a small mixing bowl, whisk together the egg, egg whites, skim milk and black pepper. Pour egg mixture into skillet, cover and cook about 4 minutes until eggs are set but still moist.

3 Spoon bell peppers, onion and ham onto half of the omelet. Fold omelet over filling and sprinkle with cheese. Cover and cook until filling is heated through and cheese starts to melt, about 2 minutes. Place omelet on a warmed serving plate.

4 Toast wheat bread, serve and enjoy! ☺

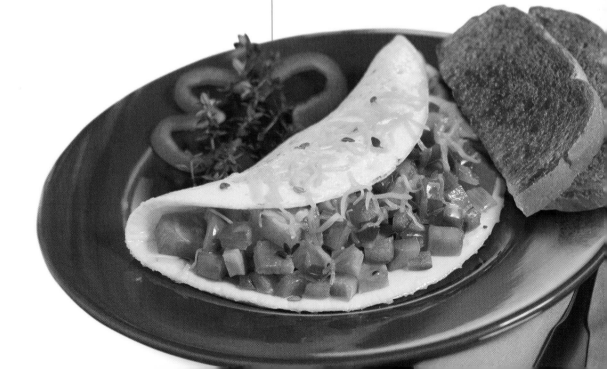

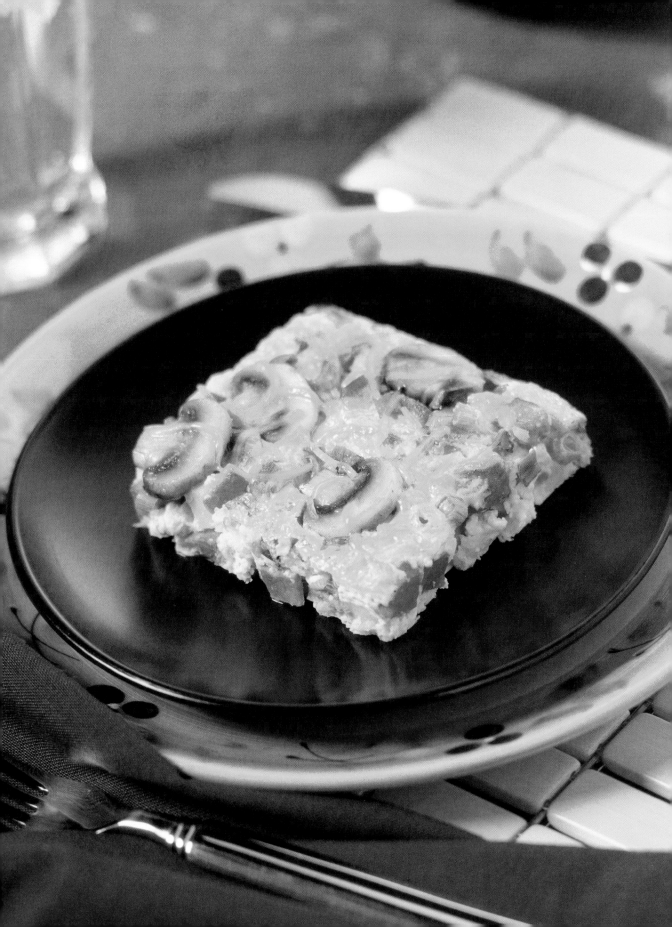

Ham and Cheese Egg Casserole

Complete breakfast of eggs, ham, potatoes and vegetables, topped with cheddar cheese

Servings: 4
Preparation Time: 50 minutes

INGREDIENTS

2   cups frozen diced potatoes

1   cup cooked lean ham, diced

1/2   cup fresh mushrooms, sliced

2   green onions, sliced

1 1/4   cup egg substitute

1/2   cup skim milk

1/2   cup reduced-fat cheddar cheese, shredded

— Tasteful Tip —

Egg substitutes, such as Egg Beaters®, can be used in place of whole eggs and egg whites. One cup egg substitute is the equivalent of approximately four whole eggs or eight egg whites.

DIRECTIONS

1 Preheat oven to 325° F.

2 Lightly coat a 9" x 13" baking dish with cooking spray.

3 Layer potatoes evenly on the bottom of the dish; top with ham, mushrooms and onions.

4 In a small mixing bowl, beat egg substitute and skim milk with a fork or whisk until well blended.

5 Pour egg mixture over ham and vegetables in baking dish and top with cheese.

6 Bake until eggs are firm and top is lightly browned, approximately 40 minutes.

7 Cut into 4 portions. Serve and enjoy! ☺

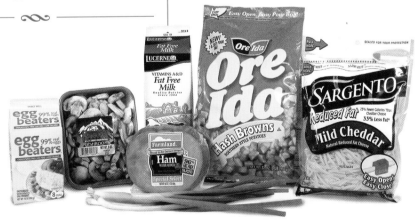

Indian Eggs

Uniquely seasoned mix of egg whites, sautéed bell peppers,
fresh tomato and chopped onions with whole-wheat pita bread

Servings: 1
Preparation Time: 15 minutes

INGREDIENTS

1 slice onion, chopped

½ green bell pepper, cut into thin strips

½ tomato, seeded and chopped

¼ tsp turmeric

¼ tsp chili powder

⅛ tsp ground black pepper

4 egg whites

½ whole-wheat pita

2 orange slices

1 Tbsp fresh cilantro, chopped

——— Tasteful Tip ———

Notice that in this meal, the carbohydrate serving is made up of partial portions of pita and orange slices. As you become more familiar with the Eating *for* Lifestyle, you'll discover countless variations and combinations of quality carbs as well as proteins.

DIRECTIONS

1 Lightly coat a small nonstick skillet with cooking spray and place over medium heat.

2 Sauté onions until golden, about 4 minutes. Add bell pepper and sauté for about 2 more minutes. Add tomatoes and sauté for another 2 minutes. Stir in turmeric, chili powder and black pepper.

3 In a small mixing bowl, lightly beat the egg whites, then pour them over vegetables in skillet and stir until set.

4 Warm pita in microwave for about 20 seconds. Place eggs and pita on a small plate with orange slices. Sprinkle eggs with cilantro. Serve and enjoy! ☺

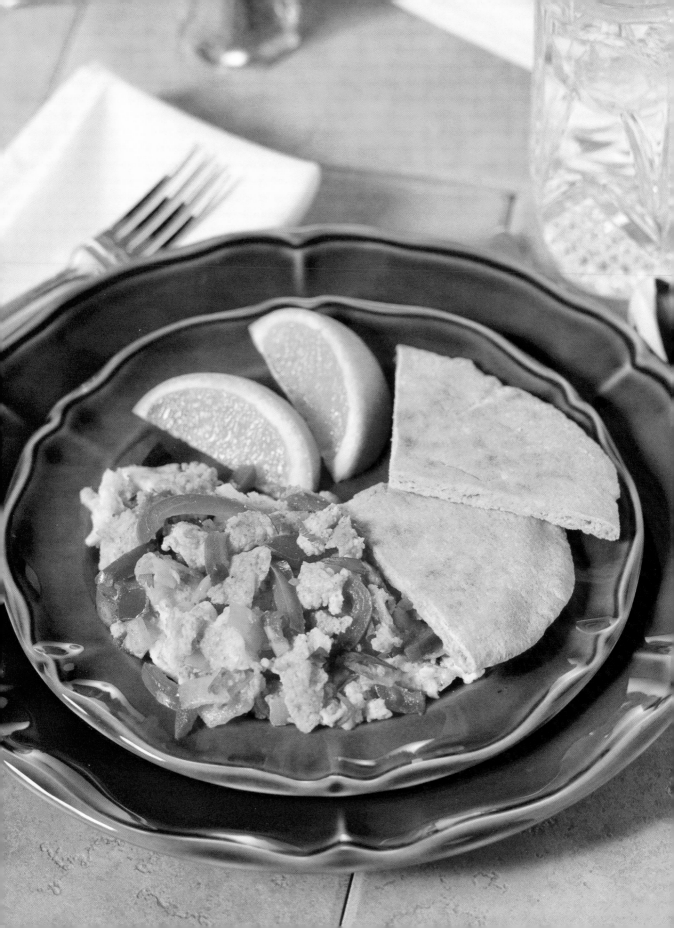

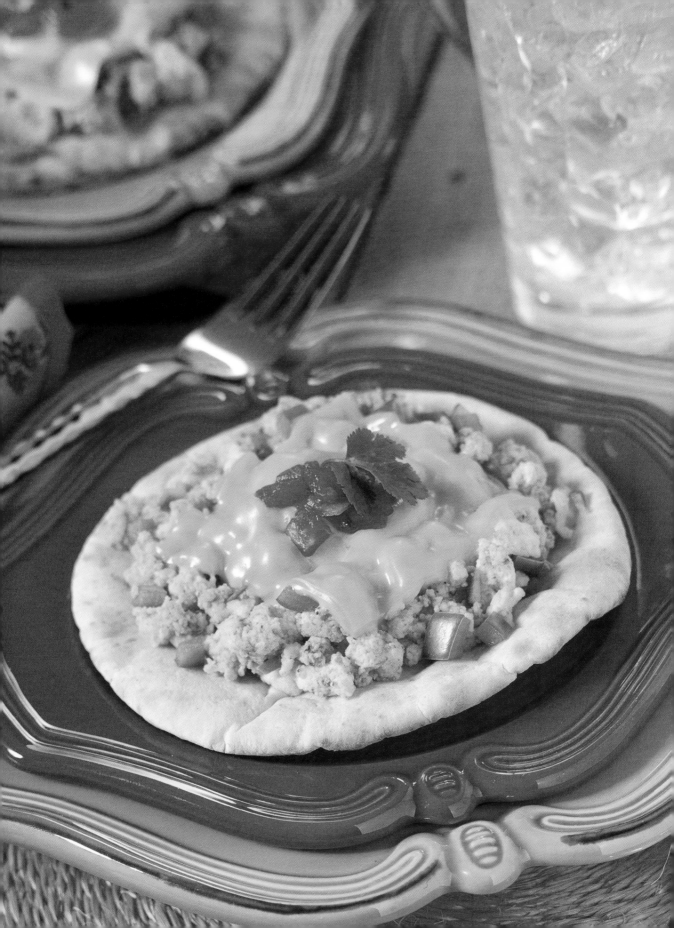

Breakfast
Pita Pizza

*Scrambled eggs with salsa, green bell pepper
and onion on a warm pita*

Servings: 1
Preparation Time: 10 minutes

INGREDIENTS

1 whole egg

3 egg whites

2 Tbsp salsa, divided

½ green bell pepper, diced

1 slice onion, chopped

1 pita

1 slice reduced-fat cheddar cheese

─────── Tasteful Tip ───────

Remember, you can use egg substitutes in place of
eggs if you prefer. For example, in this recipe, ½ cup
plus 2 Tbsp Egg Beaters® could be used in place of
the one whole egg and three egg whites.

DIRECTIONS

1 In a small mixing bowl, lightly beat
egg and egg whites. Add 1 tablespoon of
salsa, blend well.

2 Lightly coat a medium nonstick skillet
with cooking spray. Sauté diced bell
pepper and onion over medium heat
for 2 to 3 minutes until softened. Add
the egg mixture and cook with vegetables,
stirring occasionally, until set.

3 Place pita on a plate and spoon the egg
mixture on it. Top with cheddar cheese
and microwave for about 20 seconds,
until the cheese melts.

4 Top pita pizza with remaining salsa,
serve and enjoy! ☺

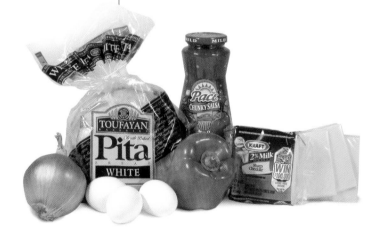

Sunny Side Up

Bright and basic morning meal!

Servings: 1
Preparation Time: 10 minutes

INGREDIENTS

1   egg white

2   whole eggs

1   slice whole-grain bread, toasted

$\frac{1}{2}$ grapefruit, sectioned

DIRECTIONS

1 Lightly coat a small nonstick skillet with cooking spray and place over medium heat.

2 Add egg white and whole eggs to skillet; cover and cook until whites are set and yolks have thickened, about 3 minutes.

3 Slide eggs onto warmed plate with toast. Serve with grapefruit half, a hot cup of coffee and enjoy! ☺

Chocolate
Oatmeal

Old-fashioned oats, all-natural peanut butter
with the added power of protein

Servings: 1
Preparation Time: 5 minutes

INGREDIENTS

1/3 cup uncooked whole-grain oats (non-instant)

1/2 cup water

1 scoop (about 24 grams of protein)
chocolate protein powder (whey or soy)

1 Tbsp natural peanut butter

Sugar substitute, to taste

1/2 cup skim milk

DIRECTIONS

1 In a bowl, combine oats, water and protein powder. Microwave on high until oats are cooked, about 2 minutes.

2 Stir in the peanut butter and add sugar substitute to taste.

3 Pour milk on top. Serve and enjoy! ☺

Turkey Bacon Melt

*Lean turkey bacon, cheese and a slice of fresh tomato,
on a toasted whole-wheat English muffin*

Servings: 1
Preparation Time: 15 minutes

INGREDIENTS

3 strips lean turkey bacon (each cut in half)

1 whole-wheat English muffin, split

2 thick slices of tomato

2 slices reduced-fat cheese

— Tasteful Tip —

For even faster preparation, you can use a toaster oven. If you have one at work, you might want to consider bringing the cooked bacon, sliced tomato, cheese slices and English muffin in separate Ziploc® bags. You can simply put it together and heat for a quick, delicious lunch.

DIRECTIONS

1 Preheat oven to 400° F.

2 Cook turkey bacon according to its package directions.

3 Place the whole-wheat English muffin halves face up on a baking sheet. Top each with a slice of tomato. Layer with cheese and top with 3 "half slices" of cooked bacon.

4 Place in the oven and bake for 3 to 5 minutes, until cheese is melted and bubbly. Serve and enjoy! ☺

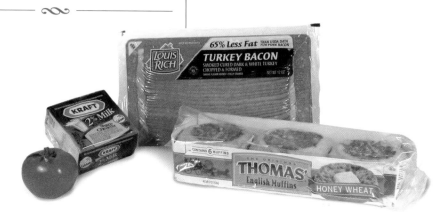

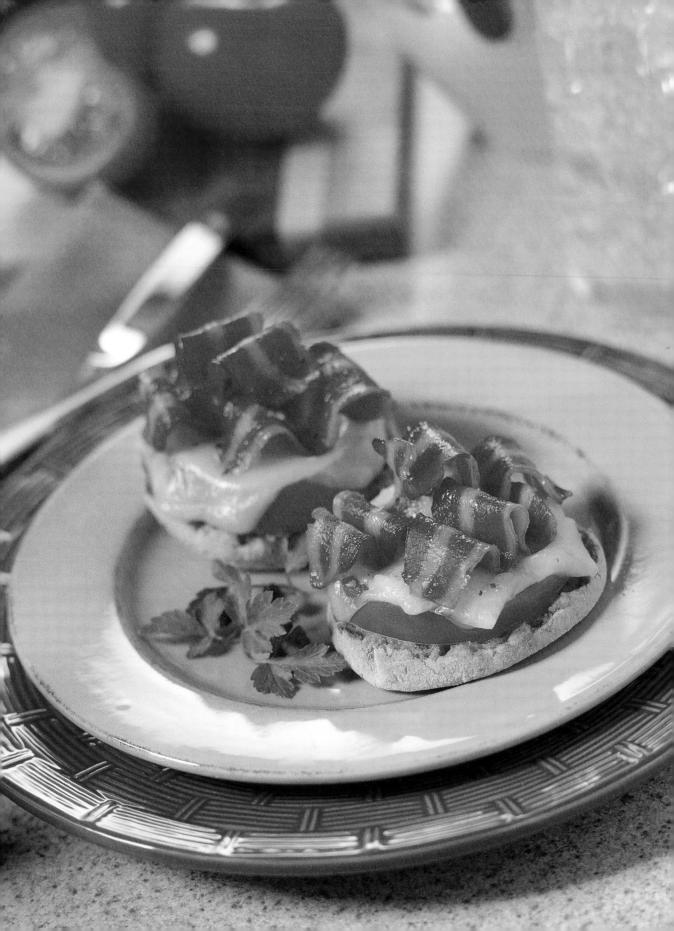

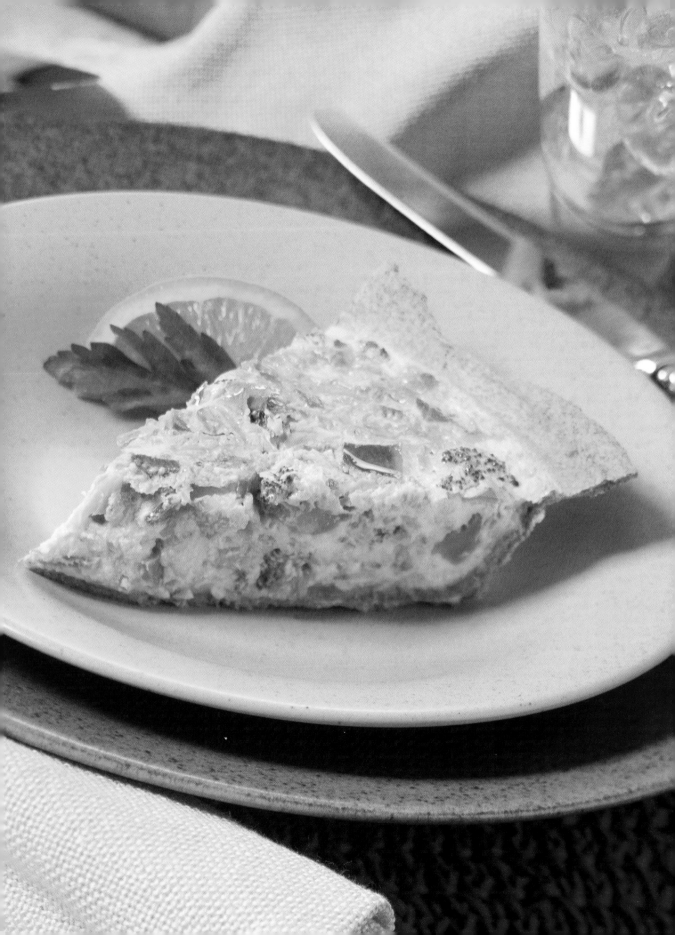

Turkey Bacon Quiche

Lean turkey bacon and broccoli quiche
with a whole-wheat tortilla crust

Servings: 4
Preparation Time: 1 hour, 10 minutes

INGREDIENTS

6 strips lean turkey bacon

3 (8-inch) whole-wheat tortillas

3 whole eggs

8 egg whites (or 1 cup egg substitute)

½ cup skim milk

½ cup low-fat sour cream

¾ cup reduced-fat cheddar cheese, shredded

1 cup broccoli florets, fresh or frozen, thawed

DIRECTIONS

1 Preheat oven to 350° F.

2 Cook turkey bacon according to its package directions. Set aside to cool.

3 Lightly coat a 9-inch pie plate with cooking spray. Overlap 2 tortillas and cut the third one in half to form a crust. (See photo above.)

4 In a large mixing bowl, beat whole eggs and egg whites with a fork or whisk until well blended. Then mix skim milk and sour cream into the eggs.

5 Chop cooled turkey bacon into bite-size pieces.

6 Add turkey bacon, cheddar cheese and broccoli to blended egg mixture; combine thoroughly.

7 Pour egg mixture into tortilla-lined pie plate; bake for approximately 50 minutes. (You'll know it's done when you tap the edge of the pie plate and the filling is set and moist. If it is still liquidy, bake a few minutes longer and test again.)

8 Allow to cool for 10 minutes before slicing into portions. Serve and enjoy! ☺

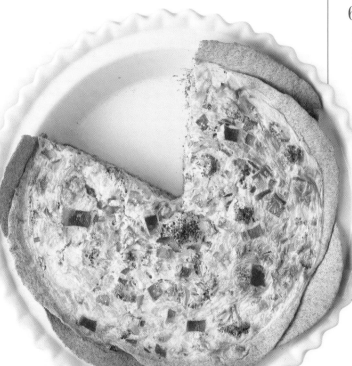

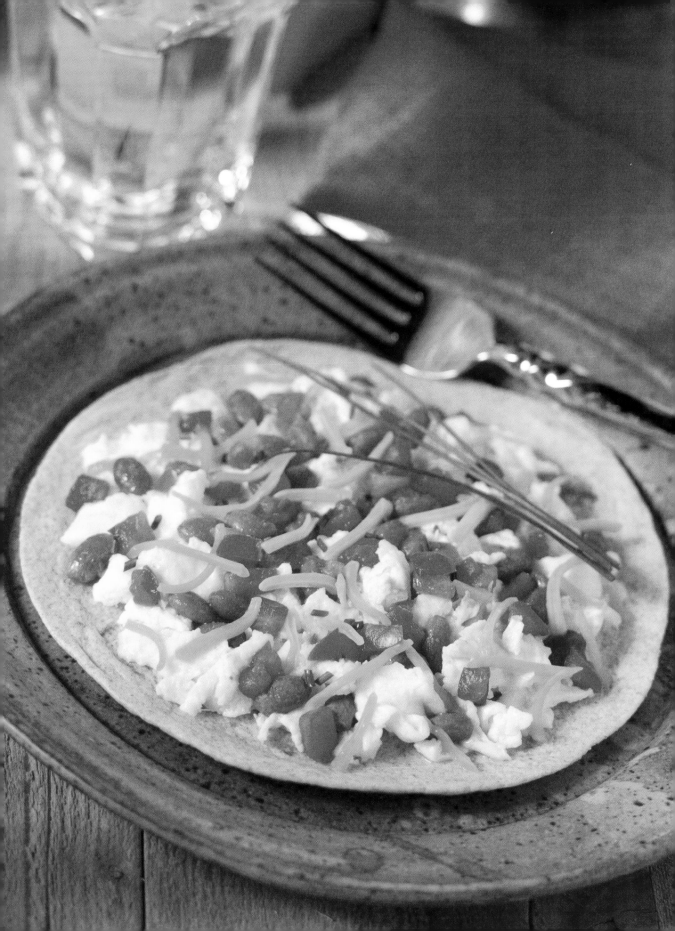

Ranchero
Eggs

Scrambled eggs and pinto beans topped with salsa
and cheddar cheese on a whole-wheat tortilla

Servings: 1
Preparation Time: 10 minutes

INGREDIENTS

1   whole egg

3   egg whites

¼   cup pinto beans, drained and rinsed

1   (8-inch) whole-wheat tortilla

2   Tbsp salsa

2   Tbsp reduced-fat cheddar cheese, shredded

1   tsp chives, chopped

1   jalapeño, seeded, chopped

DIRECTIONS

1 Lightly coat a small nonstick skillet with cooking spray and place over medium heat. In a small mixing bowl, beat the egg and egg whites; pour into skillet. Stir until eggs are set but still moist.

2 Add the beans to the skillet and stir to blend with the eggs; reduce heat to low.

3 Microwave the tortilla for 20 seconds to soften.

4 Place the tortilla on a plate, top with egg and bean mixture. Then layer with salsa, cheese, chives and jalapeño. Serve and enjoy! ☺

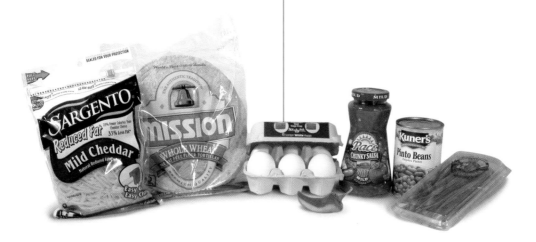

Sunrise Fiesta Pita

Scrambled eggs, sautéed vegetables and melted cheddar cheese in a whole-wheat pita

Servings: 2
Preparation Time: 15 minutes

INGREDIENTS

1 cup fresh mushrooms, sliced

½ onion, chopped

½ red bell pepper, sliced

2 whole eggs

6 egg whites

½ cup reduced-fat cheddar cheese, shredded

1 whole-wheat pita, cut in half

Hot pepper sauce, to taste

DIRECTIONS

1 Lightly coat a medium nonstick skillet with cooking spray and place over medium heat. Add mushrooms, onion and bell pepper; sauté until tender, approximately 5 minutes.

2 While the vegetables are cooking, in a medium mixing bowl, combine the eggs and egg whites; blend well.

3 Pour the egg mixture over the sautéed vegetables and cook, stirring occasionally, until set, approximately 5 minutes. Then, add cheddar cheese and cook a couple more minutes, until cheese melts.

4 Divide the mixture into two portions and spoon into pita bread halves. Top with hot pepper sauce, serve and enjoy! ☺

Vegetable Scramble

Sautéed mixed vegetables and red potato
with scrambled egg whites

Servings: 1
Preparation Time: 15 minutes

INGREDIENTS

1   portion precooked red potato, diced

½   cup frozen mixed vegetables

1   jalapeño, seeded and chopped

1   vegetable breakfast patty, thawed

3   egg whites

DIRECTIONS

1 Lightly coat a medium nonstick skillet with cooking spray and place over medium heat.

2 Add diced potato, mixed vegetables and jalapeño to the skillet. Then crumble the breakfast patty into the skillet. Sauté until heated through and vegetables are tender, about 5 minutes.

3 In a small bowl, whisk egg whites, then pour into the skillet. Stir until the eggs have set, about 3 minutes. Serve and enjoy! ☺

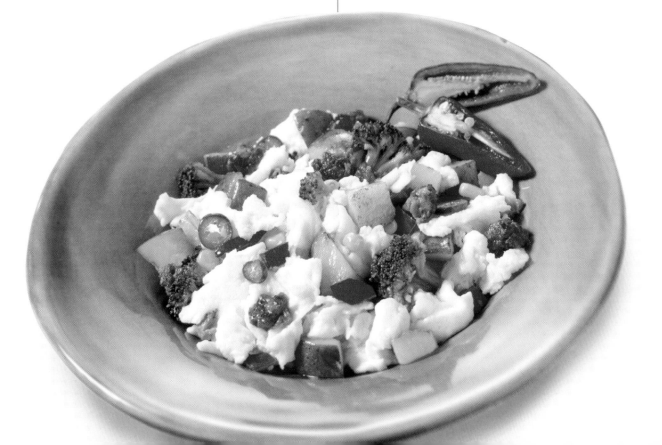

Seafood Omelet

Crab meat and shrimp with fresh tomatoes and mushrooms in an omelet with whole-wheat toast

Servings: 2
Preparation Time: 20 minutes

INGREDIENTS

¼ cup cooked crab meat, fresh, canned or frozen, thawed

¼ cup cooked shrimp, fresh, canned or frozen, thawed

¼ cup mushrooms, sliced

1 green onion, sliced

½ tomato, diced

¼ tsp ground black pepper

¼ cup fat-free sour cream

1 cup egg substitute

¼ cup reduced-fat colby-jack cheese, shredded

2 slices whole-wheat bread

———— Tasteful Tip ————

*To serve omelets on warmed plates, simply rinse the plates with hot water until warm, then dry them thoroughly.

DIRECTIONS

1 Lightly coat a medium saucepan with cooking spray and place over medium heat. Add crab meat, shrimp, mushrooms, green onion, tomato and black pepper; cook, stirring frequently, for 2 minutes.

2 Stir in sour cream and continue to cook until heated through, about 2 more minutes. Then reduce heat to low.

3 Lightly coat a small nonstick skillet with cooking spray and place over medium-low heat. Pour half of the egg substitute into skillet, cover and cook about 4 minutes, until eggs are set but still moist.

4 Fill the center of the omelet with a portion of warm seafood mixture. With a spatula, fold each side of the omelet over the filling. Sprinkle with half the cheese. Cover and cook for 1 minute or until cheese starts to melt. Place omelet on warmed plate.*

5 Make the second omelet by lightly coating the skillet again and using the remaining egg substitute, seafood mixture and cheese.

6 While the second omelet is cooking, toast the wheat bread, serve and enjoy! ☺

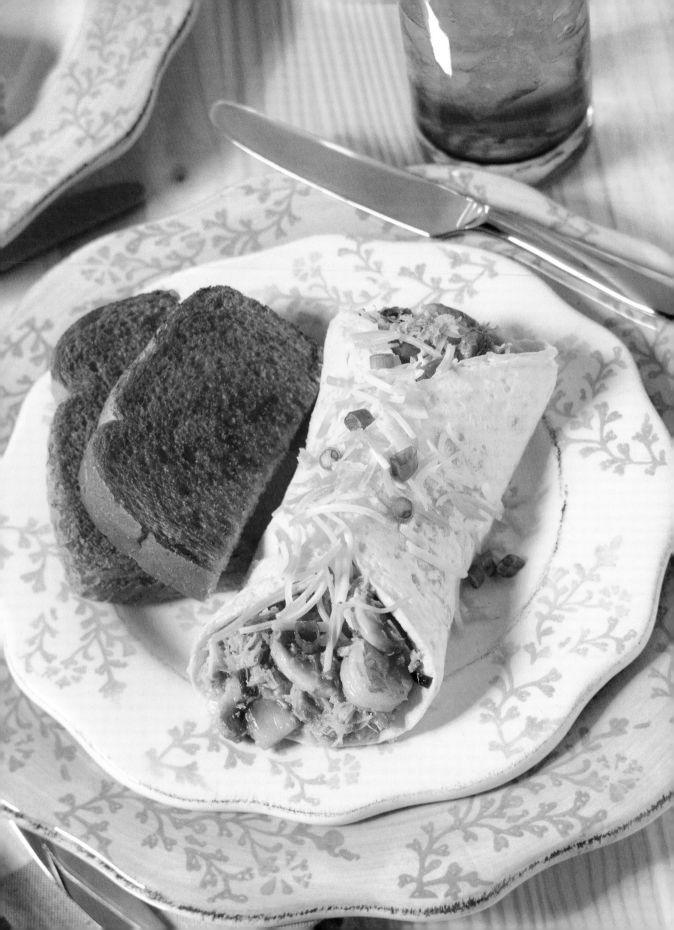

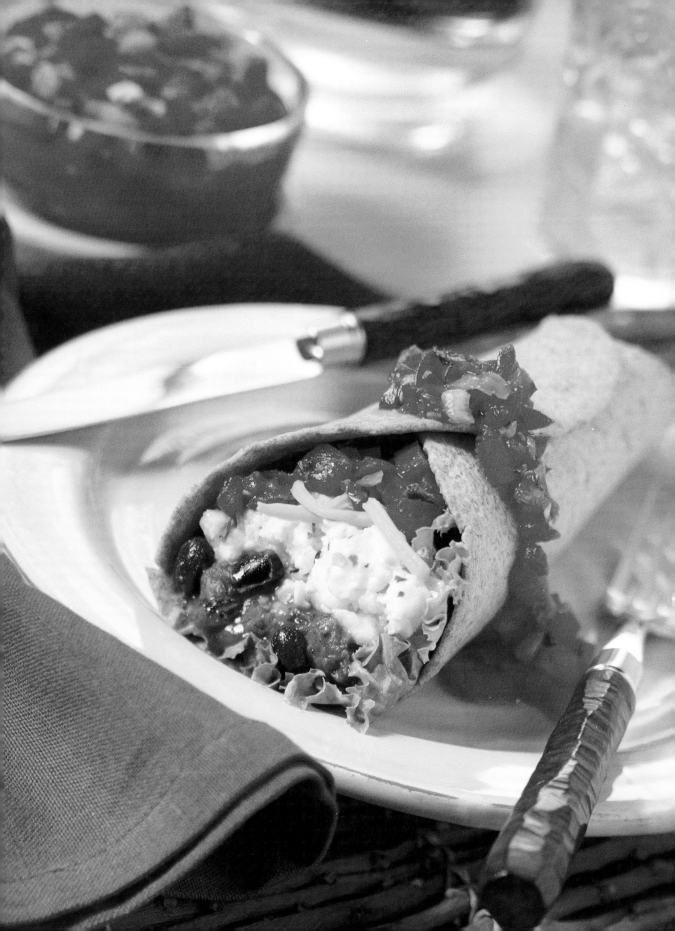

Breakfast
Burrito

*Scrambled eggs, cheddar cheese, beans
and salsa in a whole-wheat tortilla*

Servings: 1
Preparation Time: 10 minutes

INGREDIENTS

1   (8-inch) whole-wheat tortilla

1   whole egg

3   egg whites

1   lettuce leaf

2   Tbsp fat-free refried beans

1   Tbsp reduced-fat cheddar cheese, shredded

¼   cup salsa, divided

DIRECTIONS

1 Lightly coat a medium nonstick skillet with cooking spray and place over medium heat. Place tortilla in the skillet and warm for 30 seconds, turn and warm the other side for 30 seconds. Place the warmed tortilla on a small plate.

2 Whisk the egg and egg whites together. Pour into warmed skillet and cook, stirring occasionally, until set.

3 While the eggs are cooking, place the lettuce leaf on the tortilla and spread the refried beans over the lettuce leaf. Top the beans with cooked eggs, shredded cheddar cheese and 2 Tbsp of salsa.

4 Roll it up and top with remaining salsa. Serve and enjoy! ☺

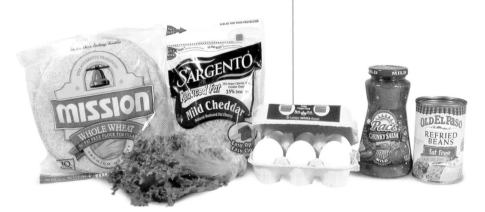

Vanilla Nut Cereal

Crunchy almonds and cinnamon over
vanilla-flavored Cream of Wheat®

Servings: 1
Preparation Time: 5 minutes

INGREDIENTS

3 Tbsp Cream of Wheat® cereal (non-instant)

¾ cup water

1 scoop (about 24 grams of protein) vanilla protein powder (whey or soy)

¼ tsp ground cinnamon

Sugar substitute, to taste

1 Tbsp slivered almonds

¼ cup skim milk

DIRECTIONS

1 In a bowl, combine Cream of Wheat, water and protein powder. Microwave on high for 1 minute. Stir, then return to microwave for 30 seconds. Stir again, and microwave for 30 more seconds if needed, to thicken.

2 Sprinkle with cinnamon, sugar substitute and slivered almonds.

3 Pour in milk, serve and enjoy! ☺

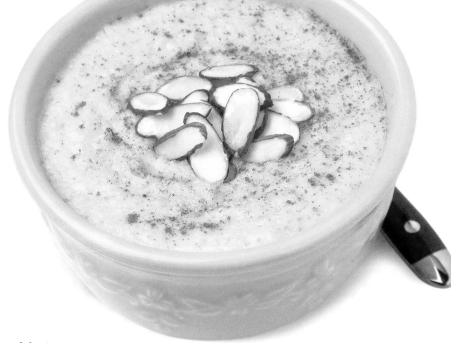

Eggs Florentine

*Egg whites, sautéed baby spinach and
crumbled feta cheese with tart blueberries*

Servings: 1
Preparation Time: 10 minutes

INGREDIENTS

1 cup fresh baby spinach

4 egg whites

2 Tbsp reduced-fat feta cheese, crumbled

$^1/_2$ cup fresh blueberries

DIRECTIONS

1 Lightly coat a small nonstick skillet with cooking spray and place over medium heat. Sauté spinach until it wilts, about 4 minutes.

2 Whisk egg whites until blended. Pour over the spinach and stir until eggs are set. Sprinkle with feta cheese and then slide onto a warmed serving plate.

3 Place blueberries on plate with eggs. Serve and enjoy!

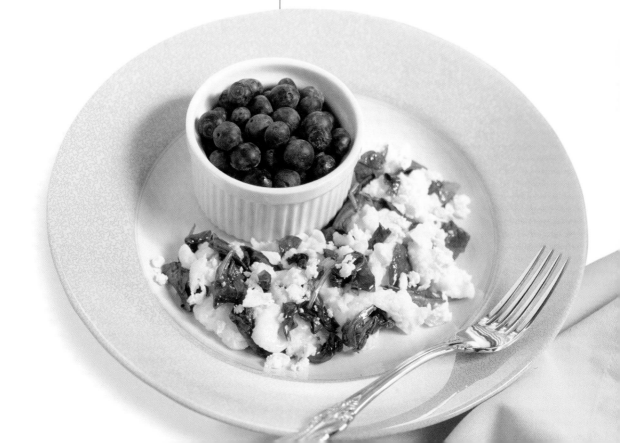

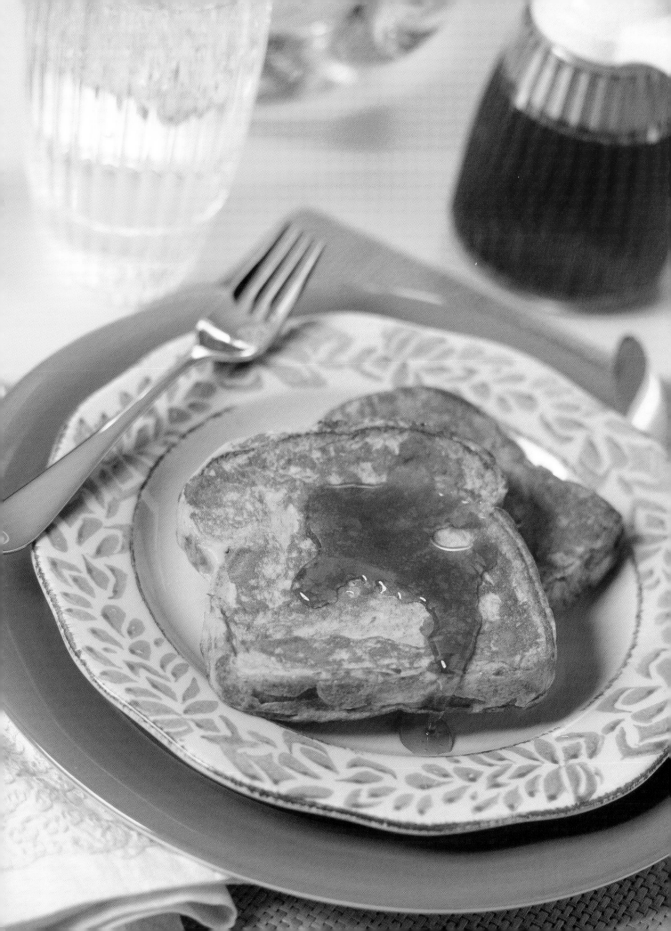

Fortified French Toast

*Protein-enriched French toast with
vanilla, cinnamon and warm maple syrup*

Servings: 1
Preparation Time: 10 minutes

INGREDIENTS

3 Tbsp vanilla Myoplex Lite® or vanilla protein
   powder (whey or soy)

¹/₂ cup egg substitute

¹/₄ tsp ground cinnamon

2 slices whole-wheat bread

¹/₄ cup sugar-free maple syrup

DIRECTIONS

1 Lightly coat a large nonstick skillet
or griddle with butter-flavored cooking
spray and place over medium heat.

2 Place Myoplex in a pie plate and slowly
pour in egg substitute while stirring with
a fork until smooth. (The batter will
be thick.) Sprinkle cinnamon on top of
the batter.

3 Dip one piece of bread in the batter and
let it soak up the egg mixture for 10 seconds. Carefully turn the bread over to coat
the other side. Repeat with second piece
of bread.

4 Place batter-soaked bread in the skillet
and spoon any remaining batter on top.
Cook 2 to 3 minutes on each side or until
golden brown. Then place on a small plate.

5 While French toast is cooking, microwave
maple syrup until warm, about 20 seconds.

6 Pour warm maple syrup over French
toast, serve and enjoy! ☺

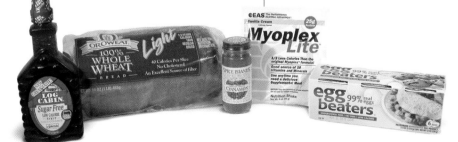

Lunches

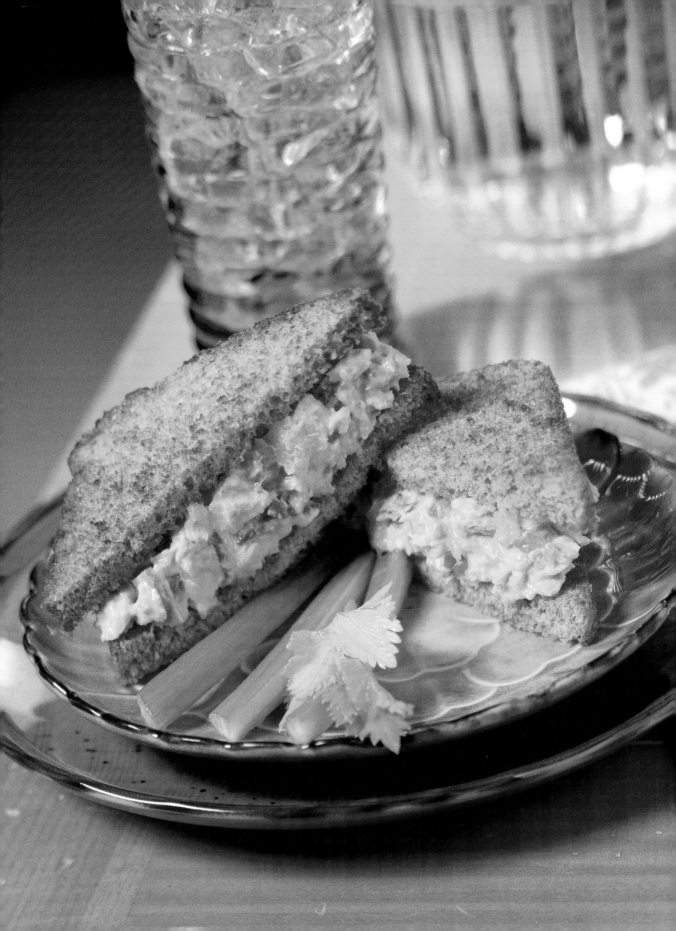

Tropical Tuna Sandwich

Tuna salad with pineapple on golden grilled wheat bread

Servings: 2
Preparation Time: 15 minutes

INGREDIENTS

1 can (6 oz) tuna, water packed, drained

2 Tbsp Miracle Whip® Free

1 Tbsp crushed pineapple, drained

1 celery stalk, chopped

2 Tbsp sweet pickle relish

1 tsp yellow mustard

$\frac{1}{8}$ tsp ground cinnamon

4 slices whole-wheat bread

—— Tasteful Tip ——

This tuna filling can be made ahead of time and stored in an airtight container for up to three days. You might consider bringing a portion with you to work along with two slices of whole-wheat bread, a pita or tortilla. Then you could make the sandwich at lunchtime for a quick, nutritious and delicious meal!

DIRECTIONS

1 In a medium mixing bowl, combine tuna, Miracle Whip, pineapple, celery, relish, mustard and cinnamon; mix well.

2 Spread a portion of tuna mixture on 2 slices of bread. Top with remaining slices of bread.

3 Lightly coat a large nonstick skillet with cooking spray. Place sandwiches in the pan and cook over medium heat for about 2 to 3 minutes on each side, until the sandwiches are warm and the bread is lightly browned.

4 Slice tuna sandwiches in half, serve and enjoy! ☺

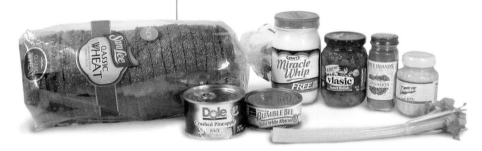

Turkey Sandwich

Roasted turkey breast, lettuce and tomato on fresh whole-grain bread

Servings: 1
Preparation Time: 5 minutes

INGREDIENTS

1 Tbsp mustard or fat-free mayonnaise

2 slices whole-grain bread

2 lettuce leaves

1 portion roasted turkey breast, sliced

$^1/_2$ tomato, sliced

DIRECTIONS

1 Spread mustard or fat-free mayonnaise evenly over bread slices.

2 Top one slice of bread with lettuce, turkey and tomato.

3 Stack with the other slice of bread and then cut sandwich in half. Serve and enjoy! 😋

—— Tasteful Tip ——

Turkey sandwiches are great "make-and-take" meals. To keep this sandwich from getting soggy, try putting the tomato and lettuce in a separate bag than the turkey and bread. Then put it all together when you're ready for lunch.

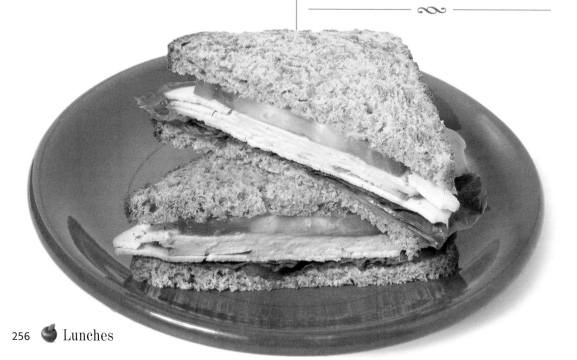

Cool Taco Salad

Taco-seasoned ground beef, lettuce and tomatoes with a creamy salsa dip

Servings: 2
Preparation Time: 20 minutes

INGREDIENTS

2 portions lean ground beef (about $1/2$ lb)

1 Tbsp water

2 tsp taco seasoning mix, divided

2 whole-wheat pitas

2 Tbsp reduced-fat cream cheese, at room temperature

2 Tbsp fat-free sour cream

2 Tbsp salsa

1 cup lettuce, shredded

1 tomato, diced

$1/4$ cup reduced-fat cheddar cheese, shredded

DIRECTIONS

1 Preheat oven to 400° F.

2 In a medium skillet, brown ground beef over medium heat until no longer pink; drain off any excess fat. Add water and 1 tsp taco seasoning to the beef and simmer for 3 minutes. Remove from heat and set aside to cool slightly.

3 Cut each pita into 8 wedges and place on baking sheet. Bake for about 7 minutes or until lightly browned.

4 While the beef is cooling, combine the remaining taco seasoning, cream cheese, sour cream and salsa in a small bowl; mix well. Divide and spread this mixture evenly on 2 small plates.

5 Spoon a portion of the beef over the sour cream mixture, and top each with half the lettuce, tomato and cheddar cheese.

6 Place 8 baked pita wedges on each plate, serve and enjoy! ☺

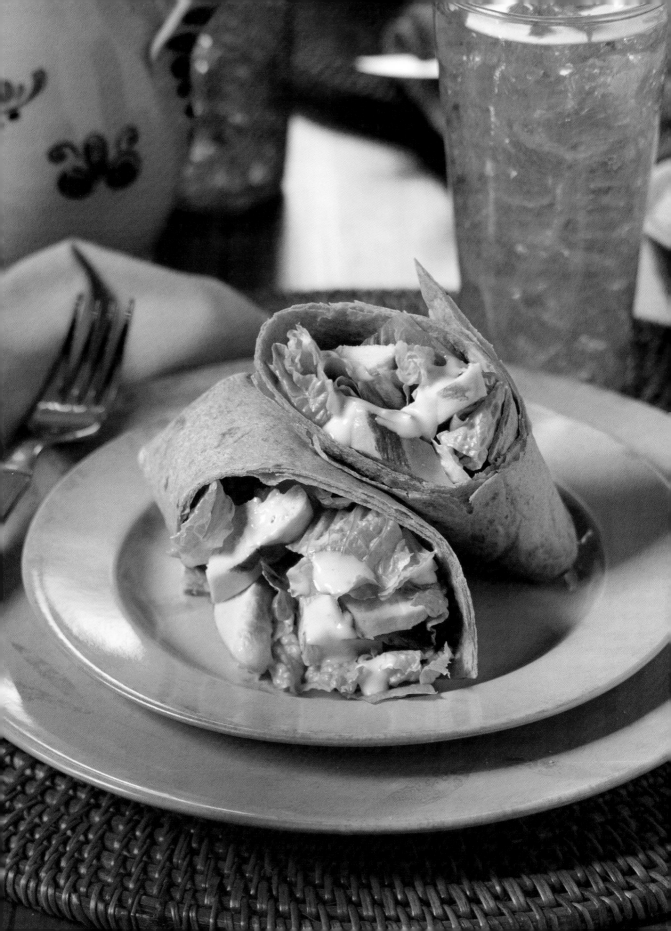

Chicken Caesar Wrap

Sliced chicken, crisp romaine lettuce
with Caesar salad dressing in a spinach tortilla

Servings: 1
Preparation Time: 10 minutes

INGREDIENTS

1   portion grilled chicken breast, sliced*

1   cup romaine lettuce, cut into bite-size pieces

1   Tbsp low-fat Caesar salad dressing

1   Tbsp reduced-fat Parmesan cheese, grated

1   (10-inch) spinach tortilla

—————— Tasteful Tip ——————

*To save time, you can use "pre-grilled" chicken breasts in recipes like this one. Quality brands include Louis Rich® Chicken Breast Strips, Tyson® Fully Cooked Roasted Chicken Breasts and Butterball® Fully Cooked Chicken Breast Chunks. Remember that preparing ahead of time helps you set the table for success!

DIRECTIONS

1 In a medium mixing bowl, toss together chicken, lettuce, Caesar dressing and Parmesan cheese.

2 Microwave tortilla for about 20 seconds to soften. Spoon chicken mixture onto tortilla.

3 Wrap tortilla around filling and cut in half. Serve and enjoy! ☺

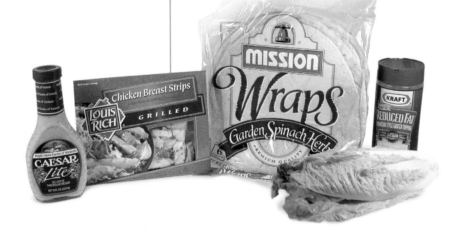

Apple Tuna Salad

Tuna with crisp apple and celery on a bed of lettuce with fresh tomato wedges

Servings: 2
Preparation Time: 10 minutes

INGREDIENTS

1 can (6 oz) tuna, water packed, drained

1/2 onion, diced

1 stalk celery, sliced

1 Tbsp dill relish

1 tsp spicy brown mustard

2 Tbsp fat-free mayonnaise

1 apple, cored and diced

4 cups lettuce leaves

2 tomatoes, cut in wedges

DIRECTIONS

1 In a medium mixing bowl, combine tuna, onion, celery, relish, mustard, mayonnaise and apple; mix well.

2 Divide lettuce and tomato wedges between two separate plates. Top with a portion of tuna mixture, serve and enjoy! ☺

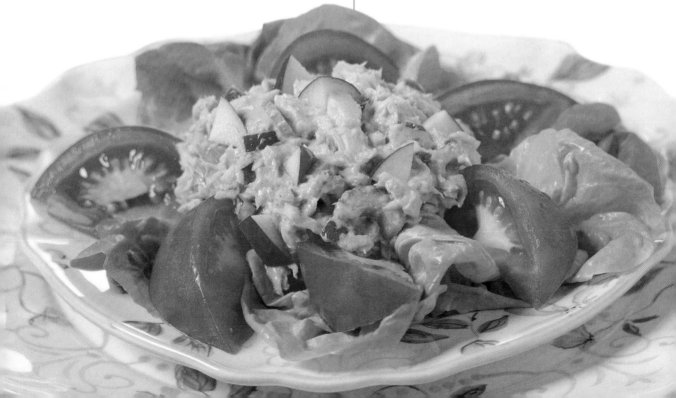

Chicken Pita Pizza

Homemade pizza for one topped with chicken,
bell peppers, zucchini and melted mozzarella

Servings: 1
Preparation Time: 15 minutes

INGREDIENTS

1   whole-wheat pita

¼   cup low-fat pizza sauce

1   portion cooked chicken breast, sliced

¼   red bell pepper, sliced

¼   yellow bell pepper, sliced

¼   small zucchini, sliced

¼   cup reduced-fat mozzarella
    cheese, shredded

DIRECTIONS

1 Preheat oven to 425° F.

2 Place the pita on a baking sheet. Spoon
pizza sauce evenly over the pita. Top with
the sliced cooked chicken, bell peppers,
zucchini and mozzarella cheese.

3 Bake for about 10 to 12 minutes or
until the cheese is melted and the pizza is
heated through.

4 Slice, serve and enjoy! ☺

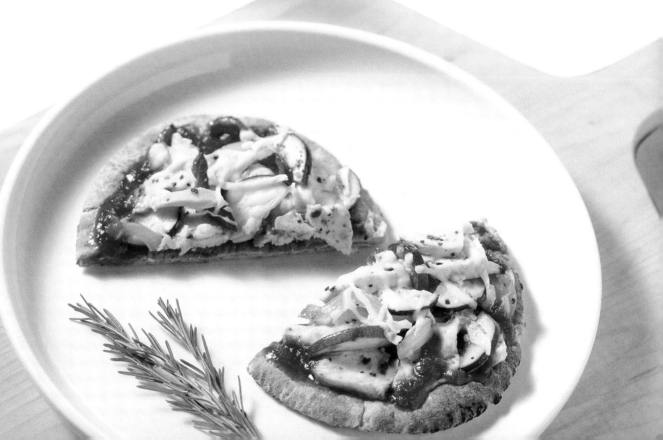

Fired Up Chicken Pita

Whole-wheat pita filled with chicken, diced cucumber, tomato and onion in yogurt dressing

Servings: 1
Preparation Time: 10 minutes

INGREDIENTS

1   portion cooked chicken breast

½   cucumber, peeled, diced

1   tomato, diced

1   slice red onion, chopped

Ground red pepper, to taste

1   Tbsp fat-free plain yogurt

Hot pepper sauce, to taste

1 pita, cut in half

DIRECTIONS

1 Slice cooked chicken breast into bite-size pieces. In a medium mixing bowl, combine chicken, cucumber, tomato, onion, red pepper, yogurt and hot pepper sauce; mix well.

2 Spoon the chicken mixture into the pita. Serve and enjoy! ☺

———— Tasteful Tip ————

To save time, you can buy precooked chicken breasts or you can cook extra chicken breasts and store them whole or sliced in Ziploc® bags in your freezer for up to two months. Simply thaw in your microwave and add to your favorite recipes.

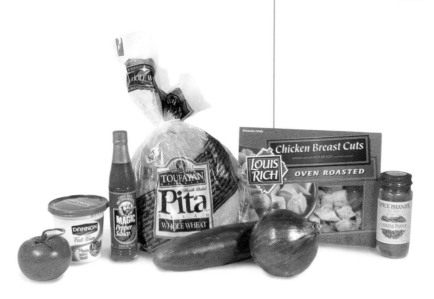

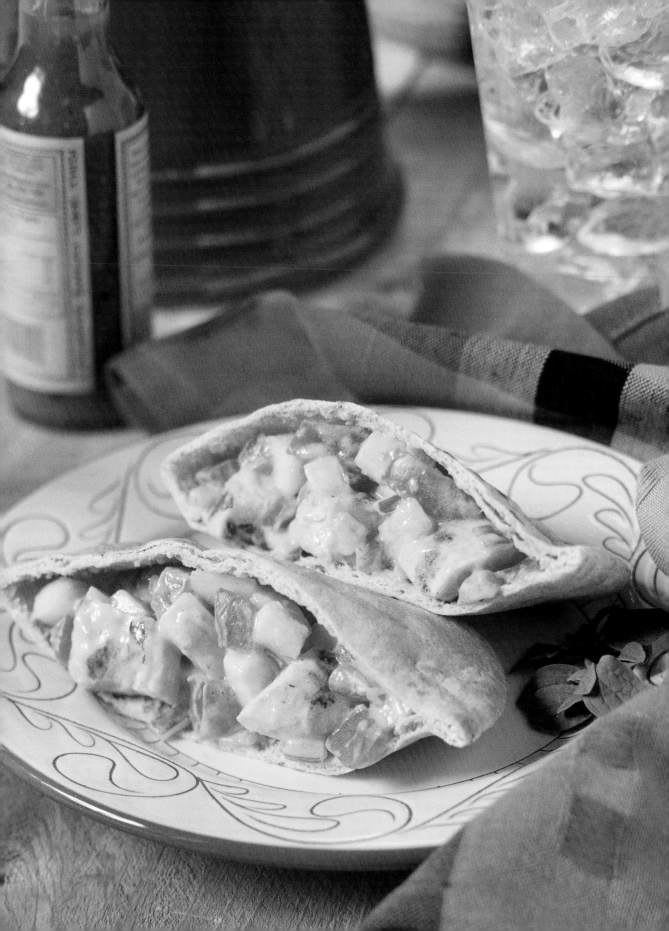

Cilantro Burrito

*Sautéed chicken, cilantro, bell pepper, salsa and
sour cream in a whole-wheat tortilla*

Servings: 1
Preparation Time: 15 minutes

INGREDIENTS

2 slices red onion

¼ red bell pepper, sliced

¼ green bell pepper, sliced

2 Tbsp fresh cilantro, chopped

1 portion cooked chicken breast, sliced

1 (8-inch) whole-wheat tortilla

2 Tbsp salsa

1 Tbsp fat-free sour cream

DIRECTIONS

1 Lightly coat a medium skillet with cooking spray and place over medium heat. Add onion, bell peppers and cilantro; sauté until the vegetables soften, about 6 minutes.

2 Add cooked chicken and sauté until heated through, about 3 minutes.

3 Microwave tortilla for 20 seconds to soften. Place chicken and vegetables on flat tortilla. Wrap the tortilla around the filling and cut in half.

4 Place burrito on a plate with salsa and sour cream for dipping. Serve and enjoy!

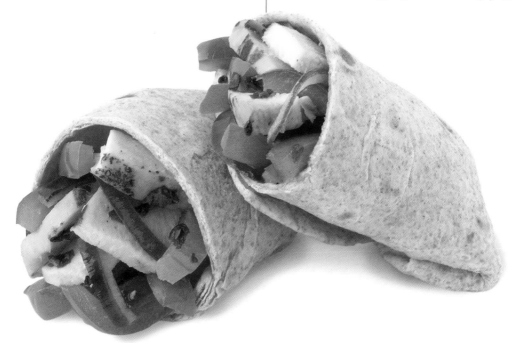

Turkey Salad

Lean turkey breast, raisins and sliced almonds in a ginger-curry dressing

Servings: 2
Preparation Time: 25 minutes

INGREDIENTS

$^1/_2$ cup low-fat plain yogurt

1 tsp curry

$^1/_2$ tsp ground ginger

$^1/_2$ tsp dried thyme

$^1/_3$ cup raisins

2 portions cooked turkey breast (about $^1/_2$ lb), chopped

1 stalk celery, sliced

2 cups mixed salad greens

2 Tbsp sliced almonds

DIRECTIONS

1 In a large mixing bowl, combine yogurt, curry, ginger and thyme. Stir in raisins, cover and refrigerate for 15 minutes.

2 Combine precooked, chopped turkey and celery with yogurt mixture.

3 Line 2 plates with mixed salad greens. Top each with a portion of turkey mixture and sprinkle with sliced almonds. Serve and enjoy! ☺

Egg Salad Sandwich

Toasted whole-grain bread topped with delicious egg salad and ripe avocado slices

Servings: 1
Preparation Time: 10 minutes

INGREDIENTS

4   hard-boiled eggs, peeled

1   Tbsp Miracle Whip® Free

1   Tbsp mustard

$\frac{1}{2}$ stalk celery, sliced

$\frac{1}{4}$ red bell pepper, chopped

1   tsp sweet pickle relish

1   Tbsp fresh parsley

1   slice whole-grain bread

1   lettuce leaf

$\frac{1}{4}$ avocado, sliced

DIRECTIONS

1 Chop 1 whole egg. Then discard the yolks from the 3 other eggs and chop the whites.

2 In a small mixing bowl, combine chopped eggs, Miracle Whip, mustard, celery, bell pepper, pickle relish and parsley.

3 Toast whole-grain bread and place on a small plate. Top with lettuce leaf, egg salad and avocado slices. Serve and enjoy! ☺

———— Tasteful Tip ————

You probably already know how to boil an egg, *but...* just in case... here's a quick reminder: First, place the eggs in a saucepan and add cold water until it fills up the pan about an inch above the eggs. Then place on the stove over high heat and bring to a boil. Cover saucepan, remove from heat and let stand for about 15 minutes. Then pour off hot water and run cold water over eggs to cool. (You probably knew all that already. If not, now you do.)

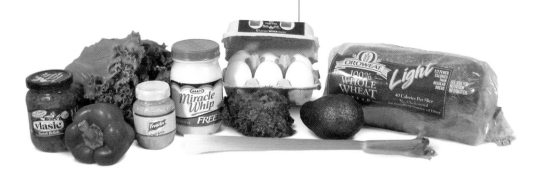

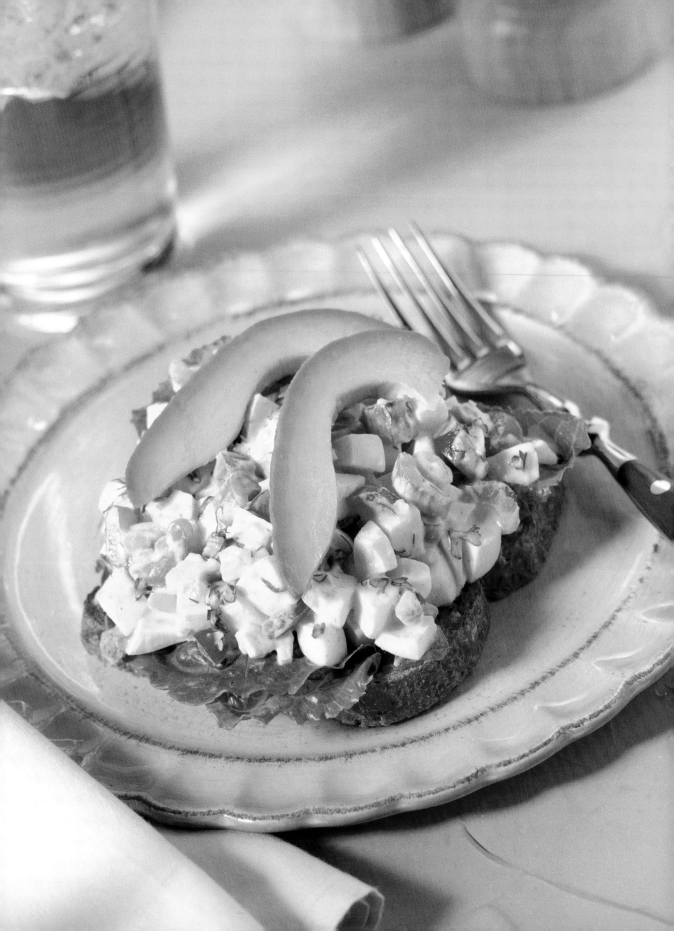

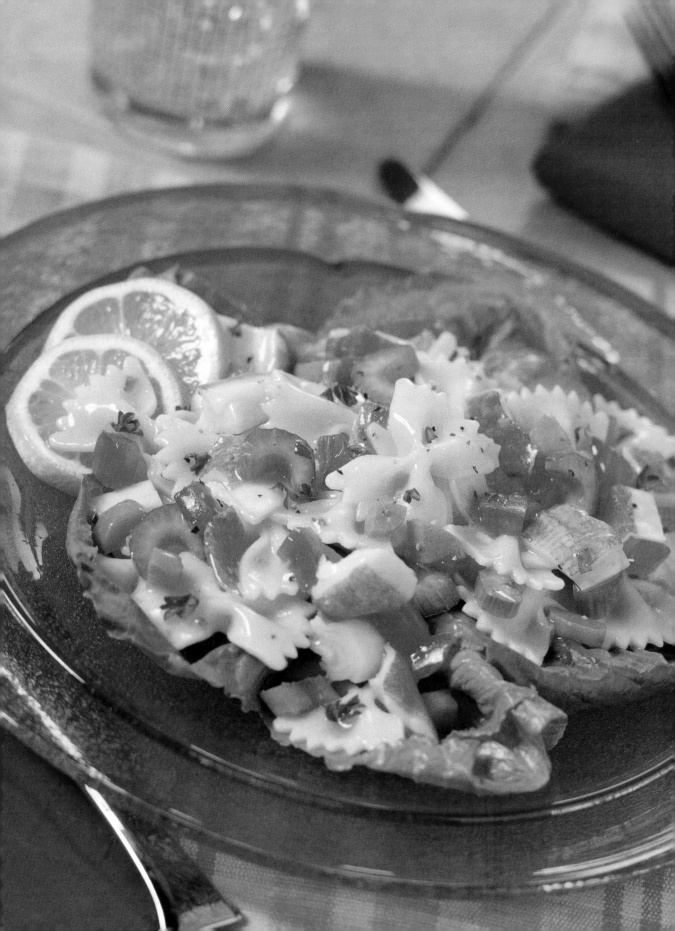

Seafood Pasta Salad

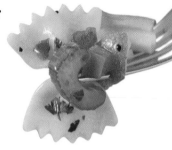

*Bow tie pasta, crab meat and tomato in a
lemon vinaigrette over romaine lettuce*

Servings: 2
Preparation Time: 20 minutes

INGREDIENTS

2   portions bow tie pasta (about 4 oz uncooked)

2   portions cooked crab meat (about 8 oz), fresh,
    canned or frozen, thawed, chopped

1   carrot, peeled and chopped

1   celery stalk, sliced

1   tomato, diced

¼   cup low-fat Italian dressing

1   lemon, halved

¼   tsp ground black pepper

1   head romaine lettuce

DIRECTIONS

1 Prepare bow tie pasta according to its
package directions. Rinse with cold running
water; drain well.

2 While pasta is cooking, combine crab
meat, carrot, celery, tomato, Italian dressing,
lemon juice and black pepper in a large
mixing bowl.

3 Add cooked pasta to crab mixture and
toss to combine.

4 Divide romaine lettuce leaves between
two separate plates. Top each with a
portion of pasta salad. Serve and enjoy!

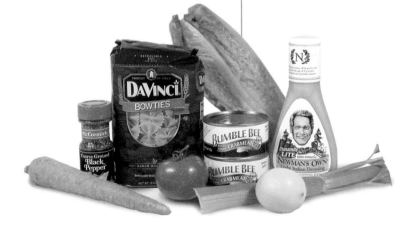

Tex-Mex Burrito

*Lean ground turkey blended with black beans and salsa
in a whole-wheat tortilla topped with cheddar cheese*

Servings: 4
Preparation Time: 15 minutes

INGREDIENTS

4 portions lean ground turkey (about 1 lb)

1 cup salsa

½ can black beans, drained and rinsed

4 (8-inch) whole-wheat tortillas

¼ cup reduced-fat cheddar cheese, shredded

DIRECTIONS

1 Lightly coat a large skillet with cooking spray and place over medium heat. Sauté ground turkey until no longer pink, about 8 minutes. Stir in salsa and beans; sauté until heated through.

2 Warm flour tortillas by placing them between two damp paper towels and microwaving on high for 45 seconds. Spoon a portion of turkey mixture onto each tortilla and roll up.

3 Sprinkle each burrito with a tablespoon of cheese. Serve and enjoy! ☺

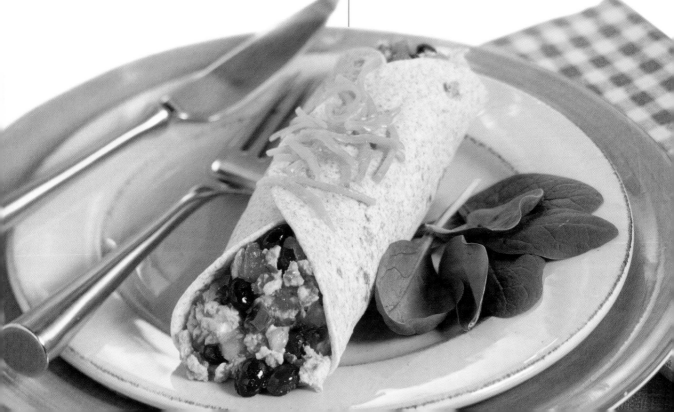

Ranch
Chicken Salad

*Fresh and crisp combination of corn, black beans,
red bell pepper and chicken in a cilantro-lime dressing*

Servings: 4
Preparation Time: 15 minutes

INGREDIENTS

¼ cup fat-free mayonnaise

¼ cup low-fat sour cream

¼ cup cilantro, chopped

1 tsp grated lime zest (peel)

1 lime, halved

½ tsp ground cumin

¼ tsp ground red pepper

4 portions cooked chicken breast
(about 1 lb), cut into
bite-size pieces

1 can (15 oz) black beans,
drained and rinsed

1 can (11 oz) whole-
kernel corn, drained

1 red bell pepper,
diced

½ red onion, chopped

2 heads Bibb lettuce,
separated into leaves,
washed

DIRECTIONS

1 In a large mixing bowl, combine mayonnaise, sour cream, cilantro, lime zest, lime juice, cumin and ground red pepper. Stir in chicken, beans, corn, bell pepper and onion.

2 Divide lettuce evenly among four plates and top with a portion of chicken salad. Serve and enjoy! ☺

Tuna Salad Wrap

Fresh tomato, crisp cucumber and tuna with ranch dressing wrapped in a whole-wheat tortilla

Servings: 1
Preparation Time: 10 minutes

INGREDIENTS

1   can (3 oz) tuna, water packed, drained

1   Tbsp fat-free ranch dressing

1   celery stalk, chopped

¼   tsp ground black pepper

1   tsp Mrs. Dash® Table Blend seasoning

1   (8-inch) whole-wheat tortilla

¼   cucumber, thinly sliced

½   tomato, diced

DIRECTIONS

1 In a medium mixing bowl, combine tuna, ranch dressing, celery, black pepper and Mrs. Dash seasoning; mix well.

2 Microwave the tortilla for about 20 seconds, to soften. Place cucumber slices on the tortilla. Top with the tuna mixture and tomato.

3 Roll it up, serve and enjoy! ☺

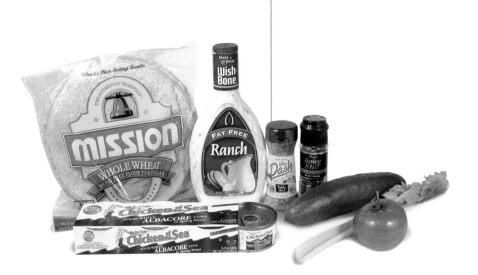

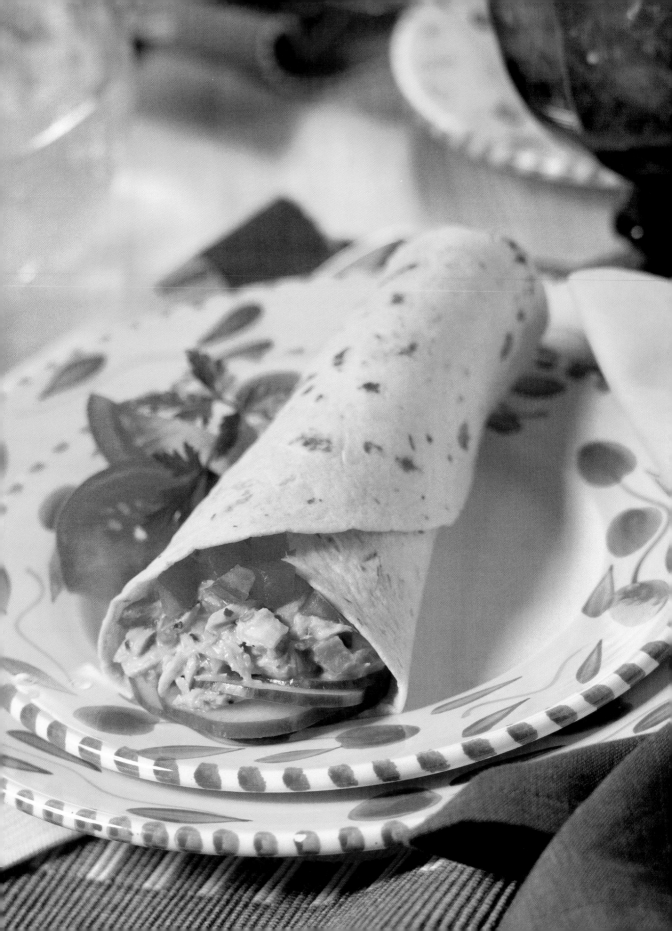

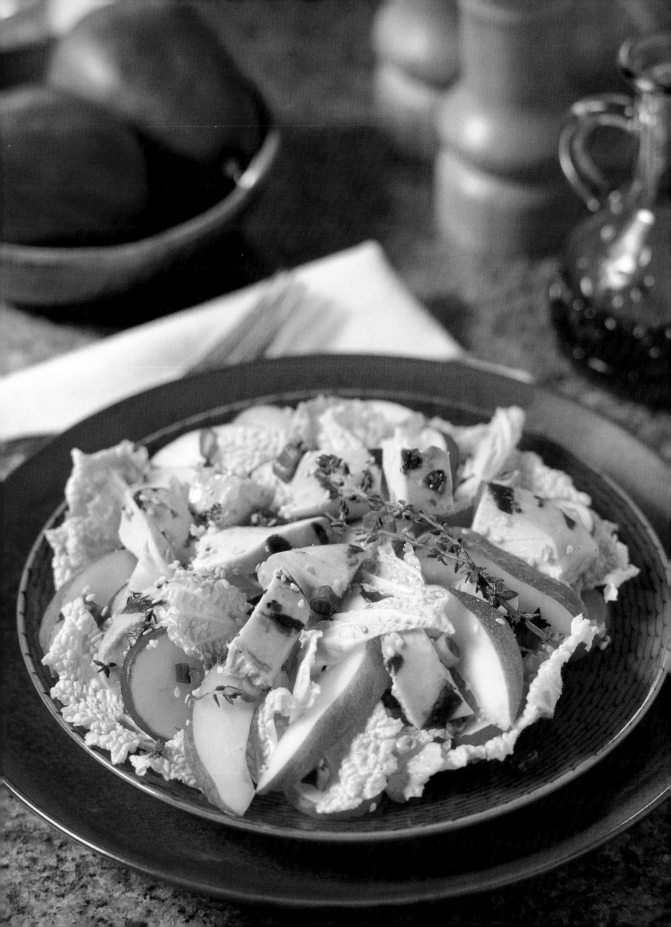

Chicken and Pear Salad

Grilled chicken breast, fresh pear slices with napa cabbage and vinaigrette dressing

Servings: 2
Preparation Time: 30 minutes

INGREDIENTS

2 portions chicken breast (about $^1/_2$ lb)

1 Tbsp sesame seeds

2 pears, cored and sliced

2 cups napa cabbage, shredded

$^1/_2$ cup radishes, sliced

2 green onions, sliced

2 Tbsp olive oil

2 Tbsp vinegar

2 Tbsp fresh parsley, minced

1 tsp fresh thyme, chopped

1 tsp grated lemon peel

DIRECTIONS

1 Preheat grill to high. Place chicken on hot grill and cook for approximately 6 minutes; turn and grill for 6 more minutes until no longer pink in the center. Remove from heat and allow to cool. Then slice into bite-size pieces.

2 While the chicken is cooking, in a medium skillet, toast sesame seeds over medium heat, stirring lightly. Remove seeds when they are golden brown, approximately 5 minutes.

3 In a large mixing bowl, combine the cooled chicken, pear slices, cabbage, radishes, green onion and sesame seeds.

4 In a small mixing bowl, combine the olive oil, vinegar, parsley, thyme and lemon peel; mix well.

5 Pour vinaigrette dressing over chicken and pear salad; toss well.

6 Divide into two portions, serve and enjoy! ☺

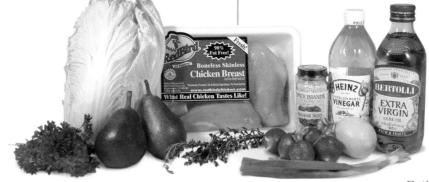

Artichoke
Chicken Salad

*Artichoke hearts and chicken with
tomato and cucumber in a light vinaigrette*

Servings: 2
Preparation Time: 15 minutes

INGREDIENTS

2 cans (5 oz each) white meat chicken
chunks, drained

1 can (14 oz) artichoke hearts in water,
drained and sliced

1 tomato, diced

1 cucumber, peeled, seeded and diced

1 Tbsp fresh parsley, chopped

1 clove garlic, minced

Ground black pepper, to taste

¼ cup fat-free Italian dressing

6 lettuce leaves

DIRECTIONS

1 In a large mixing bowl, combine chicken,
artichoke hearts, tomato, cucumber, parsley,
garlic and black pepper. Add Italian dressing;
toss to coat.

2 Place lettuce leaves on two separate plates.
Divide chicken mixture into two portions and
spoon over lettuce leaves. Serve and enjoy! ☺

——— Tasteful Tip ———

This chicken salad can be refrigerated for up to two
days in an airtight container and makes a great
"planned-over."

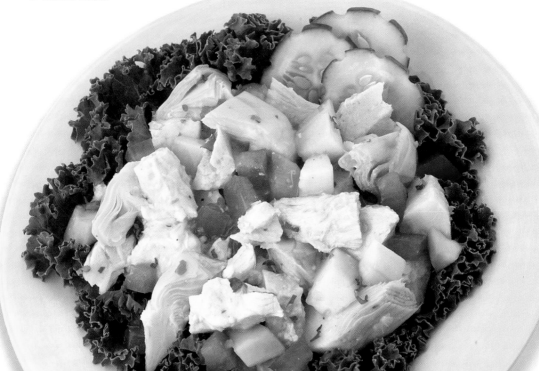

BLT Wrap

Crispy turkey bacon, sliced tomato, lettuce and cheddar cheese in a whole-wheat tortilla

Servings: 1
Preparation Time: 10 minutes

INGREDIENTS

3   strips lean turkey bacon

1   (8-inch) whole-wheat tortilla

1   Tbsp reduced-fat mayonnaise

2   lettuce leaves

3   slices tomato

¼   cup reduced-fat cheddar cheese, shredded

DIRECTIONS

1 Prepare turkey bacon according to its package directions.

2 Microwave the tortilla for about 20 seconds to soften.

3 Spread mayonnaise on warmed tortilla. Then layer with lettuce, tomato, cooked turkey bacon and cheese.

4 Wrap the tortilla around the filling, serve and enjoy! ☺

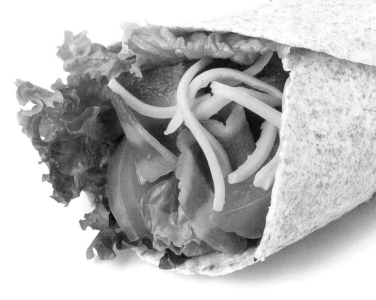

Chilled Grape Chicken Salad

Chopped chicken with chilled red and green grapes, accented with bites of apple and pecan

Servings: 2
Preparation Time: 15 minutes

INGREDIENTS

2 portions of cooked chicken, chopped (about $\frac{1}{2}$ lb)

$\frac{1}{2}$ cup seedless red grapes, chilled, halved

$\frac{1}{2}$ cup green grapes, chilled, halved

1 apple, cored and diced

$\frac{1}{2}$ cup fat-free mayonnaise

1 lemon, halved

$\frac{1}{4}$ tsp ground black pepper

2 cups baby romaine leaves

2 Tbsp chopped pecans

DIRECTIONS

1 In a medium mixing bowl, combine pre-cooked and chopped chicken, chilled red and green grapes, apple, mayonnaise, lemon juice and black pepper.

2 Place baby romaine leaves on 2 small plates. Divide chicken salad mixture into 2 portions and spoon onto lettuce. Sprinkle each salad with half the chopped pecans. Serve and enjoy! ☺

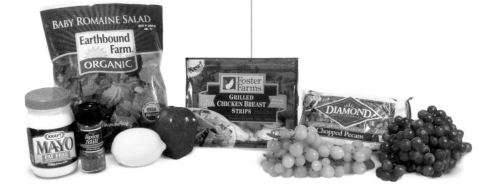

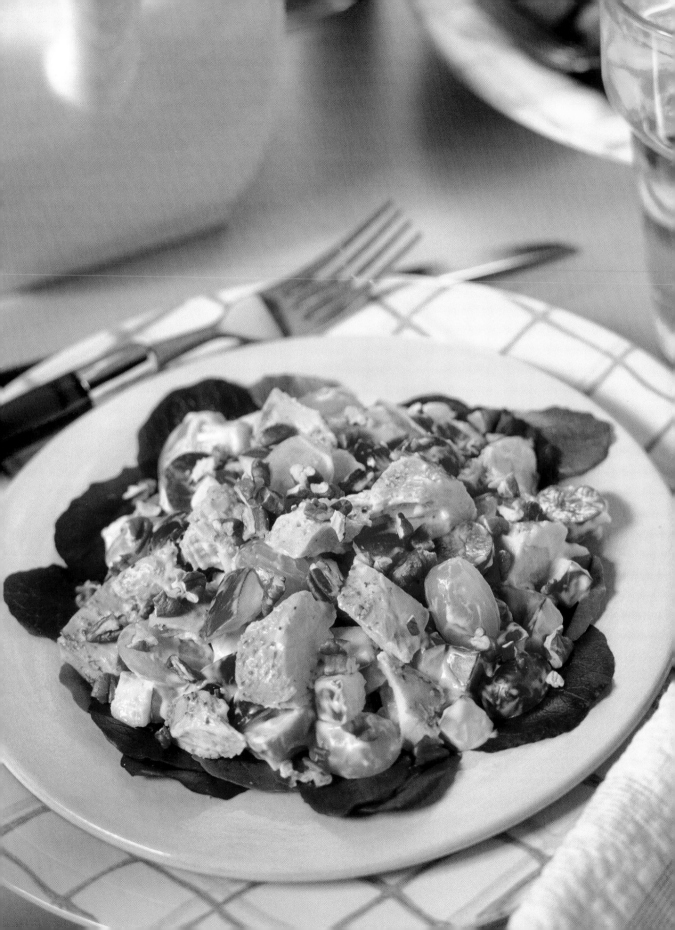

Oriental Chicken Salad

*Chunks of chicken, green onion and shredded cabbage
tossed with sesame-ginger dressing and crispy noodles*

Servings: 4
Preparation Time: 15 minutes

INGREDIENTS

4 portions cooked chicken (about 1 lb),
   cut into bite-size pieces

1 bag (16 oz) coleslaw mix

4 green onions, chopped

2 Tbsp light sesame oil

1/3 cup rice vinegar

1/4 cup lite soy sauce

1/2 tsp ground ginger

1 cup crisp chow mein noodles

DIRECTIONS

1 In a large mixing bowl, combine cooked chicken, coleslaw mix and green onions.

2 In a small mixing bowl, combine sesame oil, rice vinegar, soy sauce and ginger. Drizzle over chicken mixture and toss to coat.

3 Divide chicken salad into four portions. Top with crispy chow mein noodles, serve and enjoy! ☺

Big-Beef Sub

*Homemade sub sandwich packed with roast beef,
juicy tomato, onion and a bit of mayo... to go!*

Servings: 1
Preparation Time: 5 minutes

INGREDIENTS

1   whole-grain roll

1   Tbsp fat-free mayonnaise

2   lettuce leaves

½   tomato, sliced

1   portion lean roast beef (about 4 oz), sliced

1   slice red onion

DIRECTIONS

1 Slice roll horizontally in half and spread with fat-free mayonnaise.

2 Top with lettuce leaves, tomato slices, roast beef and onion.

3 Serve and enjoy! ☺

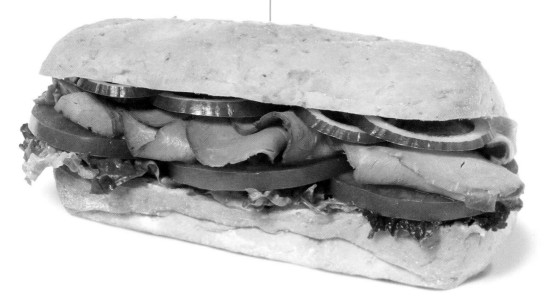

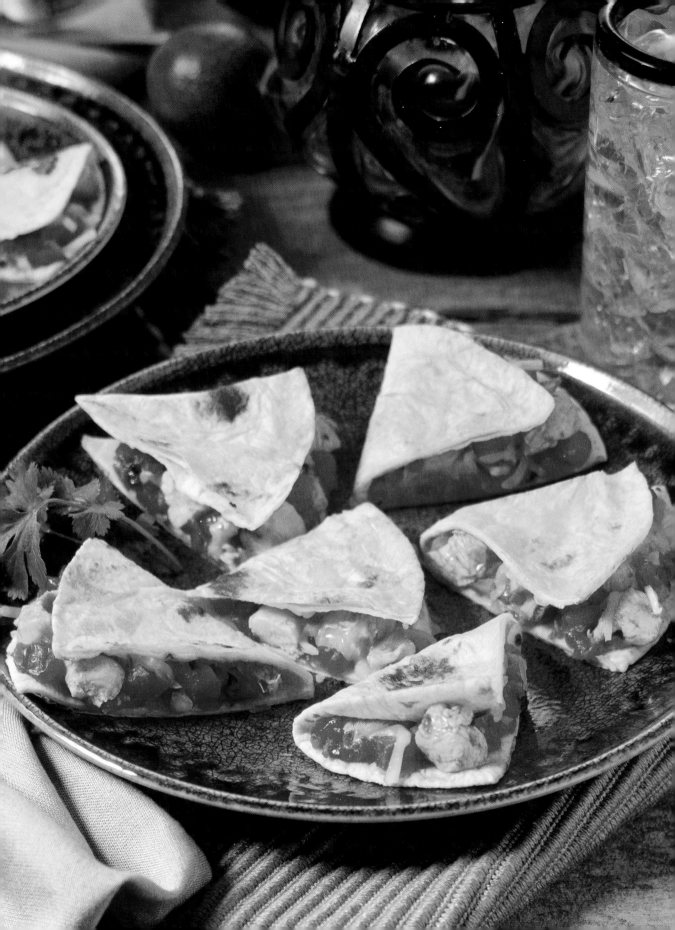

Chicken
Quesadillas

*Chopped chicken with salsa and melted cheese
in a lightly browned tortilla with sour cream*

Servings: 2
Preparation Time: 20 minutes

INGREDIENTS

2   portions chicken breast (about $1/2$ lb)

1   cup salsa

2   (8-inch) flour tortillas

$1/4$ cup reduced-fat cheddar cheese, shredded

$1/4$ cup fat-free sour cream

1 Lightly coat a medium skillet with cooking spray and place over medium heat. Slice chicken breast into $1/2$-inch cubes. Sauté chicken and salsa until chicken is no longer pink, about 10 minutes.

2 Lightly coat a large skillet with cooking spray and place over medium heat. Place a tortilla in the skillet and spread half the chicken mixture over the tortilla. Top with half the cheese. Fold tortilla over filling and cook until lightly browned, about 3 minutes. Turn and brown the other side. Remove from skillet and set aside.

3 Repeat with remaining tortilla, chicken mixture and cheese.

4 Cut quesadillas into wedges and place on small plates. Put half the sour cream on each plate for dipping. Serve and enjoy! ☺

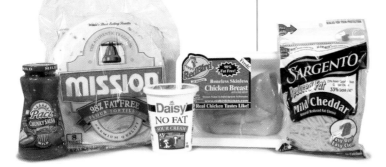

Mile High Baked Potato

A piping-hot baked potato topped with chicken, cottage cheese, broccoli and salsa

Servings: 1
Preparation Time: 15 minutes

INGREDIENTS

1 portion-size russet potato

2 tsp fat-free, reduced-sodium chicken broth

¼ cup low-fat cottage cheese

¼ cup cooked chicken, chopped

¼ cup cooked broccoli

¼ cup salsa

1 Tbsp fresh cilantro, chopped

DIRECTIONS

1 Pierce potato several times with a fork. Place in microwave and cook on high until tender (about 5 to 8 minutes). Let stand for 1 minute.

2 Use a knife to cut an "X" in the top of the cooked potato. Press ends slightly to open potato, and pour chicken broth into opening.

3 Top potato with cottage cheese, cooked chicken, broccoli and salsa. Place filled potato in microwave and cook on high for 30 more seconds.

4 Sprinkle the top with fresh cilantro, serve and enjoy! ☺

Lobster
Salad

Creamy lobster salad on a bed of lettuce with red apple slices

Servings: 2
Preparation Time: 15 minutes

INGREDIENTS

- 2 portions cooked lobster meat (about 8 oz) fresh, canned or frozen, thawed, chopped

- 4 green onions, sliced

- 1 stalk celery, sliced

- $1/8$ tsp ground black pepper

- $1/2$ cup low-fat cottage cheese

- $1/4$ cup fat-free plain yogurt

- 1 tsp Dijon mustard

- 4 lettuce leaves

- 2 red apples, cored and sliced

DIRECTIONS

1 In a small mixing bowl, combine chopped lobster, green onion, celery, black pepper, cottage cheese, yogurt and mustard; mix well.

2 Line two plates with lettuce leaves and spoon a portion of the salad on top of each.

3 Place half of the apple slices on each plate. Serve and enjoy! ☺

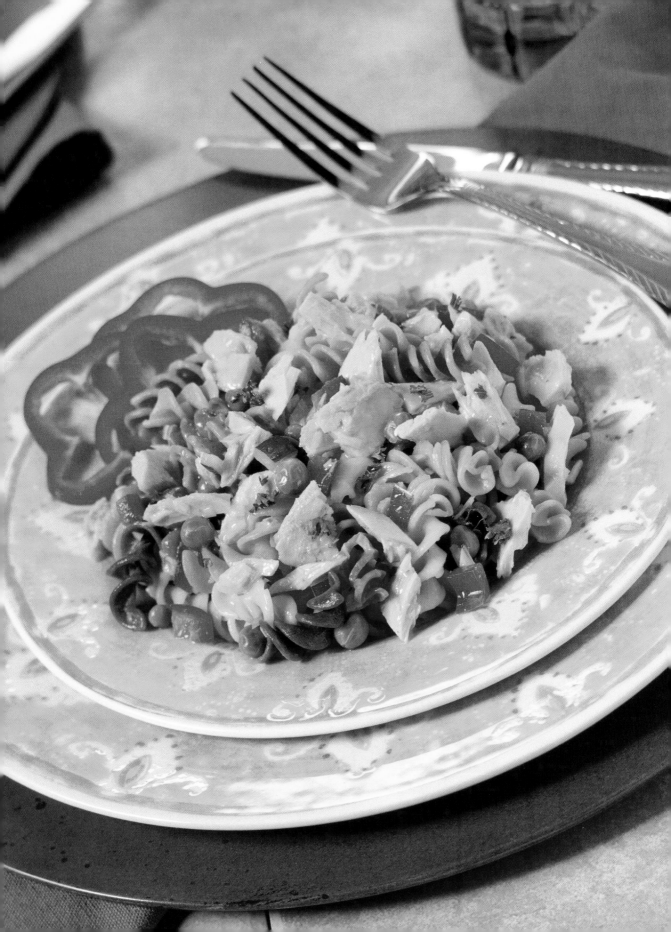

Tuna Rotini Salad

Tuna, bell pepper and peas,
tossed with rotini pasta in vinaigrette

Servings: 2
Preparation Time: 15 minutes

INGREDIENTS

2 portions rotini (about 4 oz uncooked)

1 can (6 oz) tuna, packed in water, drained

1 red bell pepper, diced

1 slice onion, chopped

½ cup frozen peas, thawed

¼ cup low-fat Italian dressing

3 Tbsp fresh parsley, chopped

DIRECTIONS

1 Prepare rotini according to its package directions.

2 Combine pasta and remaining ingredients in a large mixing bowl; toss until well combined.

3 Divide into two portions, serve and enjoy! ☺

Tasteful Tip

This meal can be served hot, right after you make it for lunch. And, you can make extra portions or "planned-overs" and store in the refrigerator and serve them for lunch the following day. You'll enjoy Tuna Rotini Salad hot or cold!

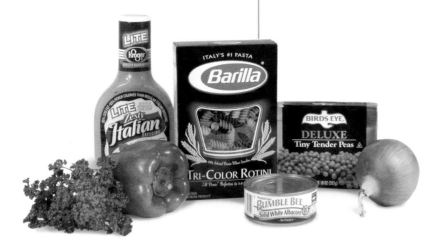

Great
Chicken Pita

Sweet, chilled chicken salad with a whole-wheat pita

Servings: 2
Preparation Time: 15 minutes

INGREDIENTS

- 2 portions cooked chicken (about $^1/_2$ lb), cut into bite-size pieces
- 1 stalk celery, sliced
- 1 slice red onion, chopped
- 1 Tbsp sliced almonds
- $^1/_4$ cup fat-free Miracle Whip®
- 1 tsp Mrs. Dash® Extra Spicy
- $^1/_2$ tsp paprika
- $^1/_2$ cup seedless red grapes, halved
- 1 whole-wheat pita, cut in half
- 1 tomato, chopped
- 2 lettuce leaves

DIRECTIONS

1 In a medium mixing bowl, combine cooked chicken, celery, red onion, almonds and Miracle Whip.

2 Stir in Mrs. Dash and paprika. Then, gently stir in red grapes.

3 Fill each pita half with a portion of chicken mixture, tomato and lettuce. Serve and enjoy! ☺

Crunchy Taco Salad

Chili-seasoned ground turkey on a bed of lettuce
topped with salsa and sour cream

Servings: 4
Preparation Time: 20 minutes

INGREDIENTS

4 portions lean ground turkey (about 1 pound)

1 can (15 oz) chili beans in chili sauce

5 cups romaine lettuce, chopped

1 cup salsa

$\frac{1}{2}$ cup reduced-fat cheddar cheese, shredded

1 tomato, diced

4 green onions, sliced

$\frac{1}{2}$ cup light sour cream

4 oz baked tortilla chips

DIRECTIONS

1 Place a large skillet over medium-high heat. Add ground turkey and cook until no longer pink, about 5 minutes.

2 Stir in chili beans and simmer until heated through and slightly thickened, about 10 more minutes.

3 Evenly divide lettuce onto 4 plates. Spoon a portion of turkey mixture over lettuce. Then top with salsa, cheddar cheese, tomato, green onion and sour cream.

4 Crumble about a fourth of the tortilla chips over each salad. Serve and enjoy!

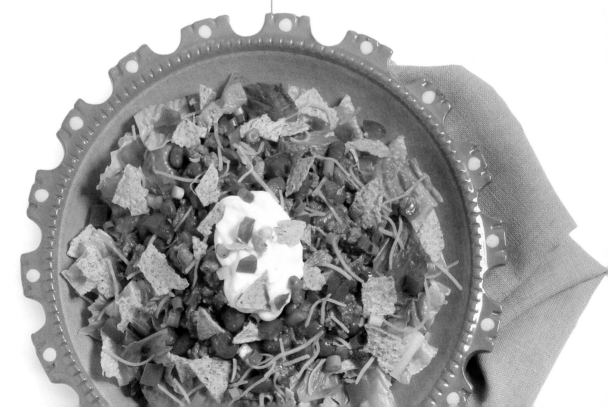

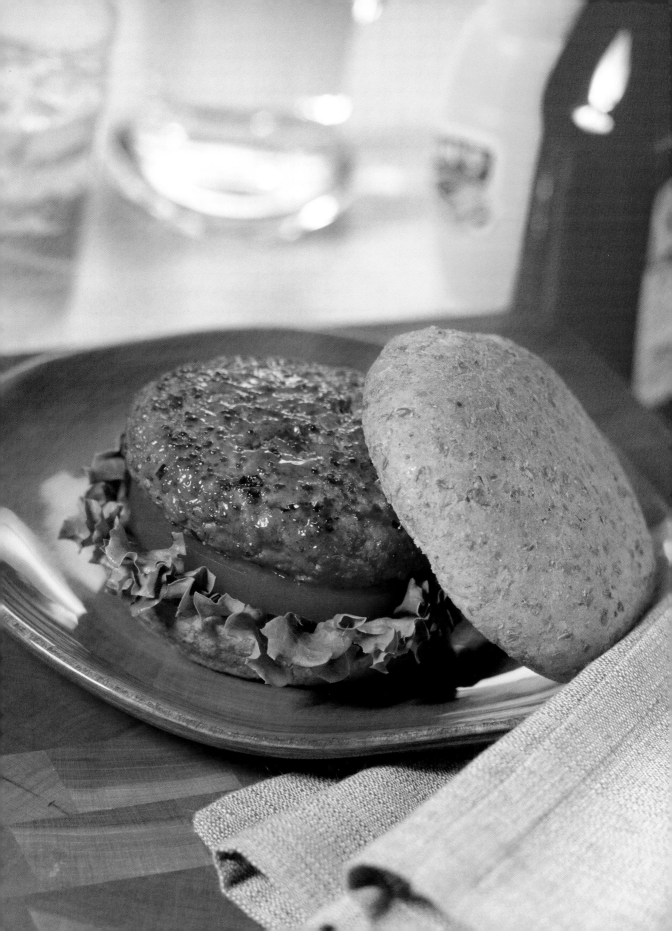

Turkey Burgers

An American classic made with lean ground turkey
with lettuce and tomato on a whole-wheat bun

Servings: 4
Preparation Time: 20 minutes

INGREDIENTS

4 portions lean ground turkey (about 1 lb)

$^1/_2$ onion, finely chopped

1 tsp horseradish

1 tsp lite soy sauce

$^1/_4$ tsp ground black pepper

1 clove garlic, minced

2 Tbsp fresh parsley, chopped

$^1/_2$ cup egg substitute

4 whole-wheat buns or rolls, split

4 lettuce leaves

4 slices tomato

Ketchup, to taste

Mustard, to taste

Tasteful Tip

An alternative to *grilling* turkey burgers (as well as chicken and fish) is to use a "George Foreman Grill®," which cooks both sides of the meat at once. This not only saves time but helps bring out the best flavors!

DIRECTIONS

1 Preheat grill to high.

2 In a large mixing bowl, combine ground turkey, onion, horseradish, soy sauce, black pepper, garlic, parsley and egg substitute. Form into 4 portion-size patties.

3 Place patties on a hot grill and cook until no longer pink in the center, approximately 6 minutes per side.

4 Place burger on whole-wheat bun with lettuce, tomato, ketchup and mustard. Serve and enjoy! ☺

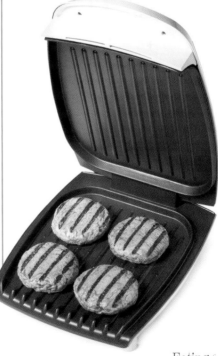

BBQ Chicken Pita Pizza

Homemade pizza with a crispy pita crust topped with chicken, onion and barbecue sauce

Servings: 1
Preparation Time: 15 minutes

INGREDIENTS

- 1 whole-wheat pita
- 2 Tbsp barbecue sauce
- 1 portion cooked chicken (about 4 oz), cubed
- 1 slice red onion, diced
- 2 tsp fresh rosemary, chopped (or ¼ tsp dried rosemary)
- ¼ cup reduced-fat mozzarella cheese, shredded

DIRECTIONS

1 Preheat oven to 425° F.

2 Place pita on a baking sheet and spoon barbecue sauce evenly over the pita. Top with chicken, onions, rosemary and cheese.

3 Bake for 10 to 12 minutes or until the cheese is melted, the pizza is heated through and the pita crisp.

4 Slice, serve and enjoy! ☺

Turkey Reuben Sandwich

*Sliced turkey breast, Swiss cheese and
sauerkraut on grilled rye bread*

Servings: 1
Preparation Time: 10 minutes

INGREDIENTS

Spicy mustard, to taste

2 slices rye bread

1 slice reduced-fat Swiss cheese

1 portion sliced turkey breast (about 4 oz)

¼ cup sauerkraut, drained

— Tasteful Tip —

This lean and delicious Reuben sandwich also tastes
great when served cold. For more variety, you can
substitute reduced-fat Thousand Island dressing in
place of mustard.

DIRECTIONS

1 Lightly coat a small skillet with cooking
spray and place over medium heat.

2 Spread spicy mustard over both slices
of bread.

3 Layer cheese, turkey and sauerkraut on
one of the bread slices. Top with remaining
bread slice (mustard-side down, of course).

4 Place the sandwich in the skillet and cook
until the bottom is golden brown, about 4
minutes. Turn and brown the other side.

5 Slice in half, serve and enjoy! ☺

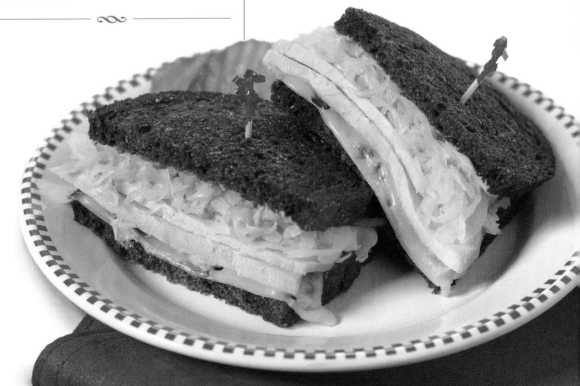

Midmeals

Cottage Berries

Fresh, sweet raspberries with cottage cheese

Servings: 1
Preparation Time: 5 minutes

INGREDIENTS

1 portion low-fat cottage cheese (about $^1/_2$ cup)

$^1/_2$ cup fresh raspberries

DIRECTIONS

1 Place low-fat cottage cheese and fresh raspberries on a small plate.

2 Serve and enjoy! ☺

Apple
& Cheese

Any apple and your choice of cheese!

Servings: 1
Preparation Time: 2 minutes

INGREDIENTS

1   portion-size apple

1   portion part-skim string cheese

DIRECTIONS

1 Place apple and string cheese on a plate (or not).

2 Serve and enjoy! 🍎

─── Tasteful Tip ───

Apples have a tremendous nutrient content and are nature's original "fast food." Red ones, green ones... even golden apples are delicious! Just be sure to pick one that's *your* portion size.

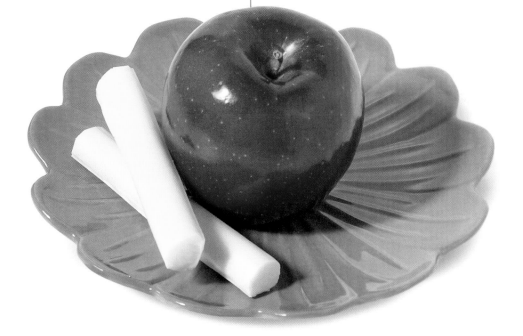

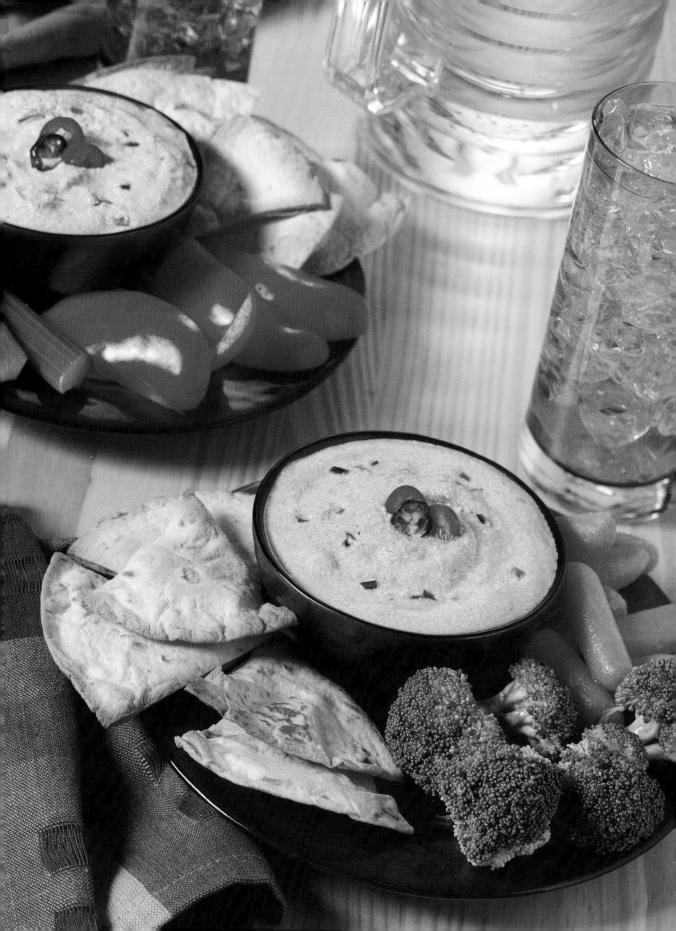

Creamy Salsa Dip

Savory and smooth dip with baked tortilla chips and fresh vegetables

Servings: 2
Preparation Time: 10 minutes

INGREDIENTS

1 cup low-fat cottage cheese

½ cup salsa

½ cup fat-free plain yogurt

1 jalapeño, seeded and chopped

2 (8-inch) flour tortillas

2 cups fresh vegetables of your choice

——— Tasteful Tip ———

This flavorful recipe is a nutritious alternative to high-fat "chips and dips." You'll really like it!

DIRECTIONS

1 Preheat oven to 400° F.

2 Blend cottage cheese, salsa, yogurt and jalapeño in a food processor or blender until smooth, about 30 seconds.

3 Cut each tortilla into 12 wedges and place on a baking sheet. Bake for about 7 minutes, until lightly browned.

4 Divide dip into 2 portions and place in 2 small bowls. Surround each with a portion of baked tortilla chips and half of the fresh vegetables. Serve and enjoy! ☺

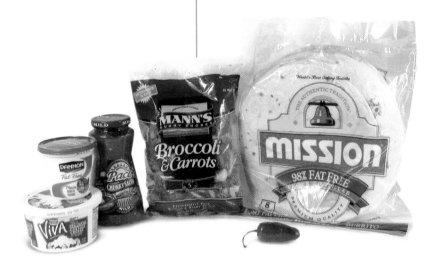

Cantaloupe
Cottage Cup

Surprisingly sweet and satisfying serving of fruit and protein

Servings: 2
Preparation Time: 5 minutes

INGREDIENTS

1 cantaloupe

2 portions low-fat cottage cheese (about 1 cup)

———— Tasteful Tip ————

You will be able to spot a nice ripe cantaloupe by following your nose! The best melons smell *very* sweet!

DIRECTIONS

1 Slice cantaloupe in half. Use a spoon to scoop out seeds from center of cantaloupe.

2 Place each cantaloupe half on a small plate. Fill the center of each with a portion of cottage cheese.

3 Serve and enjoy! ☺

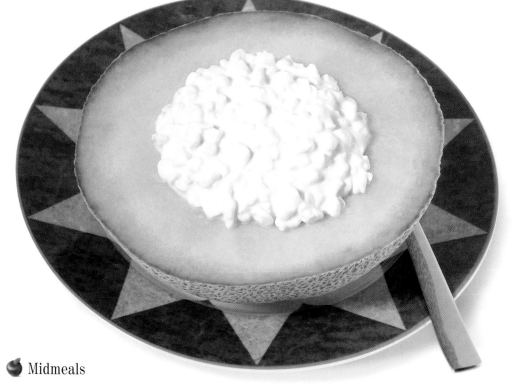

Eggs & Oranges

Quality protein and sun-kissed carbs!

Servings: 1
Preparation Time: 20 minutes

INGREDIENTS

2   whole eggs

1   portion-size orange

DIRECTIONS

1 Place eggs in a saucepan and add cold water until it fills up the pan approximately 1 inch above the eggs.

2 Place on the stove over high heat and bring to a boil. Cover saucepan, remove from heat and let stand for about 15 minutes. Then pour off hot water and run cold water over the eggs to cool. Peel shell off of cooled eggs and slice in half.

3 Slice orange into wedges, serve with hard-boiled eggs and enjoy! ☺

Greek Pinwheels

*Turkey breast, feta cheese, ripe olives with spinach,
whole-wheat wrapped and sliced*

Servings: 2
Preparation Time: 20 minutes

INGREDIENTS

¼ cup fat-free cream cheese, softened

¼ tsp dried oregano

¼ cup reduced-fat, basil- and tomato-flavored
feta cheese, crumbled

1 can (2 oz) chopped ripe olives, drained

2 (8-inch) whole-wheat tortillas

4 oz sliced turkey breast

1 cup baby spinach leaves

DIRECTIONS

1 In a medium mixing bowl, use a fork to combine cream cheese, oregano, reduced-fat feta cheese and olives.

2 Evenly spread half the cheese mixture on each tortilla. Then top with half the turkey breast and half the spinach leaves.

3 Roll up tightly, cover in plastic wrap and refrigerate until firm enough to slice, about 15 minutes.

4 Remove plastic wrap and slice each tortilla into 6 pieces. Serve and enjoy! 🍎

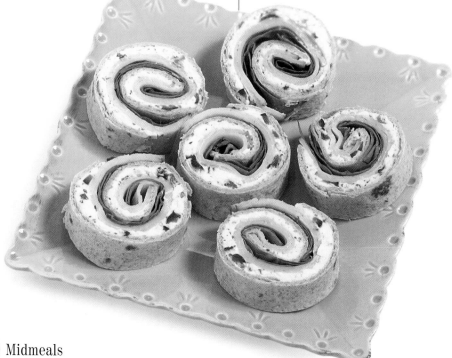

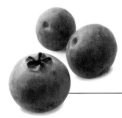

Blueberry Blend

Protein-rich cottage cheese with blueberry yogurt

Servings: 1
Preparation Time: 2 minutes

INGREDIENTS

1 portion low-fat cottage cheese (about ½ cup)

1 portion light, fat-free blueberry yogurt (about 6 oz)

DIRECTIONS

1 In a serving bowl, combine cottage cheese and blueberry yogurt.

2 Serve and enjoy! ☺

—————— Tasteful Tip ——————

Combining yogurt and cottage cheese creates a nutritious Eating *for* Life midmeal, complete with high-quality protein and carbohydrates. It's also very quick and easy!

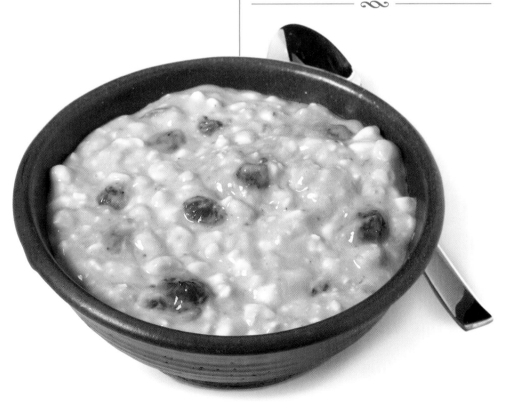

Tropical
Treat

*Mandarin oranges, crushed pineapple,
vanilla yogurt and cottage cheese in papaya*

Servings: 2
Preparation Time: 5 minutes

INGREDIENTS

2 portions low-fat cottage cheese (about 1 cup)

1 cup light fat-free, sugar-free vanilla yogurt

½ cup crushed pineapple, drained

½ cup mandarin oranges, drained

1 papaya, halved and seeded

DIRECTIONS

1 In a medium mixing bowl, combine cottage cheese and yogurt. Then add pineapple and mandarin oranges. Stir gently until well combined.

2 Divide filling into two portions and spoon into papaya halves. Serve and enjoy! ☺

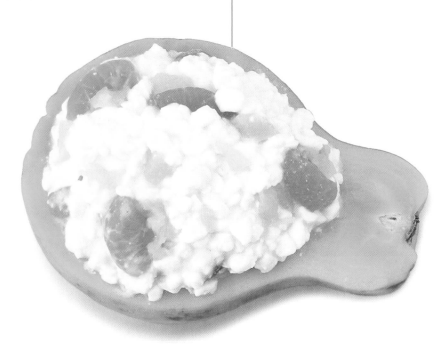

Cool
Ranch Dip

Creamy ranch-flavored dip with
baked pita wedges and fresh vegetables

Servings: 2
Preparation Time: 10 minutes

INGREDIENTS

2 portions low-fat cottage cheese (about 1 cup)

1 green onion, chopped

2 tsp Italian seasoning

¼ tsp ground black pepper

2 pitas

2 cups vegetables of your choice

DIRECTIONS

1 Preheat oven to 400° F.

2 Combine cottage cheese and green onion in blender or food processor and blend on high speed until smooth, about 30 seconds. Spoon into small mixing bowl; add Italian seasoning and black pepper, stirring to combine.

3 Cut each pita into 8 wedges and place on baking sheet. Bake for about 7 minutes, until lightly browned.

4 Divide dip into 2 portions and place in 2 small bowls. Place on serving plate with a portion of baked pita wedges and vegetables. Serve and enjoy! ☺

Orange-Vanilla Fruit Dip

Cool, creamy orange-vanilla dip with fresh strawberries

Servings: 1
Preparation Time: 5 minutes

INGREDIENTS

1   portion low-fat cottage cheese (about $^1/_2$ cup)

$^1/_2$ cup light, fat-free vanilla yogurt

1   tsp grated orange peel

1   portion fresh strawberries

DIRECTIONS

1 Combine cottage cheese, yogurt and orange peel in a blender or food processor and blend on high speed until smooth, about 30 seconds.

2 Spoon orange-vanilla dip into a small bowl and place a portion of fresh strawberries on the side for dipping. Serve and enjoy! ☺

Cottage Apple

Crisp apple wedges with
cinnamon-spiced cottage cheese

Servings: 1
Preparation Time: 3 minutes

INGREDIENTS

1 portion low-fat cottage cheese (about $^1/_2$ cup)

$^1/_8$ tsp cinnamon

sugar substitute, to taste

1 portion-size apple

DIRECTIONS

1 Place cottage cheese in a small bowl. Sprinkle with cinnamon and sugar substitute.

2 Slice apple into wedges and place on a small plate.

3 Serve and enjoy! ☺

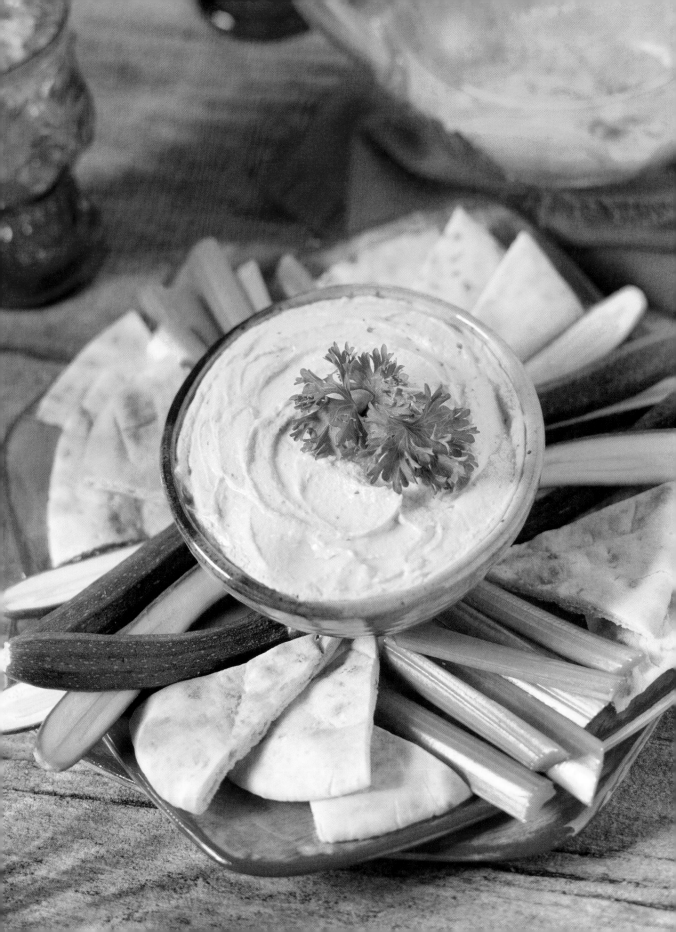

Creamy
Tuna Paté

Spicy cream cheese and tuna dip with
baked pita wedges and fresh vegetables

Servings: 2
Preparation Time: 15 minutes

INGREDIENTS

4   oz fat-free cream cheese, at room temperature

1   can (3 oz) tuna, packed in water, drained

1   Tbsp chili sauce

1   Tbsp fresh parsley, chopped

1   tsp onion, minced

Hot pepper sauce, to taste

2   pitas

2   cups fresh vegetables of your choice

DIRECTIONS

1 Preheat oven to 400° F.

2 Combine cream cheese, tuna, chili sauce, parsley, onion and hot pepper sauce in a blender or food processor and blend on high speed until smooth, about 30 seconds.

3 Cut each pita into 8 wedges and place on baking sheet. Bake for about 7 minutes or until lightly browned.

4 Divide tuna paté into 2 portions and place in 2 small bowls. Surround each with a portion of baked pita wedges and half the vegetables. Serve and enjoy! ☺

Tasteful Tip

Pita wedges can be baked ahead of time and stored in an airtight container for up to four days. "Stacy's" is a brand of Pita Chips that are ready-made. For more information, check out www.pitachip.com

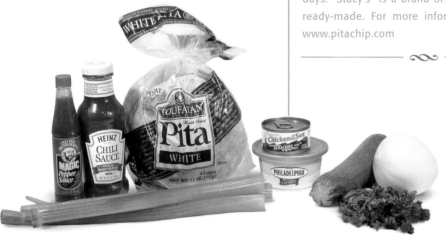

Cinnamon Apple

Spiced apple slices with cheddar cheese

Servings: 1
Preparation Time: 10 minutes

INGREDIENTS

1 portion-size apple, peeled, cored and sliced

$^1/_3$ cup water

$^1/_4$ tsp ground cinnamon

$^1/_4$ tsp ground nutmeg

2 oz reduced-fat cheddar cheese, sliced

DIRECTIONS

1 Layer apple slices in the bottom of a shallow dish. Add water and sprinkle with cinnamon and nutmeg.

2 Microwave on high for about 3 to 5 minutes, until apple slices are tender. Allow apples to cool slightly, then place them on a small serving plate.

3 Slice cheese and place next to cooked apple slices. Serve and enjoy! ☺

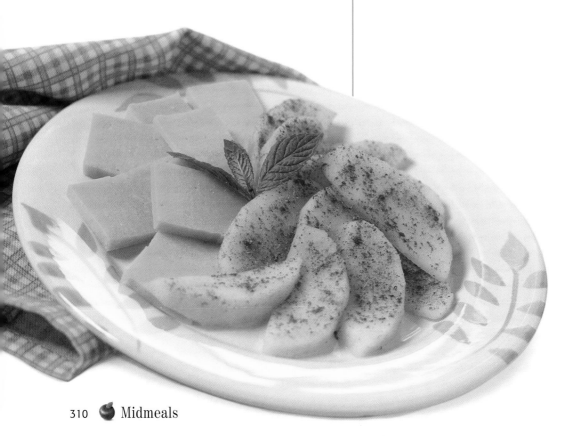

Swiss Turkey Krisp

Cheese and crisp crackers with sliced turkey

Servings: 1
Preparation Time: 2 minutes

INGREDIENTS

2 slices turkey breast (about 2 oz)

1 slice reduced-fat Swiss cheese (about 1 oz)

2 seasoned Ry Krisp® crackers

DIRECTIONS

1 Place turkey and Swiss cheese on crackers.

2 Serve and enjoy! ☺

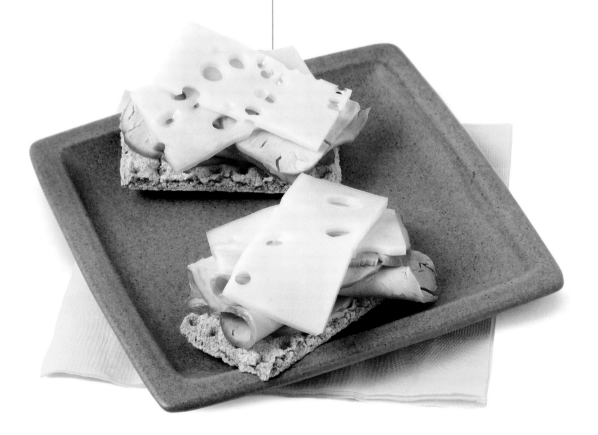

Nutrition Shakes

Strawberry Banana Smoothie

Sweet, smooth strawberries blended with banana and bursting with nutrition!

Servings: 1
Preparation Time: 3 minutes

INGREDIENTS

12 oz cold water

1   packet vanilla Myoplex® Lite

1   small banana

6   frozen strawberries

DIRECTIONS

1 Pour cold water in blender. Then add Myoplex powder and blend on medium speed for 15 seconds.

2 Add banana; blend for 30 more seconds. Add frozen strawberries and blend on high speed until smooth, about 30 more seconds.

3 Pour into a tall glass, serve and enjoy! ☺

Chocolate Mint

Satisfying sweet chocolate nutrition shake
with a hint of cool peppermint

Servings: 1
Preparation Time: 3 minutes

INGREDIENTS

12 oz cold water

1 packet chocolate Myoplex® Lite

$\frac{1}{8}$ tsp peppermint extract

6 ice cubes

DIRECTIONS

1 Pour cold water in blender. Then add Myoplex powder and blend on medium speed for 15 seconds.

2 Add peppermint extract; blend for 30 more seconds. Add ice cubes and blend on high speed until smooth, about 30 more seconds.

3 Pour into a tall glass, serve and enjoy! ☺

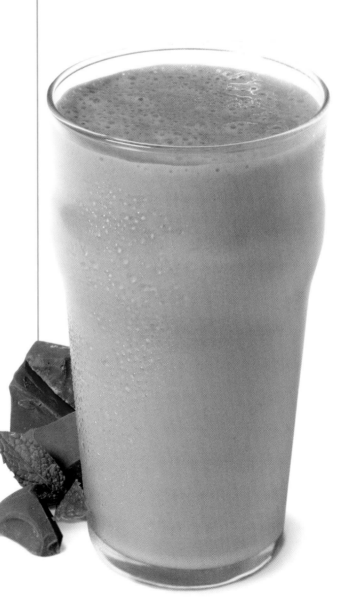

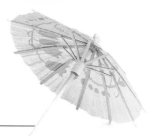

Piña Colada

Tempting tropical taste with
*   sultry and satisfying nutrition!*

Servings: 1
Preparation Time: 3 minutes

INGREDIENTS

12 oz cold water

1 packet vanilla Myoplex® Lite

½ cup unsweetened pineapple chunks

¼ tsp coconut extract

6 ice cubes

DIRECTIONS

1 Pour cold water in blender.
Then add Myoplex powder
and blend on medium speed
for 15 seconds.

2 Add pineapple chunks and
coconut extract; blend for 30
more seconds. Add ice cubes
and blend on high speed until
smooth, about 30 more seconds.

3 Pour into a tall glass, serve and enjoy! 😊

Vanilla Malt

Protein-enriched, very vanilla "soda-fountain-style" shake

Servings: 1
Preparation Time: 3 minutes

INGREDIENTS

1 cup cold skim milk

1 scoop (about 24 grams of protein) vanilla protein powder (whey or soy)

2 Tbsp malted milk powder

1 Tbsp fat-free, sugar-free vanilla instant pudding mix

6 ice cubes

DIRECTIONS

1 Place skim milk and protein powder in blender and blend on medium speed for 15 seconds. Add malted milk and blend 15 more seconds.

2 Add pudding mix and blend for about 30 seconds. Add ice cubes and blend on high speed until smooth, about 30 more seconds.

3 Pour into a tall glass. Serve and enjoy! ☺

Cookies & Cream

High-quality Myoplex® nutrition with
a bit of Cool Whip® and cookies

Servings: 1
Preparation Time: 3 minutes

INGREDIENTS

12 oz cold water

1 packet vanilla Myoplex® Lite

¼ cup Cool Whip® Lite

6 ice cubes

3 chocolate wafer cookies

DIRECTIONS

1 Pour cold water in blender. Then add
Myoplex powder and blend on medium
speed for 15 seconds.

2 Add Cool Whip and ice cubes; blend for
30 seconds on high speed. Add cookies and
blend on medium speed until mixed, about
15 more seconds.

3 Pour into a tall glass, serve and enjoy! ☺

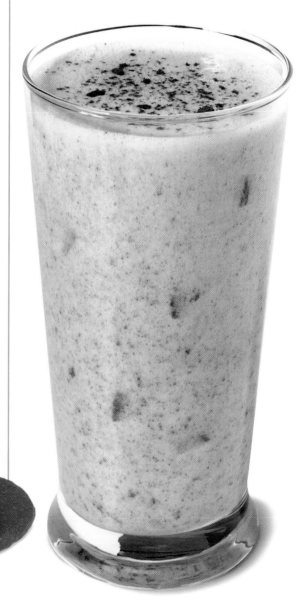

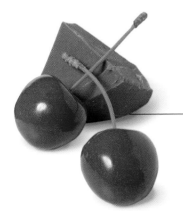

Very Cherry

Chocolate-covered-cherry-inspired nutrition shake

Servings: 1
Preparation Time: 3 minutes

INGREDIENTS

12 oz cold water

1 packet chocolate Myoplex® Lite

1/3 cup frozen cherries, unsweetened

6 ice cubes

DIRECTIONS

1 Pour cold water in blender. Then add Myoplex powder and blend on medium speed for 15 seconds.

2 Add frozen cherries; blend for 30 more seconds. Add ice cubes and blend on high speed until smooth, about 30 more seconds.

3 Pour into a tall glass, serve and enjoy! ☺

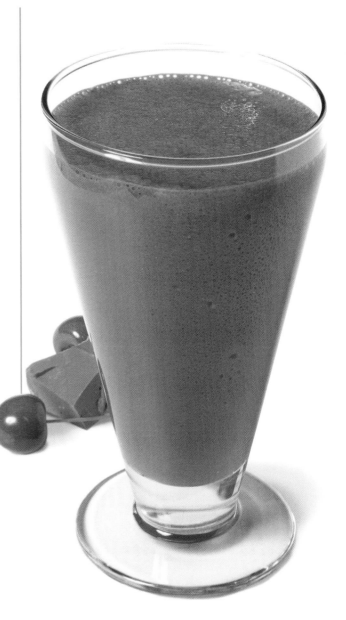

Sparkling Orange

Sun-kissed-orange smoothie with
protein and a splash of soda

Servings: 1
Preparation Time: 3 minutes

INGREDIENTS

12 oz diet orange soda

6 oz light, fat-free orange-flavored yogurt

1 scoop (about 24 grams of protein) vanilla
protein powder (whey or soy)

½ orange, peeled

6 ice cubes

DIRECTIONS

1 Pour orange soda in blender. Then add
yogurt and protein powder; blend on
medium speed for 15 seconds.

2 Add peeled orange and blend for 30 more
seconds. Add ice cubes and blend on high
speed until smooth, about 30
more seconds.

3 Pour into a tall glass,
serve and enjoy! 😊

Blackberry Smoothie

Super simple, sweet, satisfying and nutritious!

Servings: 1
Preparation Time: 3 minutes

INGREDIENTS

12 oz cold water

1 packet vanilla Myoplex® Lite

2 Tbsp frozen orange juice concentrate

10 frozen blackberries

3 ice cubes

DIRECTIONS

1 Pour cold water in blender. Then add Myoplex powder and blend on medium speed for 15 seconds.

2 Add frozen orange juice concentrate and blackberries; blend 30 more seconds. Add ice cubes and blend on high speed until smooth, about 30 more seconds.

3 Pour into a tall glass, serve and enjoy! 😊

—— Tasteful Tip ——

To make your nutrition shakes and smoothies thicker and creamier, add less water. To make them thinner, add a few ounces more water. Simple!

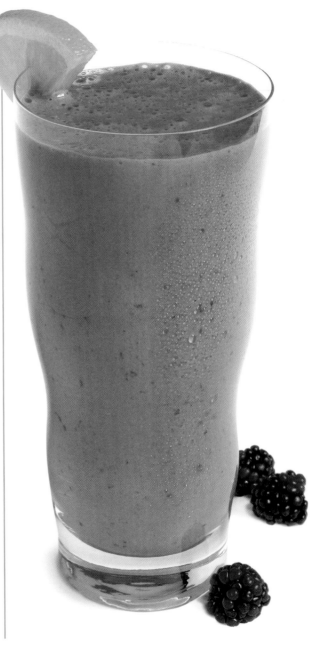

Cappuccino Strength

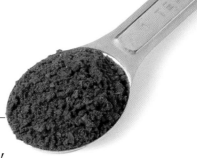

Invigorating nutrition shake with a shot of coffee!

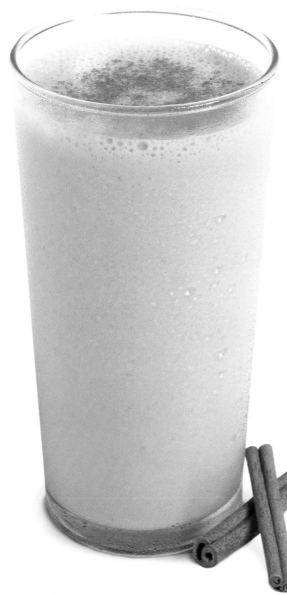

Servings: 1
Preparation Time: 3 minutes

INGREDIENTS

12 oz cold water

1 packet vanilla Myoplex® Lite

2 tsp instant coffee

¼ tsp cinnamon, divided

6 ice cubes

DIRECTIONS

1 Pour cold water in blender. Then add Myoplex powder and blend on medium speed for 15 seconds.

2 Add coffee and half the cinnamon; blend for 30 more seconds. Add ice cubes and blend on high speed until smooth, about 30 more seconds.

3 Pour into a tall glass and sprinkle with the remaining cinnamon.

4 Serve and enjoy! 😋

Iced
Chai

Delicious blend of black tea, soy milk, honey,
ginger and spices with added protein

Servings: 1
Preparation Time: 3 minutes

INGREDIENTS

$^1\!/_2$ cup cold vanilla soy milk

$^1\!/_2$ cup chai tea concentrate

1 scoop (about 24 grams of protein)
natural-flavor protein (whey or soy)

1 cup crushed ice

DIRECTIONS

1 Place soy milk, chai tea concentrate and protein powder in blender. Blend on medium speed until smooth and slightly frothy, about 30 seconds.

2 Place ice cubes in a tall glass. Pour chai tea blend over ice. Serve and enjoy! ☺

—— Tasteful Tip ——

Chai (pronounced as a single syllable and rhymes with "pie") is the word for tea in over 18 languages. When you buy chai in America, you are actually getting a version based on an ancient tea recipe from India made with black tea, milk, honey and various spices. You can usually find chai tea concentrates in the coffee section of your grocery store.

Apple Pie á la Mode

Tart cinnamon apple flavor, bursting with nutrition and topped with whipped cream

Servings: 1
Preparation Time: 3 minutes

INGREDIENTS

6 oz cold unsweetened apple juice

6 oz cold water

1 packet vanilla Myoplex® Lite

½ tsp Butter Buds®

¼ tsp cinnamon, divided

6 ice cubes

2 Tbsp Cool Whip® Free

DIRECTIONS

1 Pour cold apple juice and water into blender. Then add Myoplex powder and blend on medium speed for 15 seconds.

2 Add Butter Buds and half the cinnamon; blend for 30 more seconds. Add ice cubes and blend on high speed until smooth, about 30 more seconds.

3 Pour into a tall glass, top with a dollop of Cool Whip and a sprinkle of cinnamon. Serve and enjoy! ☺

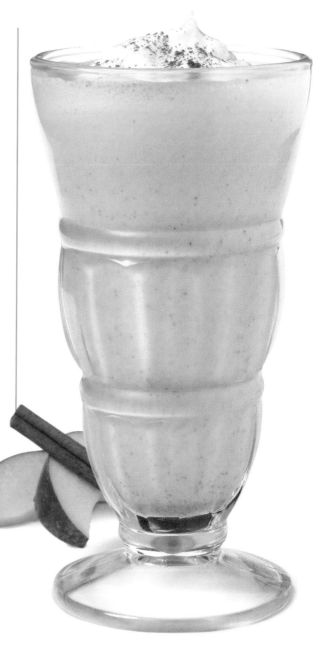

Chocolate Peanut Butter Blend

Creamy peanut butter blended into
a rich chocolate nutrition shake

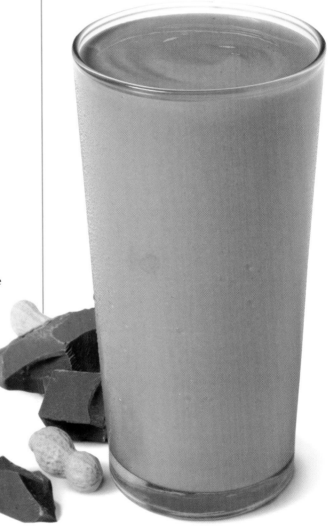

Servings: 1
Preparation Time: 3 minutes

INGREDIENTS

12 oz cold water

1 packet chocolate Myoplex® Lite

1 Tbsp natural peanut butter

6 ice cubes

DIRECTIONS

1 Pour cold water in blender. Then add Myoplex powder and blend on medium speed for 15 seconds.

2 Add peanut butter; blend for 30 more seconds. Add ice cubes and blend on high speed until smooth, about 30 more seconds.

3 Pour into a tall glass, serve and enjoy! ☺

Frosted Key Lime Pie

Nutritionally balanced and dessert delicious!

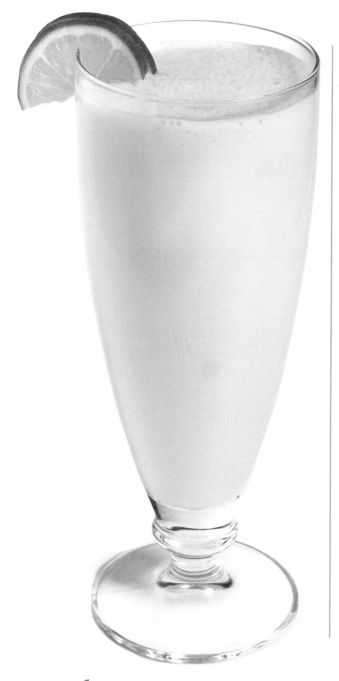

Servings: 1
Preparation Time: 3 minutes

INGREDIENTS

12 oz cold water

1 packet vanilla Myoplex® Lite

3 Tbsp frozen limeade concentrate

6 ice cubes

DIRECTIONS

1 Pour cold water in blender. Then add Myoplex powder and blend on medium speed for 15 seconds.

2 Add frozen limeade concentrate; blend for 30 more seconds. Add ice cubes and blend on high speed until smooth, about 30 more seconds.

3 Pour into a tall glass, serve and enjoy! ☺

Tasteful Tip

This delicious Key Lime Pie is made with Myoplex Lite nutrition shake mix, which contains a very high-quality blend of protein, vitamins and minerals. If you prefer a different brand of nutrition shake mix, please feel free to use that instead.

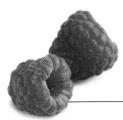

All that Razz

Tangy raspberry smoothie with a bit of lime

Servings: 1
Preparation Time: 3 minutes

INGREDIENTS

8 oz light, fat-free, sugar-free vanilla yogurt

1 scoop (about 24 grams of protein)
   vanilla protein powder (whey or soy)

1/2 cup fresh or frozen red raspberries

1 squeeze of lime juice

Sugar substitute, to taste

3 ice cubes

DIRECTIONS

1 Spoon yogurt into blender. Add protein powder and blend at low speed until smooth, about 30 seconds.

2 Add raspberries, lime juice and sugar substitute. Blend on medium speed until well mixed, about 30 seconds. Add ice and blend on high speed until smooth, about 30 more seconds.

3 Pour into a tall glass, serve and enjoy! 😊

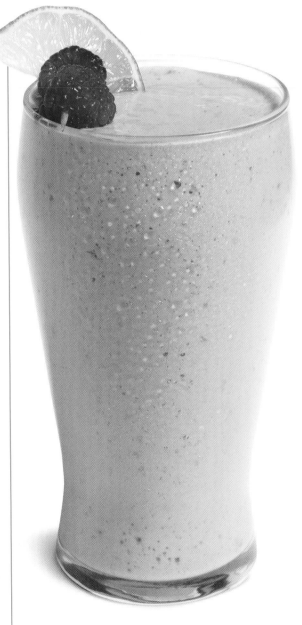

Plan to Succeed

On the following pages, you'll see how to set the table for your success by planning each of your six daily meals ahead of time. These Eating *for* Life meal plans give specific examples of what to eat each day and week. Please review the following pages carefully, keeping in mind these are *examples* and that you should create your meal plans based on *your* preferences and include your favorite foods.

Following the two weeks of examples, you'll find two weeks of blank Eating *for* Life meal plans, which give you a simple and effective structure to begin your planning process. This is your chance to begin—to actually cross that abyss between knowing and *doing*. When you take out a pencil or pen and start writing in what you're going to eat for breakfast, lunch, dinner, dessert and daily midmeals, you'll be taking a very important step forward. You will be consciously deciding to begin Eating *for* Life.

If you would like more blank Eating *for* Life meal plans to help you set the table for your success, please visit Eating*for*Life.com where you can print these forms out for free.

Eating *for* Life Meal Plan

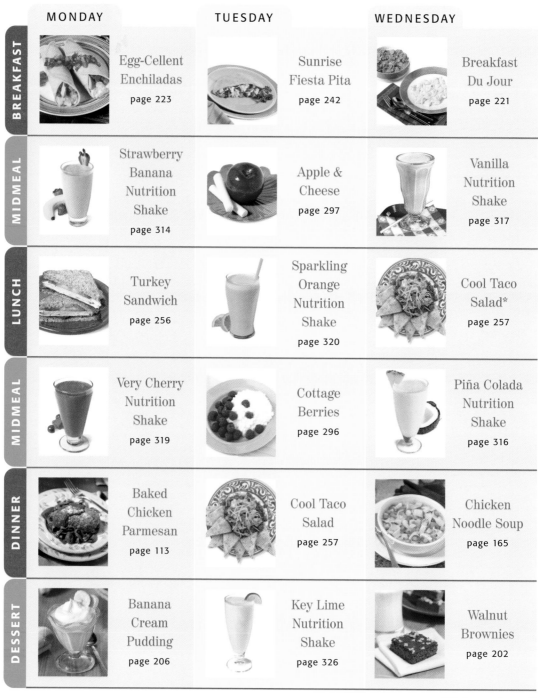

	MONDAY	TUESDAY	WEDNESDAY
BREAKFAST	Egg-Cellent Enchiladas page 223	Sunrise Fiesta Pita page 242	Breakfast Du Jour page 221
MIDMEAL	Strawberry Banana Nutrition Shake page 314	Apple & Cheese page 297	Vanilla Nutrition Shake page 317
LUNCH	Turkey Sandwich page 256	Sparkling Orange Nutrition Shake page 320	Cool Taco Salad* page 257
MIDMEAL	Very Cherry Nutrition Shake page 319	Cottage Berries page 296	Piña Colada Nutrition Shake page 316
DINNER	Baked Chicken Parmesan page 113	Cool Taco Salad page 257	Chicken Noodle Soup page 165
DESSERT	Banana Cream Pudding page 206	Key Lime Nutrition Shake page 326	Walnut Brownies page 202

* "planned-over"

Example: Week 1

	THURSDAY	FRIDAY	SATURDAY	
BREAKFAST	Denver Omelet page 227	Cappuccino Nutrition Shake page 322	Fortified French Toast page 251	
MIDMEAL	Raspberry Nutrition Shake page 327	Cottage Apple page 307	Eggs and Oranges page 301	
LUNCH	Chicken Noodle Soup* page 165	Tuna Salad Wrap page 272	Chicken Pita Pizza page 261	
MIDMEAL	Walnut Brownies* page 202	Chocolate Nutrition Bar	Cantaloupe Cottage Cup page 300	
DINNER	Spaghetti & Meatballs page 89	Grilled Salmon page 84	Filet Mignon page 103	
DESSERT	Butterscotch Bliss page 212	Vanilla Nutrition Shake page 317	Anyday Sundae page 197	

Eating *for* Life Meal Plan

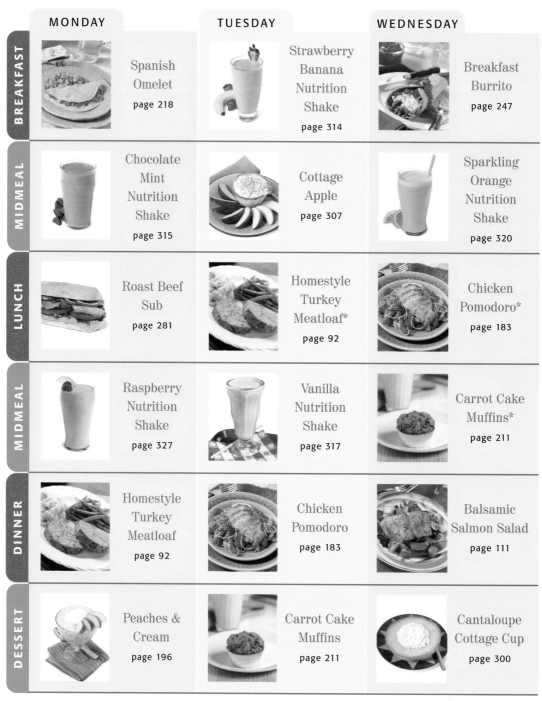

	MONDAY	TUESDAY	WEDNESDAY
BREAKFAST	Spanish Omelet — page 218	Strawberry Banana Nutrition Shake — page 314	Breakfast Burrito — page 247
MIDMEAL	Chocolate Mint Nutrition Shake — page 315	Cottage Apple — page 307	Sparkling Orange Nutrition Shake — page 320
LUNCH	Roast Beef Sub — page 281	Homestyle Turkey Meatloaf* — page 92	Chicken Pomodoro* — page 183
MIDMEAL	Raspberry Nutrition Shake — page 327	Vanilla Nutrition Shake — page 317	Carrot Cake Muffins* — page 211
DINNER	Homestyle Turkey Meatloaf — page 92	Chicken Pomodoro — page 183	Balsamic Salmon Salad — page 111
DESSERT	Peaches & Cream — page 196	Carrot Cake Muffins — page 211	Cantaloupe Cottage Cup — page 300

* "planned-over"

Example: Week 2

	THURSDAY	FRIDAY	SATURDAY	
BREAKFAST	Cappuccino Nutrition Shake page 322	Eggs and Oats page 226	Turkey Bacon Quiche page 239	BREAKFAST
MIDMEAL	Tropical Treat page 304	Strawberry Banana Nutrition Shake page 314	Cottage Berries page 296	MIDMEAL
LUNCH	Fired Up Chicken Pita page 262	Enchilada Soup* page 132	Turkey Burger page 291	LUNCH
MIDMEAL	Vanilla Nutrition Shake page 317	Chocolate Nutrition Bar	Apple & Cheese page 297	MIDMEAL
DINNER	Enchilada Soup page 132	Baked Halibut page 144	Marinated Flank Steak page 148	DINNER
DESSERT	Banana Cream Pudding page 206	Cookies & Cream Nutrition Shake page 318	Black Forest Pudding page 213	DESSERT

Eating *for* Life Meal Plan

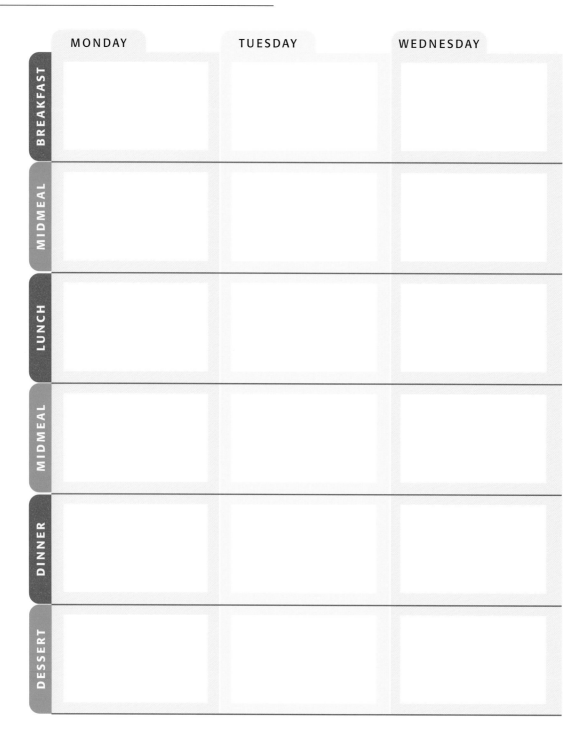

	MONDAY	TUESDAY	WEDNESDAY
BREAKFAST			
MIDMEAL			
LUNCH			
MIDMEAL			
DINNER			
DESSERT			

THURSDAY	FRIDAY	SATURDAY	
			BREAKFAST
			MIDMEAL
			LUNCH
			MIDMEAL
			DINNER
			DESSERT

Eating *for* Life **Meal Plan**

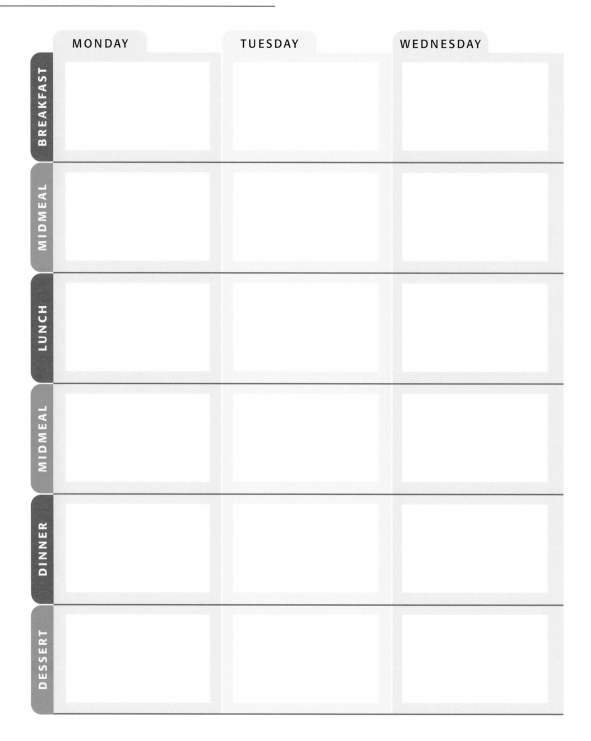

	MONDAY	TUESDAY	WEDNESDAY
BREAKFAST			
MIDMEAL			
LUNCH			
MIDMEAL			
DINNER			
DESSERT			

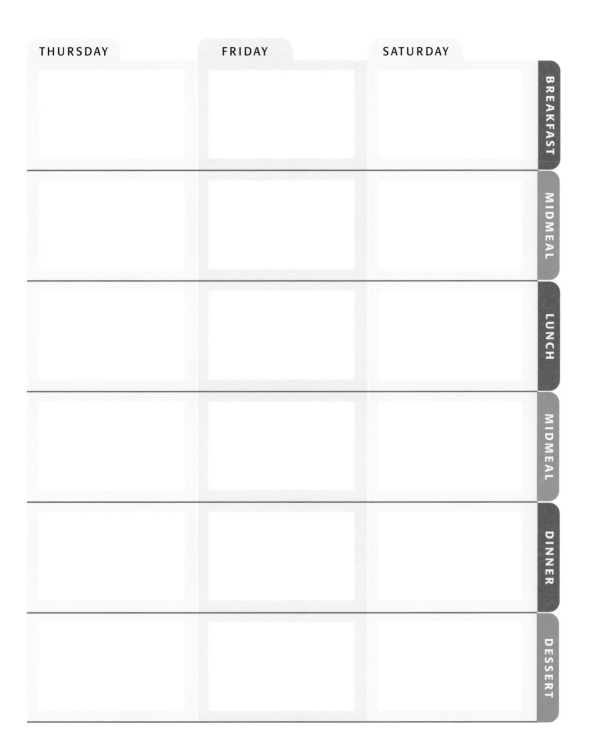

THURSDAY	FRIDAY	SATURDAY	
			BREAKFAST
			MIDMEAL
			LUNCH
			MIDMEAL
			DINNER
			DESSERT

Planning your meals ahead of time truly is one of the "must-do" aspects of Eating *for* Life. It is *the* simple step that helps you transform from eating accidentally (the wrong way) to feeding yourself with specific intent (the right way). Planning your meals doesn't require a significant investment of time. In fact, it saves time in the long run because during your busy day, you don't have to think about what you are going to eat, when and where... you just follow your plan.

Once you get the hang of this, I highly encourage you to plan not just a day but a week in advance. And with the tremendous variety of Eating *for* Life meals presented in this book, all you need to do is select a meal that looks appetizing to you and write it in on your weekly meal plan.

Now, once you have planned your meals, you'll need to make sure that you have the right ingredients you need to prepare those meals as quickly and efficiently as possible during the week. And that brings us to the Eating *for* Life grocery guide. This is a very detailed list of "authorized" foods and ingredients—the right foods and ingredients—which are included in the meal recipes in this book. Although this grocery guide is an extensive list, it's very easy to use. It is set up so that you do your grocery shopping by section—starting with the produce section, then going to the deli, then the bakery area, canned food aisles and so on.

I highly encourage you to utilize the following grocery guide and to do your shopping once a week. I go to the grocery store on Sunday so I'm prepared for the entire week. You might consider this strategy as well. For additional copies of the grocery guide, visit Eating*for*Life.com and I'll provide them to you for free.

Eating *for* Life
Grocery Guide

Vegetables

- ❑ _____ asparagus spears
- ❑ _____ avocado
- ❑ _____ bell pepper, green
- ❑ _____ bell pepper, red
- ❑ _____ bell pepper, yellow
- ❑ _____ broccoli florets
- ❑ _____ broccoli slaw (packaged)
- ❑ _____ cabbage, napa
- ❑ _____ carrots
- ❑ _____ carrots, baby
- ❑ _____ celery
- ❑ _____ coleslaw mix (packaged)
- ❑ _____ cucumber
- ❑ _____ garlic
- ❑ _____ ginger
- ❑ _____ green beans
- ❑ _____ jalapeños

- ❑ _____ lettuce, Bibb
- ❑ _____ lettuce, iceberg
- ❑ _____ lettuce, looseleaf
- ❑ _____ lettuce, romaine
- ❑ _____ lettuce, romaine salad blend (packaged)
- ❑ _____ lettuce, baby romaine salad (packaged)
- ❑ _____ lettuce, salad greens, mixed (packaged)
- ❑ _____ mushrooms, portabella
- ❑ _____ mushrooms, shiitake
- ❑ _____ mushrooms, sliced
- ❑ _____ mushrooms, whole
- ❑ _____ onions, red
- ❑ _____ onions, white
- ❑ _____ onions, green
- ❑ _____ parsnips

- ❑ _____ potatoes, new
- ❑ _____ potatoes, red
- ❑ _____ potatoes, russet
- ❑ _____ potatoes, white
- ❑ _____ radishes
- ❑ _____ shallots
- ❑ _____ snow peas
- ❑ _____ spinach leaves, baby (packaged)
- ❑ _____ squash, yellow
- ❑ _____ tomatoes
- ❑ _____ tomatoes, grape
- ❑ _____ tomatoes, Roma
- ❑ _____ yams or sweet potatoes
- ❑ _____ zucchini
- ❑ _____
- ❑ _____

Fruit

- ❑ _____ apples, red
- ❑ _____ bananas
- ❑ _____ blueberries
- ❑ _____ cantaloupe
- ❑ _____ grapefruit
- ❑ _____ grapes, green seedless

- ❑ _____ grapes, red seedless
- ❑ _____ lemon
- ❑ _____ lime
- ❑ _____ mango
- ❑ _____ oranges
- ❑ _____ papaya

- ❑ _____ peaches
- ❑ _____ pears
- ❑ _____ raspberries
- ❑ _____ strawberries
- ❑ _____
- ❑ _____

Fresh Herbs

- ❑ _____ basil
- ❑ _____ chives
- ❑ _____ cilantro
- ❑ _____ dill

- ❑ _____ mint
- ❑ _____ oregano
- ❑ _____ parsley, curly
- ❑ _____ parsley, Italian

- ❑ _____ rosemary
- ❑ _____ thyme
- ❑ _____
- ❑ _____

DELI COUNTER

- ❑ _____ ham, lean
- ❑ _____ roast beef, lean, sliced
- ❑ _____ turkey breast, roasted, sliced
- ❑ _____ turkey breast, roasted

- ❑ _____
- ❑ _____
- ❑ _____
- ❑ _____

BAKERY AREA

- ❑ _____ bread, Italian
- ❑ _____ bread, rye
- ❑ _____ bread, whole wheat
- ❑ _____ bread, whole grain
- ❑ _____ buns, whole wheat
- ❑ _____ buns, whole grain
- ❑ _____ English muffin, whole wheat

- ❑ _____ pita
- ❑ _____ pita, whole wheat
- ❑ _____ roll, whole grain
- ❑ _____ tortillas, spinach (10")
- ❑ _____ tortillas, corn
- ❑ _____ tortillas, flour (6")
- ❑ _____ tortillas, flour (8")
- ❑ _____ tortillas, whole wheat (8")

- ❑ _____
- ❑ _____
- ❑ _____
- ❑ _____
- ❑ _____
- ❑ _____
- ❑ _____
- ❑ _____

CANNED FOODS

- ❑ _____ applesauce, unsweetened
- ❑ _____ artichoke hearts in water
- ❑ _____ beans, black
- ❑ _____ beans, cannellini
- ❑ _____ beans, chili
- ❑ _____ beans, chili in sauce
- ❑ _____ beans, kidney
- ❑ _____ beans, pinto
- ❑ _____ beans, refried, fat free
- ❑ _____ beef consommé
- ❑ _____ broth, beef, low fat, reduced sodium
- ❑ _____ broth, chicken, fat free, reduced sodium
- ❑ _____ broth, vegetable, reduced sodium
- ❑ _____ capers
- ❑ _____ cherry peppers
- ❑ _____ chicken, white meat
- ❑ _____ chow mein noodles

- ❑ _____ corn, whole kernel
- ❑ _____ cranberry sauce, whole berry
- ❑ _____ cream of mushroom soup, condensed, low fat, reduced sodium
- ❑ _____ evaporated milk, fat free
- ❑ _____ green chilies, diced
- ❑ _____ green chilies, whole
- ❑ _____ green enchilada sauce
- ❑ _____ hominy, white
- ❑ _____ mandarin oranges
- ❑ _____ maraschino cherries
- ❑ _____ marinara pasta sauce, low fat
- ❑ _____ olives, ripe, chopped
- ❑ _____ olives, ripe, sliced
- ❑ _____ pasta sauce, low fat
- ❑ _____ pineapple, tidbits
- ❑ _____ pineapple, chunks

- ❑ _____ pineapple, crushed
- ❑ _____ pizza sauce, low fat
- ❑ _____ pumpkin puree
- ❑ _____ sauerkraut
- ❑ _____ tomato juice
- ❑ _____ tomato paste
- ❑ _____ tomato sauce
- ❑ _____ tomato sauce, no salt added
- ❑ _____ tomatoes, crushed
- ❑ _____ tomatoes, diced
- ❑ _____ tomatoes, pureed
- ❑ _____ tuna, albacore, water packed
- ❑ _____ water chestnuts, sliced
- ❑ _____
- ❑ _____
- ❑ _____
- ❑ _____
- ❑ _____

PACKAGED FOODS

Grains

- ❑ _____ bulgur wheat
- ❑ _____ couscous, plain
- ❑ _____ oats, old fashioned, whole grain
- ❑ _____ pearl barley
- ❑ _____ rice, brown
- ❑ _____ rice, jasmine
- ❑ _____

Pasta

- ❑ _____ bow tie
- ❑ _____ Ditalini
- ❑ _____ egg noodles, wide
- ❑ _____ fettuccini
- ❑ _____ fettuccini, spinach
- ❑ _____ penne, whole wheat
- ❑ _____ rigatoni, whole wheat
- ❑ _____ rotini
- ❑ _____ rotini, tri-color
- ❑ _____ rotini, whole wheat
- ❑ _____ spaghetti
- ❑ _____
- ❑ _____
- ❑ _____

General

- ❑ _____ chai tea concentrate
- ❑ _____ chocolate wafer cookies
- ❑ _____ Cream of Wheat
- ❑ _____ graham crackers
- ❑ _____ instant pudding mix, banana, fat free, sugar free
- ❑ _____ instant pudding mix, butterscotch, fat free, sugar free
- ❑ _____ instant pudding mix, chocolate, fat free, sugar free
- ❑ _____ instant pudding mix, pistachio, fat free, sugar free
- ❑ _____ instant pudding mix, vanilla, fat free, sugar free
- ❑ _____ Kellogg's Complete Oat Bran Flakes
- ❑ _____ Knorr Hunter Mushroom Gravy Mix
- ❑ _____ Knorr Roasted Chicken Gravy Mix
- ❑ _____ Knorr Vegetable Soup Mix
- ❑ _____ malted milk
- ❑ _____ Myoplex Lite (chocolate)
- ❑ _____ Myoplex Lite (vanilla)
- ❑ _____ peanut butter, natural
- ❑ _____ protein powder (whey or soy), chocolate
- ❑ _____ protein powder (whey or soy), vanilla
- ❑ _____ raisins
- ❑ _____ Ry Krisp, seasoned
- ❑ _____ stuffing mix, herb flavored
- ❑ _____ teriyaki marinade
- ❑ _____ tortilla chips, baked
- ❑ _____ whey protein, naturally flavored
- ❑ _____
- ❑ _____

BAKING AISLE

- ❑ _____ almonds, sliced
- ❑ _____ baking powder
- ❑ _____ baking soda
- ❑ _____ breadcrumbs, Italian seasoned
- ❑ _____ breadcrumbs, plain
- ❑ _____ brown sugar substitute
- ❑ _____ canola oil
- ❑ _____ cherry pie filling, sugar free
- ❑ _____ cocoa powder, unsweetened
- ❑ _____ cooking spray
- ❑ _____ cooking spray, butter flavored
- ❑ _____ cornstarch
- ❑ _____ extract, almond
- ❑ _____ extract, coconut
- ❑ _____ extract, peppermint
- ❑ _____ extract, vanilla
- ❑ _____ flour, all purpose
- ❑ _____ flour, oat
- ❑ _____ flour, soy
- ❑ _____ flour, whole wheat
- ❑ _____ nuts, chopped
- ❑ _____ olive oil, extra virgin
- ❑ _____ pecans, chopped
- ❑ _____ pistachios, chopped
- ❑ _____ pine nuts
- ❑ _____ Ready Crust, reduced fat graham cracker crust
- ❑ _____ sesame oil, toasted
- ❑ _____ sesame oil, light
- ❑ _____ Splenda, granular
- ❑ _____ sugar substitute
- ❑ _____ walnut pieces
- ❑ _____ wheat germ
- ❑ _____
- ❑ _____

SPICES AND SEASONINGS AISLE

- ❏ _____ allspice
- ❏ _____ basil, dried
- ❏ _____ bay leaves
- ❏ _____ black pepper
- ❏ _____ blackened redfish seasoning
- ❏ _____ Butter Buds
- ❏ _____ Cajun seasoning
- ❏ _____ chili powder
- ❏ _____ cinnamon, ground
- ❏ _____ coriander, dried
- ❏ _____ cumin, ground
- ❏ _____ curry
- ❏ _____ five-spice powder
- ❏ _____ fresh red chili powder
- ❏ _____ ginger, ground
- ❏ _____ Greek seasoning
- ❏ _____ Hungarian paprika
- ❏ _____ Italian seasoning

- ❏ _____ lemon-pepper seasoning
- ❏ _____ McCormick Montreal Chicken seasoning
- ❏ _____ McCormick Montreal Steak seasoning
- ❏ _____ McCormick Rotisserie Chicken seasoning
- ❏ _____ Mrs. Dash Extra Spicy
- ❏ _____ Mrs. Dash Original Blend
- ❏ _____ Mrs. Dash Table Blend
- ❏ _____ Mrs. Dash Tomato-Basil-Garlic
- ❏ _____ nutmeg, ground
- ❏ _____ oregano, dried
- ❏ _____ paprika
- ❏ _____ poultry seasoning

- ❏ _____ pumpkin pie spice
- ❏ _____ red pepper flakes
- ❏ _____ red pepper, ground (cayenne)
- ❏ _____ salt
- ❏ _____ sesame seeds
- ❏ _____ Spike seasoning
- ❏ _____ taco seasoning
- ❏ _____ thyme, dried
- ❏ _____ turmeric
- ❏ _____ wasabi, powdered
- ❏ _____ white pepper, ground
- ❏ _____
- ❏ _____
- ❏ _____
- ❏ _____
- ❏ _____

CONDIMENTS

- ❏ _____ barbecue sauce
- ❏ _____ chili garlic sauce
- ❏ _____ chili sauce
- ❏ _____ chocolate syrup
- ❏ _____ hoisin sauce
- ❏ _____ horseradish
- ❏ _____ hot pepper sauce
- ❏ _____ ketchup
- ❏ _____ maple syrup, sugar free
- ❏ _____ mayonnaise, fat free
- ❏ _____ mayonnaise, reduced fat
- ❏ _____ Miracle Whip Free
- ❏ _____ mustard, Dijon
- ❏ _____ mustard, spicy brown
- ❏ _____ mustard, yellow
- ❏ _____ relish, dill
- ❏ _____ relish, sweet pickle
- ❏ _____ salad dressing, Caesar, low fat
- ❏ _____ salad dressing, honey-Dijon, lite

- ❏ _____ salad dressing, Italian, fat free
- ❏ _____ salad dressing, Italian, low fat
- ❏ _____ salad dressing, Newman's Own Light Balsamic Vinaigrette
- ❏ _____ salad dressing, ranch, fat free
- ❏ _____ salsa
- ❏ _____ soy sauce, lite
- ❏ _____ teriyaki marinade
- ❏ _____ vinegar, balsamic
- ❏ _____ vinegar, cider
- ❏ _____ vinegar, rice
- ❏ _____ vinegar, white
- ❏ _____ Worcestershire sauce
- ❏ _____
- ❏ _____
- ❏ _____
- ❏ _____
- ❏ _____

BEVERAGES

- ❏ _____ apple juice, unsweetened
- ❏ _____ bottled water
- ❏ _____ coffee, instant
- ❏ _____ diet orange soda
- ❏ _____ sherry, dry*
- ❏ _____ vermouth, dry*
- ❏ _____ wine, red*
- ❏ _____ wine, white*
- ❏ _____
- ❏ _____
- ❏ _____

*For cooking purposes only ☺

HOUSEHOLD

- ❏ _____ aluminum foil, heavy duty
- ❏ _____ foil muffin liners
- ❏ _____ food storage containers
- ❏ _____ plastic wrap
- ❏ _____ Ziploc bags, gallon size
- ❏ _____ Ziploc bags, sandwich size
- ❏ _____
- ❏ _____

DAIRY CASE

General

- ❏ _____ buttermilk, low fat
- ❏ _____ egg substitute
- ❏ _____ eggs
- ❏ _____ milk, skim
- ❏ _____ Reddi-wip, fat free
- ❏ _____ sour cream, fat free
- ❏ _____ sour cream, low fat
- ❏ _____ soy milk, vanilla
- ❏ _____ yogurt, blueberry, light, fat free
- ❏ _____ yogurt, orange flavored, light, fat free
- ❏ _____ yogurt, plain, fat free
- ❏ _____ yogurt, raspberry, light, fat free
- ❏ _____ yogurt, vanilla, light, fat free
- ❏ _____
- ❏ _____
- ❏ _____

Cheese

- ❏ _____ blue, crumbled
- ❏ _____ cheddar, reduced fat, shredded
- ❏ _____ cheddar, reduced fat, block
- ❏ _____ cheddar, reduced fat, sliced
- ❏ _____ colby-jack, reduced fat, shredded
- ❏ _____ feta, basil and tomato flavored, reduced fat, crumbled
- ❏ _____ feta, reduced fat, crumbled
- ❏ _____ Monterey Jack, reduced fat, block
- ❏ _____ mozzarella, reduced fat, shredded
- ❏ _____ Parmesan, fresh
- ❏ _____ Parmesan, reduced fat, grated
- ❏ _____ provolone, reduced fat, sliced
- ❏ _____ ricotta, low fat
- ❏ _____ string
- ❏ _____ Swiss, reduced fat, sliced
- ❏ _____ cottage cheese, fat free
- ❏ _____ cottage cheese, low fat
- ❏ _____ cream cheese, reduced fat
- ❏ _____
- ❏ _____

MEAT AND SEAFOOD COUNTER

Poultry

- ❑ _____ chicken breast (cooked)
- ❑ _____ chicken breast, boneless, skinless
- ❑ _____ chicken breast, tenders
- ❑ _____ turkey bacon, lean
- ❑ _____ turkey breast, slices
- ❑ _____ turkey, ground, lean
- ❑ _____
- ❑ _____

Fish/Seafood

- ❑ _____ crab meat (cooked)
- ❑ _____ halibut, fillets
- ❑ _____ halibut, steaks
- ❑ _____ lobster meat (cooked)
- ❑ _____ orange roughy fillets
- ❑ _____ salmon fillets
- ❑ _____ shrimp (cooked)
- ❑ _____ shrimp (raw)
- ❑ _____ swordfish fillet
- ❑ _____ tuna steak, yellowfin
- ❑ _____
- ❑ _____

Meats

- ❑ _____ beef, boneless bottom round roast
- ❑ _____ beef, filet mignon
- ❑ _____ beef, flank steak
- ❑ _____ beef, lean, ground
- ❑ _____ beef, top loin steak
- ❑ _____ beef, top round steak
- ❑ _____ beef, top sirloin
- ❑ _____ buffalo, lean, ground
- ❑ _____ Canadian bacon
- ❑ _____ pork tenderloin
- ❑ _____
- ❑ _____
- ❑ _____

FREEZER CASE

- ❑ _____ blackberries
- ❑ _____ blueberries
- ❑ _____ broccoli florets
- ❑ _____ cherries
- ❑ _____ Cool Whip Free
- ❑ _____ Cool Whip Lite
- ❑ _____ green beans
- ❑ _____ green beans, cut Italian
- ❑ _____ limeade concentrate
- ❑ _____ mixed vegetables
- ❑ _____ orange juice concentrate
- ❑ _____ peas
- ❑ _____ potatoes, diced
- ❑ _____ potatoes O'Brien
- ❑ _____ raspberries
- ❑ _____ soybeans in pod
- ❑ _____ strawberries
- ❑ _____ vegetable breakfast patties
- ❑ _____
- ❑ _____

MISCELLANEOUS

- ❑ _____
- ❑ _____
- ❑ _____
- ❑ _____
- ❑ _____
- ❑ _____
- ❑ _____
- ❑ _____
- ❑ _____
- ❑ _____

Appendix A
Success Stories

Real-World Proof

By now, I have no doubt that you have discovered Eating *for* Life makes sense. It's scientifically safe and sound. And it works. But how well does it work? The proof is in the pudding, so to speak. It is reflected in real-world results that you are about to see with your own eyes. Men and women, young and old, of all shapes and sizes, from all walks of life, have discovered and applied the principles of Eating *for* Life and in doing so, they have transformed from ordinary to extraordinary in terms of health and fitness.

Each of these individuals offers unique insight as well as inspiration. Many began by following my original 12-week Body-*for*-LIFE Program (which includes the Eating *for* Lifestyle) and some have now been eating this way for years. They, and the hundreds of thousands of others who've succeeded, *prove* that we all have the power to change, and no one can take that away.

Each and every one of these individuals has gone on to inspire others. They made a change and now they are making a difference. And I couldn't be more proud of each and every one of them!

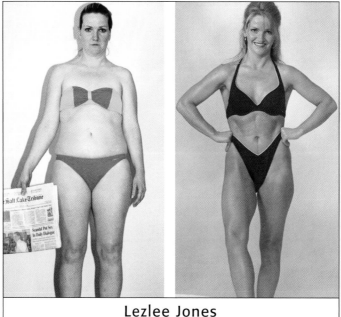

Lezlee Jones
Age 38 • Bountiful, UT • Hairstylist
Lost over 30 lbs of Fat, Increased Energy

BEFORE TYPICAL DAY'S EATING:

8:00 a.m.	Orange juice
4:00 p.m.	Cheese and crackers
7:00 p.m.	Pasta and a garden salad
8:00 p.m.	Ice cream sandwich

AFTER TYPICAL DAY'S EATING:

7:00 a.m.	Protein pancakes, ice water
10:00 a.m.	Cottage cheese, apple, iced tea
1:00 p.m.	Chicken salad, broccoli, water
4:00 p.m.	Nutrition shake
7:00 p.m.	Salmon, brown rice, water
9:00 p.m.	Chocolate protein pudding

Favorite Eating *for* Life Meal: Ranch Chicken Salad (page 271)

Favorite Free Day Food: Popcorn with butter

Toughest Eating Obstacle Overcome: Accepting the idea that eating six times a day would help me lose fat. I was convinced I had to diet and starve to get in shape.

Current Exercise Routine: Daily morning walks and lifting free weights three times a week.

Favorite Benefit of the Eating *for* Lifestyle: I have been able to eat this way for four years now, and it continues to help me feel good, healthy and confident about myself. That makes me a happier person *and* a better mom!

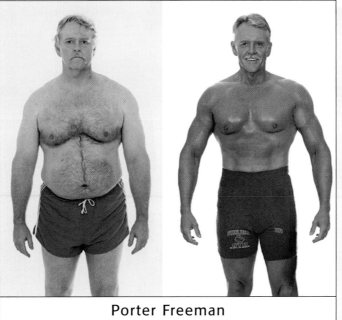

Porter Freeman
Age 53 • Golden, CO • BFL Spokesperson
Lost 54 Pounds of Fat, Gained Energy

BEFORE	TYPICAL DAY'S EATING:
11:00 a.m.	2 cups coffee
1:00 p.m.	2 eggs, 2 pancakes, bacon, sausage, coffee
5:00 p.m.	Chicken fried steak, fries, diet soda
7:00 p.m.	Cookies, diet soda
10:00 p.m.	Baby back ribs, fries, coleslaw, 2 cold beers
2:00 a.m.	Patty melt, fries, 2 cold beers

AFTER	TYPICAL DAY'S EATING:
7:00 a.m.	Egg-white omelet with 1 yolk, oatmeal, water
10:00 a.m.	Nutrition shake
1:00 p.m.	Chicken salad, pear, broccoli, water
4:00 p.m.	Nutrition bar, water
7:00 p.m.	Baked chicken, sweet potato, spinach, water
10:00 p.m.	Cottage cheese, yogurt, water

Favorite Eating *for* Life Meal: Tangy BBQ Chicken (page 122)

Favorite Free Day Food: Blueberry granola pancakes

Toughest Eating Obstacle Overcome: It was hard to stop drinking all those cold beers! Being in the bar business, I had friends who would say, "Let's have a couple of beers." I had to learn to tell them, "No thanks… I've decided to change my lifestyle!"

Current Exercise Routine: I perform shadow boxing, running or swimming every morning and 45 minutes of lifting weights three days a week.

Favorite Benefit of the Eating *for* Lifestyle: I'm alive! At over 260 pounds, I was killing myself with food. Now I eat healthy, I am healthy, and I have been doing this for over six years!

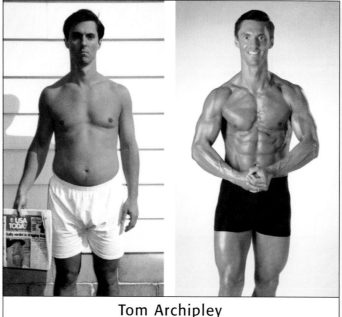

Tom Archipley

Age 36 • Okemos, MI • Executive
Lost 31 Pounds of Fat, Gained Strength and Energy

BEFORE TYPICAL DAY'S EATING:

7:00 a.m.	2 bowls Raisin Bran with milk and honey, coffee
10:00 a.m.	Snickers bar, Coke
12:30 p.m.	Quarter-pounder with cheese, large fries, Coke
3:00 p.m.	Hostess fruit pie or Doritos
7:00 p.m.	Spaghetti, bread and butter, milk

AFTER TYPICAL DAY'S EATING:

7:00 a.m.	Oatmeal with skim milk, 4 egg whites and 1 whole egg, water
9:30 a.m.	Nutrition shake
12:00 p.m.	Chicken breast, pear, water
3:00 p.m.	Nutrition shake
6:00 p.m.	Lean pork loin, brown rice, steamed asparagus, water
9:00 p.m.	Cottage cheese with yogurt

Favorite Eating *for* Life Meal: Caribbean Pork Tenderloin (page 136)

Favorite Free Day Food: Pepperoni pizza and carrot cake

Toughest Eating Obstacle Overcome: Making that initial decision to change was my sticking point. I "half assed" it for years. Once I made that *commitment*, I mean *really* decided to change, I felt an overwhelming rush of positive energy.

Current Exercise Routine: Body-*for*-LIFE

Favorite Benefit of the Eating *for* Lifestyle: The great feeling that comes from setting worthy health goals and achieving them is something I love!

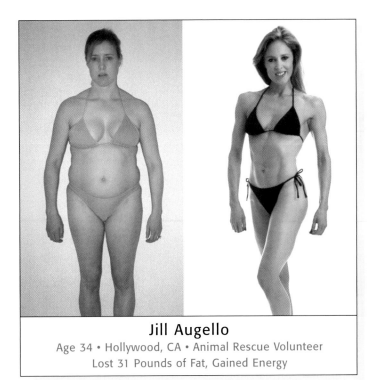

Jill Augello
Age 34 • Hollywood, CA • Animal Rescue Volunteer
Lost 31 Pounds of Fat, Gained Energy

Favorite Eating *for* Life Meal: Turkey Bacon Quiche (page 239)

Favorite Free Day Food: Taco Bell burrito

Toughest Eating Obstacle Overcome: I didn't really know how to cook before this. Now, I am able to prepare healthy meals, and I enjoy my time in the kitchen. I try new recipes often and have fun with it!

Current Exercise Routine: Body-*for*-LIFE

Favorite Benefit of the Eating *for* Lifestyle: This new style of eating gives me energy, which I totally lacked before. I no longer suffer from stomachaches and mood swings, which were an everyday part of my life before. I am now a healthy, happy person inside *and* out.

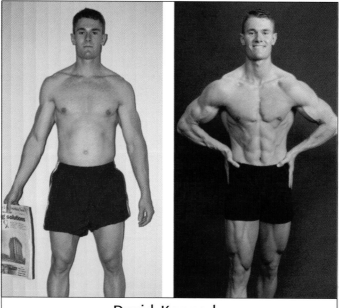

David Kennedy
Age 28 • Broomfield, CO • Science Editor for *This* Book
Lost 17 Pounds of Fat, Gained Strength

BEFORE TYPICAL DAY'S EATING:	
7:00 a.m.	HoneyNut Cheerios with milk, banana, toast, orange juice
9:00 a.m.	PowerBar, Gatorade
1:00 p.m.	Foot-long turkey Subway sandwich, chips, iced tea
7:00 p.m.	Spaghetti, salad, garlic bread, milk
9:00 p.m.	HoneyNut Cheerios, milk

AFTER TYPICAL DAY'S EATING:	
6:00 a.m.	Egg-white omelet, whole-wheat toast with natural peanut butter, green tea, water
9:00 a.m.	Chocolate nutrition shake
12:00 p.m.	Tuna salad in a pita, water
3:00 p.m.	Cottage cheese, blueberries, water
6:00 p.m.	Chicken fajitas, asparagus, water
9:00 p.m.	Chocolate protein pudding

Favorite Eating *for* Life Meal: Deluxe Turkey Dinner (page 141)

Favorite Free Day Food: HoneyNut Cheerios and *lots* of milk!

Toughest Eating Obstacle Overcome: I was convinced that I needed to eat high carbohydrates and low fat in order to get lean and strong. Now I eat smaller, balanced meals frequently throughout the day, and this has made all the difference in the world!

Current Exercise Routine: Body-*for*-LIFE

Favorite Benefit of the Eating *for* Lifestyle: Going swimming and being able to take off my shirt without feeling embarrassed. Now I am proud of the way I look!

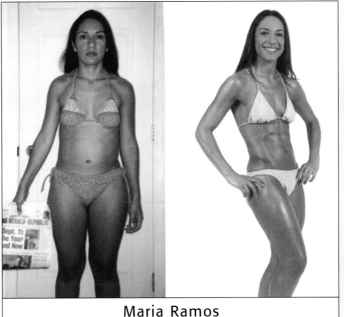

Maria Ramos

Age 24 • Yakima, WA • Case Assistant
Lost 12 Pounds of Fat, Transformed Dress Size from 8 to 4

BEFORE TYPICAL DAY'S EATING:

9:00 a.m.	Latte and bagel with cream cheese
12:00 p.m.	Hamburger, fries, soda
3:00 p.m.	Candy bar, soda
6:30 p.m.	Fried beef tacos with sour cream and salsa, soda
9:00 p.m.	Cookies and milk

AFTER TYPICAL DAY'S EATING:

7:30 a.m.	Breakfast burrito on whole-wheat tortilla, water
10:00 a.m.	Nutrition shake
12:30 p.m.	Grilled chicken salad, apple, water
3:00 p.m.	Nutrition shake
6:00 p.m.	Chicken enchilada with pico de gallo, water
9:00 p.m.	Nutrition bar, water

Favorite Eating *for* Life Meal: Shrimp Scampi (page 167)

Favorite Free Day Food: Cheesy enchiladas with Spanish rice

Toughest Eating Obstacle Overcome: Having to tell my family, "I love you, but I can't eat like 'this' (fatty family favorite foods) anymore!"

Current Exercise Routine: I perform aerobics and free weights each morning.

Favorite Benefit of the Eating *for* Lifestyle: The energy! I don't feel fatigued after a meal. I have never been able to eat right before. Now I feel healthy, and this is my *lifestyle*.

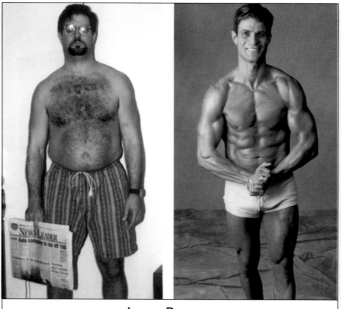

Jerry Braam
Age 40 • Springfield, MO • Respiratory Practitioner
Lost 54 Pounds of Fat, Gained Strength

BEFORE TYPICAL DAY'S EATING:	
(Worked the evening shift and woke up about 10:30 a.m.)	
1:30 p.m.	2 Taco Bell Burritos, Pepsi
5:30 p.m.	2 fried chicken breasts, macaroni and cheese, Pepsi
9:30 p.m.	Snickers bar, Pepsi
11:15 p.m.	3 slices pizza, 2 beers
1:15 a.m.	Cheese omelet, hash browns, biscuits and gravy, milk, coffee

AFTER TYPICAL DAY'S EATING:	
9:30 a.m.	Nutrition shake
12:00 p.m.	Chicken breast, spinach salad, wheat toast, water
2:30 p.m.	Nutrition bar, water
5:00 p.m.	Grilled salmon, sweet potato, steamed asparagus, ice water
7:30 p.m.	Turkey breast, brown rice, water
9:00 p.m.	Cottage cheese, apple, water

Favorite Eating *for* Life Meal: Chocolate Peanut Butter Blend nutrition shake (page 325)

Favorite Free Day Food: I love pizza!

Toughest Eating Obstacle Overcome: I tried almost all the fad diets. I realized they manipulate, trick and deceive your body until it can't handle any more because it's been forced out of balance. I had to rebalance my body. That was a "recovery" process which took a full 12 weeks. Now, over a year later, I'm still on track and I feel balanced *and* strong!

Current Exercise Routine: Body-*for*-LIFE

Favorite Benefit of the Eating *for* Lifestyle: I'm now confident that I have the knowledge to be healthy for life. And, I truly enjoy helping others discover balance and health in their lives.

 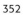

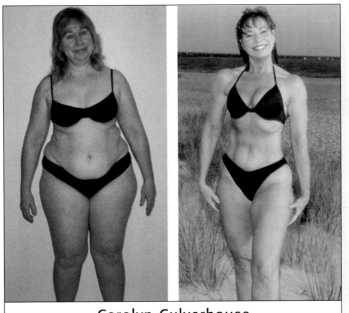

Carolyn Culverhouse
Age 53 • Wilmington, NC • Registered Nurse
Transformed from a Size 20 to 4 in 9 Months

BEFORE	TYPICAL DAY'S EATING:
6:30 a.m.	Leftover fast food
9:00 a.m.	Crackers, Coke
11:30 a.m.	TV dinner
2:00 p.m.	Hamburger, fries, Coke
5:00 p.m.	Chinese takeout, Coke
8:00 p.m.	Ice cream or chocolate

AFTER	TYPICAL DAY'S EATING:
6:00 a.m.	Egg-white omelet, banana, water
9:00 a.m.	Cottage cheese, apple, water
12:00 p.m.	Chicken salad with beans, water
3:00 p.m.	Chocolate nutrition shake
6:00 p.m.	Soft tacos with lean ground beef, tomato and lettuce, water
8:30 p.m.	Protein pudding

Favorite Eating *for* Life Meal: Cool Taco Salad (page 257)

Favorite Free Day Food: Dreyer's Dreamery ice cream

Toughest Eating Obstacle Overcome: Through years of trying to diet, I began to suffer and struggle with binge eating. It took a few months of Eating *for* Life to help me gain control.

Current Exercise Routine: I do 25 minutes of running three days a week and 45 minutes of lifting weights three days a week.

Favorite Benefit of the Eating *for* Lifestyle: I feel so much better now. When I was dieting, I was always so hungry, and I just couldn't do it for very long. Now I don't starve myself. I eat often, and I eat healthy foods. This is something I can do for life.

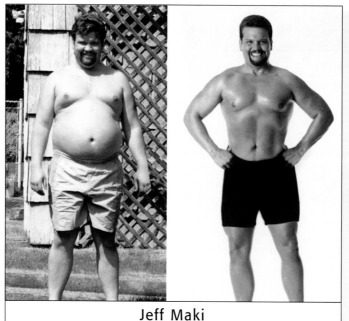

Jeff Maki

Age 43 • Marysville, WA • Public Relations Director
Lost Over 50 Pounds of Fat, Gained Health

<table>
<tr><td>BEFORE TYPICAL DAY'S EATING:</td><td colspan="2">AFTER TYPICAL DAY'S EATING:</td></tr>
<tr><td>Skipped breakfast</td><td>8:00 a.m.</td><td>Scrambled egg whites, whole-wheat toast, water</td></tr>
<tr><td>Skipped lunch</td><td>11:00 a.m.</td><td>Vanilla nutrition shake</td></tr>
<tr><td>2:00 p.m.   3 servings of teriyaki pork, 4 egg rolls, soda</td><td>2:00 p.m.</td><td>Tuna fish sandwich, water</td></tr>
<tr><td>6:00 p.m.   3 cheeseburgers, soda</td><td>5:00 p.m.</td><td>Vanilla nutrition shake</td></tr>
<tr><td>9:00 p.m.   2 slices of pie with ice cream</td><td>8:00 p.m.</td><td>Fish, baked potato, green beans, water</td></tr>
<tr><td></td><td>10:30 p.m.</td><td>Vanilla nutrition shake</td></tr>
</table>

Favorite Eating *for* Life Meal: Homestyle Turkey Meatloaf (page 92)

Favorite Free Day Food: Potato chips with sour cream and minced clam dip

Toughest Eating Obstacle Overcome: Controlling my portion sizes was tough at first. I was so used to eating very large amounts of food. After a few weeks of eating portion-controlled meals, however, my stomach adjusted. Now I'm rarely hungry or full—I just feel *satisfied*.

Current Exercise Routine: Body-*for*-LIFE

Favorite Benefit of the Eating *for* Lifestyle: I know I have renewed my health, and I will live to enjoy the future with my wife and 5-year-old son, Jason.

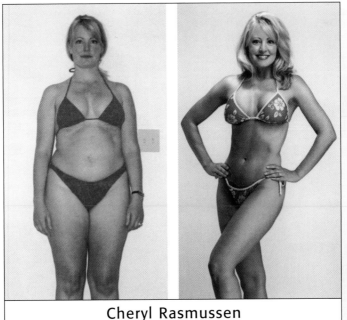

Cheryl Rasmussen

Age 35 • Los Gatos, CA • Program Marketing Manager
Reduced Dress Size from 14 to 6, Increased Energy

BEFORE TYPICAL DAY'S EATING:

8:30 a.m.	Pancakes with syrup, bacon, milk
10:30 a.m.	Starbucks coffee
12:30 p.m.	Cheeseburger, fries, Diet Coke
3:00 p.m.	Granola bar, Diet Coke
7:30 p.m.	Pasta, sourdough bread, water
10:30 p.m.	Bowl of cereal, milk

AFTER TYPICAL DAY'S EATING:

7:00 a.m.	Oatmeal, protein powder, water
10:00 a.m.	Chocolate nutrition shake
1:00 p.m.	Tuna salad, apple, water
3:30 p.m.	Cottage cheese with yogurt
6:00 p.m.	Chicken breast, sweet potato, steamed squash, water
9:00 p.m.	Chocolate nutrition shake

Favorite Eating *for* Life Meal: Mom's Chicken Enchiladas (page 114)

Favorite Free Day Food: Thai chicken pizza

Toughest Eating Obstacle Overcome: At first, I found it difficult to remember to eat every three hours, and I also felt that eating six times a day would work against me. This way of eating was so different from the crash dieting I had done in the past.

Current Exercise Routine: I perform 20 to 30 minutes of running or kick boxing three days a week and 45 minutes of lifting weights three days a week.

Favorite Benefit of the Eating *for* Lifestyle: I'm never hungry, and I enjoy the increase in energy!

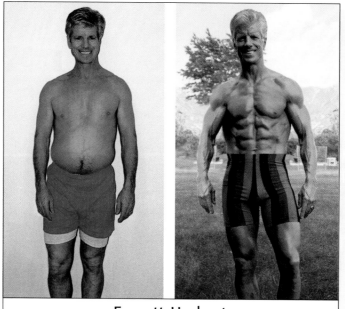

Everett Herbert

Age 56 • Salt Lake City, UT • Contractor
Lost 16 Pounds of Fat, Gained Energy

BEFORE TYPICAL DAY'S EATING:

Skipped breakfast

10:00 a.m.	Biscuits and gravy, bacon, eggs
3:00 p.m.	One dozen "mini doughnuts"
7:00 p.m.	White rice with soy sauce, spicy broccoli, pasta

AFTER TYPICAL DAY'S EATING:

7:00 a.m.	Nutrition shake
10:00 a.m.	Nutrition bar, water
1:00 p.m.	Chicken sandwich, string beans, iced tea
4:00 p.m.	Nutrition shake
7:00 p.m.	Chicken salad, wheat bread, water
10:00 p.m.	Cottage cheese, fruit, water

Favorite Eating *for* Life Meal: Zesty Italian Chicken (page 80)

Favorite Free Day Food: Hershey's chocolate-almond bar and Twizzlers® licorice ropes

Toughest Eating Obstacle Overcome: I was addicted to the *way* I was eating before. It was tough to give that up; it was a really bad set of habits. The key was making a *complete* change and not a "little adjustment." I developed a whole new lifestyle.

Current Exercise Routine: I do 45 minutes of lifting weights four days per week.

Favorite Benefit of the Eating *for* Lifestyle: I am healthy, energetic and I feel *younger*.

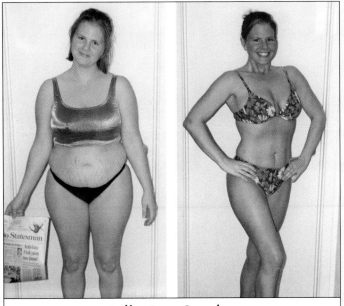

Julie Ann Sproles
Age 28 • Meridian, ID • Mother
Lost 43 Pounds, Gained Control

BEFORE	TYPICAL DAY'S EATING:
8:00 a.m.	Coffee
12:30 p.m.	2 peanut butter and banana sandwiches, chips
5:00 p.m.	3 bowls of Fruity Pebbles
10:30 p.m.	8 chocolate chip cookies

AFTER	TYPICAL DAY'S EATING:
8:30 a.m.	Strawberry nutrition shake
11:00 a.m.	Turkey sandwich, water
1:00 p.m.	Grilled chicken, fruit, water
3:00 p.m.	Hard-boiled eggs, an orange, ice water
5:00 p.m.	Nutrition shake
7:30 p.m.	Chicken fajitas, water

Favorite Eating *for* Life Meal: Chicken Fajitas (page 169)

Favorite Free Day Food: Fruity Pebbles

Toughest Eating Obstacle Overcome: When I would get overstressed or upset, I used to over-eat. This was hard to stop. But as I began Eating *for* Life, two years ago, I learned how good food, in the right amounts, could help balance my mood and reduce stress.

Current Exercise Routine: Hiking, spinning classes, RollerBlading, weightlifting or walking the dog with my children.

Favorite Benefit of the Eating *for* Lifestyle: I now have a healthy "relationship" with food. I am in control of it; it is no longer in control of me. And I feel *very* good about that!

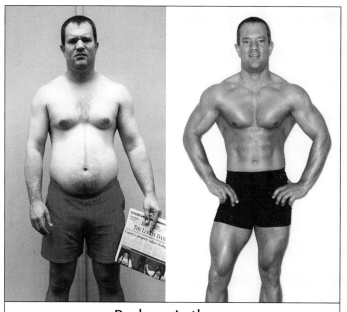

Rodney Latham
Age 34 • Lufkin, TX • Respiratory Therapist
Lost 28 Pounds of Fat, Gained Muscle

BEFORE TYPICAL DAY'S EATING:		AFTER TYPICAL DAY'S EATING:	
Skipped breakfast		7:00 a.m.	4 egg whites, 1 whole egg, whole-wheat toast, water
11:30 a.m.	2 cheeseburgers, fries and a Coke	10:00 a.m.	Chocolate nutrition shake
3:00 p.m.	Chips and a Coke	1:00 p.m.	Sirloin steak, potato, broccoli, water
7:00 p.m.	Chicken fried steak, mashed potatoes and gravy, Coke	4:00 p.m.	Nutrition bar, water
		7:00 p.m.	Grilled salmon, wild rice, asparagus, water
		9:30 p.m.	Chocolate nutrition shake

Favorite Eating *for* Life Meal: Lemon-Peppered Salmon Fillet (page 131)

Favorite Free Day Food: Mexican food

Toughest Eating Obstacle Overcome: Planning my meals was hard at first. Now, I plan all my meals the night before, and I've found it saves me a lot of time the next day.

Current Exercise Routine: I perform weight training three days a week and 20 minutes of aerobics (on the stairstepper) three days a week, followed by a 10-minute walk.

Favorite Benefit of the Eating *for* Lifestyle: I feel better. I'm more productive. I get things done. And I'm stronger. At 34, I feel like I should have felt when I was 24!

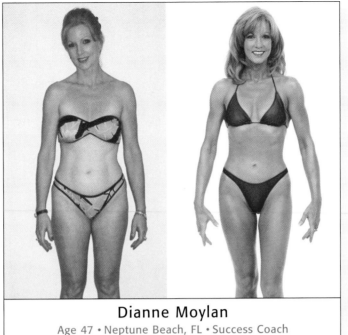

Dianne Moylan

Age 47 • Neptune Beach, FL • Success Coach
Lost 17 Pounds of Fat, Gained Energy

9:30 a.m.	Pop-Tart, 3 cups coffee
1:00 p.m.	Wendy's spicy chicken sandwich, tall Coke
5:30 p.m.	Cookies, coffee
7:30 p.m.	Macaroni and cheese, fried chicken
9:00 p.m.	4 rum and Cokes

5:15 a.m.	Protein pancakes, water
8:00 a.m.	Nutrition shake
11:00 a.m.	Chicken, potatoes, salad, water
2:00 p.m.	Nutrition shake
5:00 p.m.	Salmon, potatoes, broccoli, water
8:00 p.m.	Cottage cheese, yogurt, blueberries, water

Favorite Eating *for* Life Meal: Golden Pancakes (page 220)

Favorite Free Day Food: Chili con carne

Toughest Eating Obstacle Overcome: Initially, I struggled with giving up alcohol. However, it became the easiest thing of all to give up. Once I decided to give it up, that was it. There was no debate—I just wasn't going to do it.

Current Exercise Routine: Body-*for*-LIFE

Favorite Benefit of the Eating *for* Lifestyle: Looking and feeling *years* younger. Whenever someone guesses my age, they say "30 something." I tell them that I'm 47, and they can't believe it!

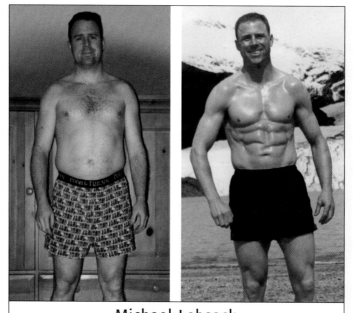

Michael Lebsack

Age 34 • Spokane, WA • U.S. Coast Guard Officer
Lost 24 Pounds of Fat, Gained Muscle

BEFORE TYPICAL DAY'S EATING:	
7:30 a.m.	Bagel, 4 cups of coffee
1:00 p.m.	Cheeseburger, fries, cola
3:00 p.m.	Candy bar, Snapple
7:00 p.m.	Lasagna and soda
10:00 p.m.	Ice cream

AFTER TYPICAL DAY'S EATING:	
7:30 a.m.	Nutrition shake, 1 cup coffee
10:00 a.m.	Cottage cheese, apple, water
12:30 p.m.	Salmon, rice, vegetables, water
3:00 p.m.	Nutrition bar, water
6:00 p.m.	Grilled chicken breast, baked potato, salad, water
9:00 p.m.	Nutrition shake

Favorite Eating *for* Life Meal: Blueberry Blend (page 303)

Favorite Free Day Food: French toast and eggs with maple syrup

Toughest Eating Obstacle Overcome: Learning to "set the table for my success" by having several basic favorite meals I eat day in and day out. Meals that are simple and easy to make (less than 5 minutes) and taste good help me stay on track.

Current Exercise Routine: Three days of rigorous racquetball or handball and three days of weight training.

Favorite Benefit of the Eating *for* Lifestyle: I feel great! I have balanced out my energy and don't have the ups and downs I struggled with when I wasn't eating right.

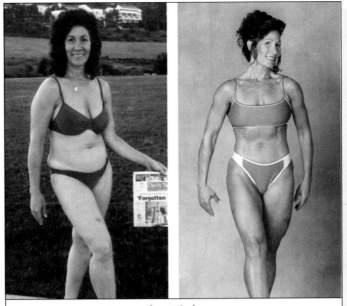

Pamela Hickerson

Age 49 • Malibu, CA • Sales and Marketing
Lost 25 Pounds of Fat, Gained Energy

BEFORE TYPICAL DAY'S EATING:

8:00 a.m.	Bagel with cream cheese, coffee
10:30 a.m.	Frosted fudge brownie, soda
1:00 p.m.	Kentucky Fried Chicken, soda
3:00 p.m.	Gummy bears or jellybeans, soda
7:00 p.m.	Pasta alfredo, bread and butter, glass red wine
9:00 p.m.	Ice cream

AFTER TYPICAL DAY'S EATING:

6:30 a.m.	Whole-wheat toast, egg whites, black coffee, water
9:30 a.m.	Cottage cheese with yogurt, water
12:00 p.m.	Turkey sandwich on whole-wheat bread, spinach, water
3:00 p.m.	Cottage cheese, orange, water
6:00 p.m.	Beef, rice, vegetables, water
8:30 p.m.	Chocolate protein "Fudgesicle"

Favorite Eating *for* Life Meal: Chicken Fajitas (page 169)

Favorite Free Day Food: Pizza with goat cheese and a glass of red wine

Toughest Eating Obstacle Overcome: Giving up fast food was really tough. I'd drive by a fast-food restaurant, and it was almost as if it was calling my name. "Pam… just one little bag of French fries won't hurt!" What really helped was visualizing myself in a bikini. And then I'd say to myself, "Those fries aren't going to help you look good in that!"

Current Exercise Routine: My routine includes weight lifting, running up the hill by my house overlooking the beach and playing with my children.

Favorite Benefit of the Eating *for* Lifestyle: My mood is more balanced. And I wear that bikini!

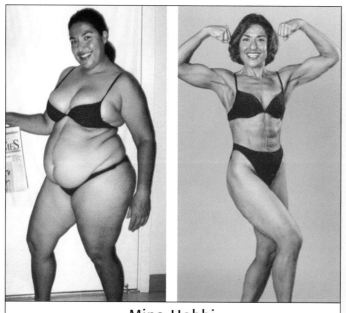

Mina Hobbi
Age 49 • Scottsdale, AZ • Fitness Coach
Lost 85 Pounds of Fat in Less than One Year

BEFORE TYPICAL DAY'S EATING:		**AFTER** TYPICAL DAY'S EATING:	
8:00 a.m.	Ben & Jerry's ice cream	7:00 a.m.	Strawberry nutrition shake
10:00 a.m.	McDonald's hash browns, Coke	10:00 a.m.	Nutrition bar, water
11:00 a.m.	Potato chips, 2 cans Coke	12:30 p.m.	Chicken breast, brown rice, broccoli and cauliflower, water
1:00 p.m.	Burger, fries, Coke	3:00 p.m.	Baked potato, cottage cheese, salsa, cauliflower, water
2:30 p.m.	Milky Way bar		
5:30 p.m.	Pizza, Coke	5:00 p.m.	Vegetables, protein dip, water
9:00 p.m.	Ice cream	8:00 p.m.	Strawberry nutrition shake

Favorite Eating *for* Life Meal: Cajun Chicken (page 191)

Favorite Free Day Food: Hamburger and French fries

Toughest Eating Obstacle Overcome: I was a binge eater. When I had a bad day or felt emotionally down, I'd eat. Then I'd feel guilty for overeating, and I'd eat more hoping I'd feel better. It was a vicious cycle.

Current Exercise Routine: I do spinning and lifting weights six days per week and a lot of walking.

Favorite Benefit of the Eating *for* Lifestyle: I am no longer depressed. I am healthy now!

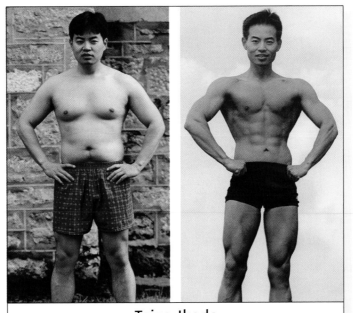

Taizo Ikeda

Age 34 • Montreal, QB, CAN • Project Administrator
Lost 25 Pounds of Fat, Gained Muscle Definition

BEFORE TYPICAL DAY'S EATING:

10:00 a.m.	Doughnut, coffee
1:00 p.m.	Burger, fries, cola
7:00 p.m.	Spaghetti
9:00 p.m.	Beer

AFTER TYPICAL DAY'S EATING:

7:00 a.m.	Nutrition shake
10:00 a.m.	Cottage cheese, fresh fruit, water
12:30 p.m.	Chicken breast, brown rice, broccoli, water
3:00 p.m.	Nutrition shake
6:00 p.m.	Fish, brown rice, broccoli, water
9:00 p.m.	Protein drink

Favorite Eating *for* Life Meal: Chocolate Peanut Butter Blend nutrition shake (page 325)

Favorite Free Day Food: Chinese food

Toughest Eating Obstacle Overcome: Social events where I'm surrounded by food used to be hard for me. Planning ahead has really helped. Now when I know there's a social event coming up that I want to attend, I plan to have my free day around it.

Current Exercise Routine: Body-*for*-LIFE

Favorite Benefit of the Eating *for* Lifestyle: I feel more in control of my life!

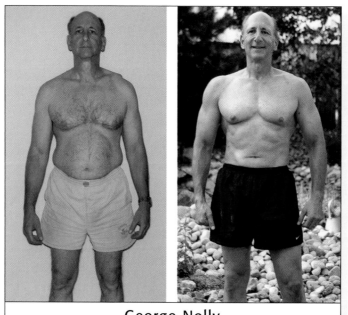

George Nolly
Age 55 • Aurora, CO • Airline Pilot
Lost 25 Pounds of Fat, Gained Strength

BEFORE	TYPICAL DAY'S EATING:
7:00 a.m.	Bowl of cereal, bagel, banana
10:00 a.m.	Egg McMuffin
1:00 p.m.	Quarter Pounder with Cheese, Coke
7:00 p.m.	Beef, fried rice, milk

AFTER	TYPICAL DAY'S EATING:
7:00 a.m.	Ham and cheese omelet, oatmeal, water
10:00 a.m.	Nutrition shake
1:00 p.m.	Cottage cheese with yogurt, water
4:00 p.m.	Chicken breast, rice, broccoli, water
7:00 p.m.	Salmon, potato, vegetables, water
9:30 p.m.	Celery stalks, peanut butter, water

Favorite Eating *for* Life Meal: Rotisserie Seasoned Chicken (page 101)

Favorite Free Day Food: Pizza

Toughest Eating Obstacle Overcome: I was used to eating until I felt really stuffed. I soon discovered that within 10 to 20 minutes of eating a proper portion size, *slowly*, I'd feel *satisfied* but not stuffed.

Current Exercise Routine: Aerobic exercise every morning; weight lifting three days a week.

Favorite Benefit of the Eating *for* Lifestyle: I enjoy great health and energy! Also, as a pilot, I adapt to changing time zones (I routinely fly between New York and Tokyo) with much less difficulty than my flying partners.

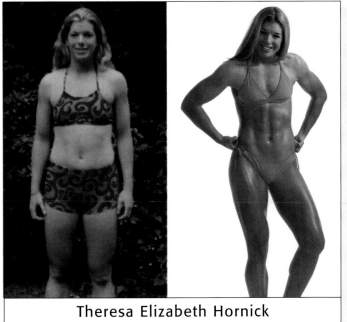

Theresa Elizabeth Hornick
Age 22 • Quantico, VA • 2nd Lt. U.S. Marine Corps
Reduced Bodyfat, Gained Energy

BEFORE TYPICAL DAY'S EATING:	
9:30 a.m.	Oatmeal and bagel with peanut butter
12:30 p.m.	Chocolate chip cookie, Italian hoagie, pasta salad
3:30 p.m.	Apple or banana
6:30 p.m.	Chicken salad
9:30 p.m.	Peanut butter frozen yogurt

AFTER TYPICAL DAY'S EATING:	
7:00 a.m.	Omelet, oatmeal, fruit, water
10:30 a.m.	Nutrition bar, water
1:00 p.m.	Turkey wrap, lettuce, tomato, water
3:30 p.m.	Nutrition shake
6:30 p.m.	Chicken breast, potato, vegetables, diet soda
9:30 p.m.	Protein pudding

Favorite Eating *for* Life Meal: Herbed Chicken (page 162)

Favorite Free Day Food: M&M's

Toughest Eating Obstacle Overcome: The most difficult thing I had to overcome was breaking the habit of just eating whatever I wanted. This became easier as I realized that I could actually control how energetic I wanted to be by controlling what I was eating.

Current Exercise Routine: My routine includes lifting weights, swimming, hiking and running.

Favorite Benefit of the Eating *for* Lifestyle: I have more confidence and focus. I look better, too!

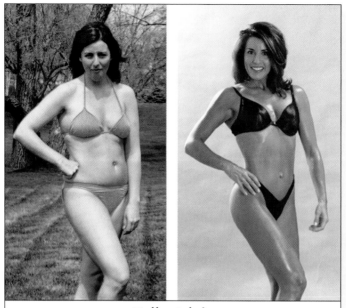

Kelly Adair
Age 41 • Omaha, NE • Mother
Lost 25 Pounds of Fat, Gained Energy

BEFORE TYPICAL DAY'S EATING:

Skipped breakfast

10:00 a.m.   M&M's

12:30 p.m.   Pizza, soda

6:00 p.m.   Chinese carryout, soda

AFTER TYPICAL DAY'S EATING:

7:30 a.m.	Oatmeal with chocolate protein powder, water
10:00 a.m.	Nutrition bar, water
12:30 p.m.	Salmon, pasta, broccoli, water
3:00 p.m.	Cottage cheese with yogurt, water
6:00 p.m.	Chicken, yam, broccoli, water
9:30 p.m.	Oatmeal with chocolate protein powder, water

Favorite Eating *for* Life Meal: Grilled Salmon (page 84)

Favorite Free Day Food: Cookie dough

Toughest Eating Obstacle Overcome: I used to crave chocolate all the time! Eating balanced, nutritious meals has really helped satisfy those cravings.

Current Exercise Routine: I do 20 minutes of intense aerobics on the stairstepper three days a week, and I lift weights three days a week

Favorite Benefit of the Eating *for* Lifestyle: Energy! I also do not get those painful "sugar headaches" anymore. I've been eating this way for five years now, and I feel good.

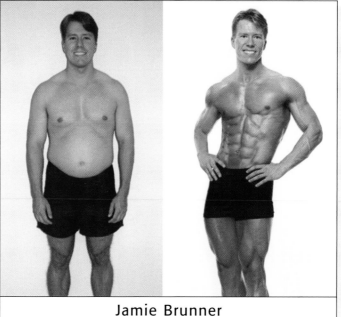

Jamie Brunner
Age 28 • Edmonton, AB, CAN • Business Owner
Lost 20 Pounds of Fat, Gained Energy

BEFORE TYPICAL DAY'S EATING:	
Skipped breakfast	
10:00 a.m.	2 cans soda
12:00 p.m.	Burger, fries, Coke
3:00 p.m.	2 cans soda
7:00 p.m.	Macaroni and cheese, soda
10:00 p.m.	Chips, popcorn, soda

AFTER TYPICAL DAY'S EATING:	
7:00 a.m.	Nutrition shake
10:00 a.m.	Nutrition bar, water
1:00 p.m.	Barbecue chicken pita with lettuce, tomato and light mayo, water
3:00 p.m.	Vegetables with protein dip
6:00 p.m.	Salmon, spinach salad, water
9:00 p.m.	Protein pudding

Favorite Eating *for* Life Meal: Balsamic Salmon Salad (page 111)

Favorite Free Day Food: Double-scoop chocolate ice cream cone

Toughest Eating Obstacle Overcome: Starting the day with a healthy breakfast took a lot of getting used to.

Current Exercise Routine: 20 minutes of aerobics; 20 minutes of lifting weights, six days a week.

Favorite Benefit of the Eating *for* Lifestyle: Shedding the roll of fat that used to hang over my belt. The ability to button up the top button on my dress shirt. Not sweating in public. Freedom to wear clothes that look good. The simple stuff. Eating right. Looking good. *Feeling great.*

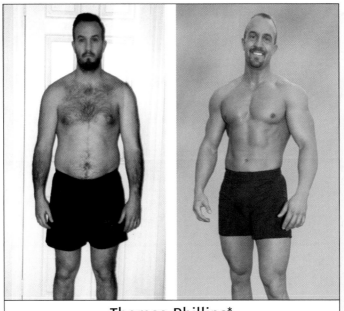

Thomas Phillips*
Age 32 • Tinton Falls, NJ • Teacher
Lost 28 Pounds of Fat, Gained Strength

*No relation to Bill Phillips

BEFORE	TYPICAL DAY'S EATING:
7:00 a.m.	2 bowls of cereal, toast with jelly, coffee with cream and sugar
11:30 a.m.	2 grilled cheese sandwiches, cookies, whole milk
3:30 p.m.	2 bowls of cereal, peanut butter and jelly sandwich
8:00 p.m.	4 slices pizza, 2 sodas

AFTER	TYPICAL DAY'S EATING:
7:00 a.m.	Omelet, toast, water
9:30 a.m.	Nutrition bar, ice water
11:30 a.m.	Grilled chicken, broccoli, brown rice, iced tea
1:30 p.m.	Nutrition shake
4:30 p.m.	Grilled salmon, sweet potato, spinach, water
8:00 p.m.	Nutrition shake

Favorite Eating *for* Life Meal: Chicken Pita Pizza (page 261)

Favorite Free Day Food: Chocolate ice cream

Toughest Eating Obstacle Overcome: Breaking free from the cravings for sugary junk food was hard for the first few weeks. It took *a lot* of effort, but I did it. I've been "craving free" for 14 months and plan to eat this way, for life.

Current Exercise Routine: Body-*for*-LIFE

Favorite Benefit of the Eating *for* Lifestyle: The energy—I have so much positive energy!

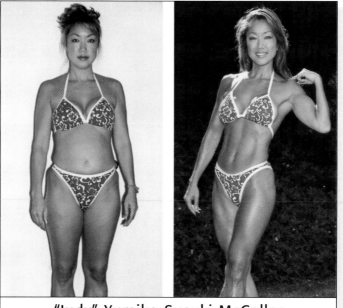

"Judy" Yumiko Susuki-McCollor

Age 42 • Kahului, Maui • Wife/Mother
Decreased from Size 6 to 2, Gained Health

BEFORE TYPICAL DAY'S EATING:		**AFTER** TYPICAL DAY'S EATING:	
10:30 a.m.	Rice, eggs, sausage	6:00 a.m.	Nutrition shake
Skipped lunch		8:30 a.m.	Omelet (egg whites, 1 whole egg, vegetables, cheese), water
2:30 p.m.	Jamba Juice smoothie	11:30 a.m.	Nutrition bar, water
7:00 p.m.	Noodles or rice, steak, bread	2:30 p.m.	Grilled chicken sandwich, water
		5:30 p.m.	Grilled salmon, baked sweet potato, asparagus and zucchini, water
		8:30 p.m.	Nutrition shake

Favorite Eating *for* Life Meal: Baked Halibut (page 144)

Favorite Free Day Food: Sushi with white rice

Toughest Eating Obstacle Overcome: I travel back and forth from Japan, where many of the restaurants just serve noodles. I go and order a portion of buckwheat noodles and then go home and eat a piece of chicken or a can of tuna to get my portion of protein.

Current Exercise Routine: Morning cardio on the treadmill or VersaClimber three days a week; 45 minutes of lifting weights three days a week.

Favorite Benefit of the Eating *for* Lifestyle: I feel younger and healthier!

Now It's Your Turn!
(Record your success here)

BEFORE PHOTO	**AFTER PHOTO**

Name: _____

BEFORE TYPICAL DAY'S EATING:

____ a.m. _____

____ a.m. _____

____ p.m. _____

____ p.m. _____

AFTER TYPICAL DAY'S EATING:

____ a.m. _____

____ a.m. _____

____ p.m. _____

____ p.m. _____

____ p.m. _____

____ p.m. _____

Favorite Eating *for* Life Meal: _____

Favorite Free Day Food: _____

Toughest Eating Obstacle Overcome: _____

_____

Current Exercise Routine: _____

_____

Favorite Benefit of the Eating *for* Lifestyle: _____

_____

Appendix B
Nutrition Definitions

Amino acids: These are nutrients that are derived from protein-containing foods. Amino acids are the building blocks from which proteins like muscle tissue, hormones, neurotransmitters, antibodies and enzymes are made. There are 21 amino acids in all, nine of them essential as they can only be obtained from the food we eat. Meat, eggs, cheese, soy as well as protein powders and nutrition shakes contain the complete proteins, which means they provide the nine essential amino acids.

Antioxidants: Vitamins and other nutrients that help protect your body from damaging "free radicals." Many fruits and vegetables are rich in natural antioxidants and may help prevent diseases like cancer.

Appetite: This is your *desire* for food in order to satisfy your physiological need.

Assimilation: This term is used to describe the conversion of the food you eat into an actual component of your body. For example, when you eat a protein-rich food like beef, your body breaks down that protein into amino acids, which can then be "assimilated" into new muscle tissue.

Authorized foods: These are foods that are approved and recommended for the Eating *for* Lifestyle. They're "authorized" due to their nutrient content, as well as the amount of calories they provide. They are also called "Right Foods."

Balanced nutrition: This is a cornerstone of Eating *for* Life. It is the best possible nutrition; balanced in the six nutrients essential to good health: protein, carbohydrates, essential fats, vitamins, minerals and water.

Binge: This is "uncontrollable" eating, typically on junk foods like crackers, cookies, candies and other "bingeables."

Bingeables: These are foods that you want to keep out of sight! They're the foods that, like the famous potato chip commercial boasted, "You can't eat just one!" Bingeables are often carbohydrate foods, such as chips, crackers, cookies, candies and sweetened cereals. Bingeables can include high-fat foods, such as ice cream and cheese as well. The best way to avoid bingeing on these unauthorized *wrong* foods is to not even keep them in your kitchen or in your desk drawer, car, etc.

Body composition: This term basically means the amount of your bodyweight that is made up of fat versus lean body mass (skeletal muscle, bone, viscera, etc.). Body composition analysis is an important way to measure your overall state of health.

Breakfast: Your first Eating *for* Life meal of the day.

Calories: This term basically means how much usable "chemical energy" a food contains. Protein and carbohydrates provide four calories per gram; fat provides nine calories per gram. When you eat more calories than your body needs to fuel your daily metabolic needs, your body stores the extra calories as fat.

Cancer: This term is used to describe a condition where cells in a part of the body begin to grow out of control. All cancers develop from a single cell that has undergone mutations in its DNA, causing it to reproduce uncontrollably. Studies have confirmed a link between how you eat and cancer. For example, eating plentiful amounts of fresh fruits and vegetables, whole grains and essential fats has been shown to help *reduce* your risk for certain cancers. On the other hand, consuming too many unhealthy fats and processed carbohydrates may *increase* your risk for certain cancers.

Carbohydrate: This is an essential nutrient found in foods that supplies the body with glucose/blood sugar. Carbohydrates such as sugars increase blood sugar levels more quickly than carbs such as brown rice and barley, which produce a more gradual increase in blood glucose levels.

Cholesterol: This is a type of fat that, although most widely known as a "bad fat" associated with heart disease, is a vital component in the production of many hormones in the body. There are different types of cholesterol: namely, HDL and LDL (HDL being the "good" form and LDL being the "bad" form). The body makes its own cholesterol, regardless of whether you eat high-fat foods or not. High cholesterol levels, which contribute to heart disease, are typically caused when the body is storing an excess amount of bodyfat.

Crash: This is a term that can describe the dramatic downturn in your blood sugar and energy levels coming off a "food high." For example, many refined carbohydrate foods (like white bread, candy or alcohol) can dramatically affect your blood sugar levels when not eaten in combination with protein or fat. When your blood sugar is overly elevated, it strongly stimulates insulin secretion, which removes excess sugar from the blood. Many times, however, your body will overreact and create too much insulin, which will then pull too much sugar out of your blood, causing your blood sugar and energy levels to "crash."

Craving: This term can be used to describe the psychological desire to eat. For some people, merely thinking about going on a "diet" (restricting food intake) causes an increase in cravings. For others, stress (both physical and emotional) and other "triggers" can increase cravings.

Dessert: Your sixth and final Eating *for* Life meal of the day.

Diabetes: This is a condition in which the pancreas fails to manufacture the insulin needed to convert glucose (sugar) into energy *or* when the body can't utilize the insulin that is produced. In either case, blood sugar rises to dangerous levels and, if left untreated, can lead to kidney damage, blindness, heart disease and even death. There are two main kinds of diabetes: Type-1, formerly called juvenile or insulin-dependent diabetes, is usually first diagnosed in children or teenagers. Type-2 diabetes, formerly called adult-onset diabetes or non-insulin-dependent diabetes, is the most common form today. It usually occurs in people who are overweight and can often be controlled through exercise and eating right.

Diet: In today's terms, this typically means restricting food intake by any one of dozens of popular (and often unhealthy) methods for the purpose of weight loss. Dieting is a short-term solution at best and a dangerous approach in many cases.

Dinner: Your fifth Eating *for* Life meal of the day.

Eating *for* Lifestyle: A style of eating in which healthy, nutritious, delicious foods are enjoyed six times a day. Meals include breakfast, lunch, dinner, dessert, as well as a morning midmeal and an afternoon midmeal. Each meal is made up of a portion of protein and carbohydrates and regularly includes fresh fruits and vegetables.

Empty calories: This term refers to calories that are derived from "wrong foods"—foods that don't serve any important nutritional purpose, such as those from saturated fat, trans fats, added sugars and other heavily processed carbohydrates.

Essential nutrients: These are the six nutrients that the body absolutely needs in order to support life, repair, renew and fuel metabolism. These six essential nutrients are protein, carbohydrates, essential fats, vitamins, minerals and water.

Fast food: This term, generally, as it's used in this book, refers to low-nutrient, highly processed foods, which are provided away from home but not in a formal "sit-down" restaurant. Fast food is crap, generally.

Fat: This is the most calorie-dense nutrient. It contains nine calories per gram, whereas protein and carbohydrates contain four. Saturated fat, such as fatty beef or cheese, is generally bad for you. Unsaturated fat, such as olive oil and fish oils, contain essential fats, which are nutrients that are good for the body when consumed as a part of the Eating Right Recipe.

Favorites: This term is used to describe Eating *for* Life meals that match your personal preference and are often prepared and consumed weekly. Favorites are often foods that make you feel good, that provide a great sense of satisfaction and/or that you enjoy preparing.

Free day: One day each week of the Eating *for* Lifestyle where you can eat any foods you might be craving, regardless of their nutritional content or value.

Frequent feeding: Eating often throughout the day, every two to three hours, in order to increase energy levels and control hunger and cravings.

Fructose: This is the main type of sugar found in fruit. It's a little sweeter than sucrose (table sugar).

Glucose: This is the form of sugar the body uses as its primary fuel source. All carbohydrate foods are broken down into glucose through the process of digestion, although at varying rates.

Glycemic index (GI): This is a measure of the extent to which a food raises the blood sugar (glucose) level as compared with white bread, which has a GI of 100. Glucose (dextrose) scores a 138, brown rice an 81 and fructose (fruit sugar) is down at 31.

Glycogen: This is what carbohydrates are called when they are digested and stored in your body within muscle cells and the liver.

HDL: This is an abbreviation for "high-density lipoprotein." It's one of the subcategories of cholesterol—typically thought of as the "good" cholesterol. You may be able to raise your HDL cholesterol levels by eating quality unsaturated fats like olive oil. Exercise has also been shown to increase HDL levels.

Hunger: This is physiological—it's the body sending a message that it needs food. Hunger is satisfied by eating.

Indigestion: This is a term used to describe a feeling of discomfort after eating, often characterized by gas, heartburn or abdominal pain. Indigestion can be brought on by eating while stressed, by eating fatty or spicy foods, by poor eating habits in general.

Insulin: This is a hormone secreted by the pancreas that aids the body in maintaining proper blood sugar levels. Insulin secretion speeds the transport of nutrients through the bloodstream and into muscle *or fat* for storage. When chronically elevated, as with a high-carbohydrate diet, insulin can cause you to gain bodyfat and may lead to the development of type-2 diabetes.

Junk food: This term refers to unhealthy food that is often "fun" to eat but bad for you. It is often highly processed, full of fat and sugar and low in nutrients. Examples include fast food, candy, cookies, chips and soda.

Ketone: This is a byproduct of fat metabolism. In extreme conditions, the body can adapt and utilize ketones as a form of "emergency fuel" when there's not enough blood glucose.

Ketosis: A condition where the body is producing high levels of ketones. Following a low-carbohydrate diet is generally intended to produce the metabolic state of ketosis. During ketosis, the brain is forced to utilize one of its "least-favorite" fuel sources, ketones. (Its favorite is glucose.)

LDL: This is an abbreviation for "low-density lipoprotein" and is a subcategory of cholesterol, typically thought of as the "bad" cholesterol. Levels of LDL cholesterol can be elevated by eating too much saturated fat and by not exercising enough.

Lipid: This is simply another name for dietary fats or triglycerides.

Lunch: Your third Eating *for* Life meal of the day.

Macronutrients: These are nutrients that are eaten in large (macro means "big") quantities on a regular basis. These include proteins, carbohydrates, fats and water. All of these macronutrients are necessary to sustain life.

Meal: As it pertains to Eating *for* Life, a meal is a portion of protein and a portion of carbohydrates. Often, meals also include a serving of vegetables.

Metabolic rate: This is basically the amount of calories your body burns up each day to keep you walking, talking, breathing, moving, thinking… living. Your metabolic rate is influenced by numerous factors, including: genetics, age, muscle mass (the more muscle you have, the higher your metabolic rate), how often you eat, how much exercise you do and your overall state of health.

Micronutrient: These are dietary nutrients that we ingest in relatively small (micro means "small") amounts compared to macronutrients. Examples of micronutrients include vitamins and minerals. Many micronutrients are essential dietary nutrients that perform vital functions in the body. Micronutrients are typically ingested in gram quantities or less.

Midmeal: This is an Eating *for* Life meal that is eaten *between* breakfast and lunch, and between lunch and dinner. Unlike "snacks," midmeals contain a portion of *both* quality protein and carbohydrates and serve the purpose of balancing energy, helping control your appetite and cravings. Midmeals also help provide your body a steady supply of nutrients needed to keep you healthy and strong.

Minerals: These essential nutrients contain no calories, but they are vitally important for optimal health. Minerals must come from the foods we eat—the body doesn't make them on its own. Among the minerals that are vitally important to your body and need to be consumed in relatively large amounts are calcium, potassium and iron. Other minerals need to be consumed in only "trace" amounts, and these include selenium, copper and chromium.

Neurotransmitter: This is a substance that is released at the end of one nerve cell when a nerve impulse arrives there. Neurotransmitters diffuse across the gap to the next nerve cell and alter the membrane of that cell in such a way that it becomes less or more likely to fire. Examples include adrenaline and serotonin. Adrenaline is responsible for the "fight-or-flight" response and is an excitatory neurotransmitter; serotonin is the opposite. Both protein and carbohydrates are vitally important for proper neurotransmitter formation and function.

Nutrient dense: This is a term used to describe foods that are rich with one or more essential nutrient. Salmon is an example of a nutrient-dense food because it provides high-quality protein, essential fats, calcium and other key micronutrients.

Nutrients: These are the essential components of food that provide the body with the materials it needs to renew itself, create energy, fuel the metabolism and keep you going strong. There are six essential nutrients: protein, carbohydrates, fats, vitamins, minerals and water.

Nutrition bar: A candy bar-like food that contains protein, carbohydrates, vitamins, minerals and other key nutrients and which can be used to replace a regular-food meal. Be careful when shopping for nutrition bars, however, as many contain too much fat and sugar. A good nutrition bar should be low in sugar and saturated fat, rich in vitamins and minerals, and balanced in protein and carbohydrates.

Nutrition shake: A food that contains protein, carbohydrates, vitamins, minerals, water and other key nutrients and which can be used to replace a regular-food meal for purposes of increasing nutrient intake.

Obesity: This is a medical term that's used to describe a level of bodyfat that is a disease. Oftentimes, "obesity" means that a person has 30 pounds of excess bodyfat.

Osteoporosis: This is a condition in which bones become fragile and more likely to break due to a loss of calcium. More than 10 million Americans suffer from osteoporosis and almost 34 million more are estimated to have low bone mass, placing them at increased risk for osteoporosis.

Planned-overs: These are Eating *for* Life meals that, unlike "leftovers," are *intentionally* prepared in advance and usually consist of recipes that can be made in large quantities and which can be kept in the refrigerator or freezer for longer periods of time. Examples include soups, chicken and pasta dishes, and other dinners that can be frozen or refrigerated and quickly reheated for future lunches and/or dinners.

Polyphenols: These are antioxidant nutrients found in some fruits, vegetables, extra-virgin olive oil, as well as in tea, coffee and wine. Scientific studies suggest polyphenols may help prevent diseases such as cancer and heart disease.

Portion: The amount of an "authorized" carbohydrate or protein food that each meal should contain. A portion of protein is generally the size of the palm of *your* hand. A portion of carbohydrates is approximately the size of your clenched fist.

Protein: An essential nutrient found in foods such as beef, chicken, turkey, fish, eggs, soy, dairy products, protein powders and nutrition shakes. Protein provides the amino acids your body needs to repair muscles after exercising. It is also essential for the immune system and mental performance. A gram of protein contains four calories. Protein from animal sources contain the nine essential amino acids. Protein from vegetable sources contain some but not all of the essential amino acids.

Recommended Dietary Allowance (RDA): The level of essential nutrients that the Food and Nutrition Board of the National Academy of Science's National Research Council has determined, through scientific studies, are needed by the body to support a disease-free state. Many scientific experts believe that the optimal intake of many vitamins and minerals exceeds the RDA.

Right Foods: This is the first ingredient in the Right Recipe of the Eating *for* Lifestyle. The right foods are those that provide the high-quality, essential nutrition your body needs. In my book Body-*for*-LIFE, I called these the "authorized" foods, which are the ones that are a-okay to include in each of your daily meals. These foods get the green light because of the amount of nutrients they contain compared to calories—they offer the most nutrients per calorie. Right foods are included in each and every one of the 150 Eating *for* Life meal recipes featured in this book.

Right Amounts: This is the second ingredient in the Right Recipe of the Eating *for* Lifestyle. The right amount of carbohydrates or protein you should eat in each meal is best gauged by counting "portions," not calories. A portion is an amount of protein roughly equal to the size of the palm of your hand and a carb is about the size of your clenched fist.

Right Combos: This is the third ingredient in the Right Recipe of the Eating *for* Lifestyle. Eating the right combos simply means choosing a portion of protein and carbohydrates and including that in each of your Eating *for* Life meals. For example, chicken breast (protein) and brown rice (carbohydrate). And in some of your daily meals, include a serving of vegetables. An example of this would be a dinner with a chicken breast, brown rice and broccoli. Throughout the 150 meal recipes featured in this book, you'll see an array of ways to combine protein, carbohydrates and vegetables.

Right Times: This is the fourth and final ingredient in the Right Recipe of the Eating *for* Lifestyle. To eat at the right times means to eat the right foods, in the right amounts, in the right combinations, *six times a day*. When you eat every few hours, you'll have more energy, less hunger pangs and cravings and you'll just flat out feel better—a lot better.

Satisfied: You've eaten enough food to satisfy your cravings, your hunger and appetite.

Saturated fats: These are bad fats. They are called "saturated" because they contain no open spots on their "carbon skeletons." Saturated fats include myristic acid, palmitic acid, stearic acid, arachidic acid and lignoceric acid. These bad fats have been shown to cause disease. Sources of these fats include animal foods and hydrogenated vegetable oils, such as margarine.

Serotonin: A neurotransmitter in the brain that affects your mood and appetite. Carbohydrate foods are essential for the production of serotonin. Often, when carbohydrates are restricted, serotonin levels are reduced, which may cause side effects such as irritability, sleeping disturbances, "fogginess" and, in some cases, depression.

Serving: This is the amount of vegetables you eat as part of at least two Eating *for* Life meals a day—usually about an amount you can hold in your cupped hand, but you can eat more if you desire.

Stuffed: You ate too much! Overly full, sluggish and perhaps sick to your stomach.

Sugar substitute: This includes a variety of products that can be used in place of sugar. Most are available in packets and granular or "spoonful" form. The packets contain a very small amount of concentrated powder that equals 2 teaspoons of sugar taste for very few calories. They can be used to sweeten coffee, tea, cereal, fresh fruit, etc. The granular or spoonful forms are better for use in recipes, and it measures cup for cup like sugar. Splenda (or sucralose) is generally better for baking.

Supplement: This is a term used to describe a preparation such as a tablet, pill or powder that contains nutrients or herbs. Supplements are often used to ensure optimal daily nutrient intake.

Syndrome X: This is a term used to describe a combination of health conditions that place a person at high risk for heart disease—the number one cause of death in the United States. This syndrome is especially dangerous for women since it increases their risk of dying by 13 times, while in men it doubles their risk. The four key components of Syndrome X are obesity (especially abdominal obesity), diabetes, elevated triglyceride levels (one of the fats in the blood) and high blood pressure. Fortunately, Syndrome X is both preventable and curable. Lifestyle modifications, including regular exercise and nutritious eating, which result in losing unhealthy bodyfat, are the keys to preventing this disease.

Unauthorized food: This is a food that is not okay to eat on the six days a week you're following the Eating *for* Lifestyle. Unauthorized foods include junk food, candy and foods that are high in saturated fat or low in nutrients. Generally, foods are unauthorized because they do not support your health and contain too many calories compared to how many nutrients are in them.

Unsaturated fats: These are "good" fats. They are called unsaturated because they have one or more open "carbon spots." Unsaturated fats can be divided into two categories: polyunsaturated fats and monounsaturated fats. Unsaturated fats have been shown to help reduce cholesterol and triglyceride levels in the blood. This category of fats includes the essential fatty acids linoleic and linolenic. The main sources of these fats are from plant foods, such as safflower, sunflower and olive oil.

Vitamins: These are nutrients that contain no calories, yet are vital to life. These essential nutrients, found in fruits and vegetables in particular, are essential to the body's production of energy and virtually all of its metabolic processes. There are 13 essential vitamins, which can be divided into two general categories: water soluble, such as vitamin C and a variety of B vitamins; and fat soluble, such as vitamins A, D, E and K. Water-soluble vitamins need to be provided *daily* from the foods or supplements you eat. Fat-soluble vitamins can be stored in the body.

Whole food: This is a regular or "solid" food, such as cottage cheese or an apple, as opposed to a "liquid" food, such as a nutrition shake. For example, on Eating *for* Life, a typical day might include having four whole-food meals and two nutrition shake meals.

Wrong foods: These are foods that are just not good for you. Wrong foods (also called "unauthorized foods") don't have enough nutrients for the total amount of calories, sugar and fat that they provide. Eat the "wrong foods," if you really enjoy them, on your one free day each week, but steer clear of them on your six Eating *for* Lifestyle days.

Appendix C

Cooking Terms & Tips

Al dente: This is an Italian phrase, pronounced "al-DEN-tay," used to describe pasta that is not completely cooked through. I prefer pasta cooked this way because of its firm texture and taste.

Bake: This means to cook food in an oven. For best results, preheat the oven to the suggested temperature before putting in the food.

Balsamic vinegar: This is an especially "tangy-sweet"-tasting, dark-colored vinegar, which can spark the flavor of many foods like salad dressings, marinades, vegetables and even fresh fruit. Like fine wine, it is made from grapes (although unfermented and thus alcohol free). Some balsamic vinegars are aged 15 years or more and can be quite expensive. "Younger" bottles are more affordable.

Beat: Here's where you vigorously mix ingredients with a fork, whisk or electric mixer to add air and make the mixture extra smooth.

Blend: Combining two or more ingredients until smooth or evenly mixed together. This is usually done with a spoon, electric mixer or a blender.

Boil: This means to heat a liquid until bubbles rise rapidly and break on the surface. At sea level, liquids boil at 212°F. At higher elevations, liquids boil at a slightly lower temperature, and boiled foods such as potatoes, pasta and hard-boiled eggs take a little longer to cook.

Bow tie pasta: This pasta is also called "farfalle," which is Italian for "butterfly."

Bread: When this term is used as a verb, it means to coat food (i.e., fish, meat, vegetables) by dipping into a liquid like beaten egg whites, then into a dry mixture, often breadcrumbs, before cooking.

Broil: This is when you cook food in the oven directly under the heat source. Often it helps to use a broiler pan with a slotted top so fat drips away, producing a leaner-cooked meat. When you preheat the broiler, be sure that you do not preheat the broiler pan or your meal may get stuck to it!

Broth: This is the clear liquid that is produced when chicken, beef, fish or vegetables are cooked in water. It is used to make flavorful soups and sauces. In Eating *for* Life recipes, this term also refers to canned or packaged broth that is low fat or fat free and reduced sodium.

Brown: To cook food quickly over high heat in a hot skillet, broiler or oven, causing the surface of the food to "brown" while keeping the inside moist.

Bulgur: This is a whole-grain carbohydrate in the form of wheat kernels that have been steamed, dried and crushed. It has a nutty flavor and a soft texture and is often used to make "tabbouleh," which is a mint, parsley and bulgur salad.

Cajun seasoning: There are many different blends, most contain the Cajun classic trio of black, white and red pepper that gives it a spicy kick. It may also include garlic, onion, salt or other spices. You can add Cajun seasoning to chicken, fish and beef before cooking.

Capers: These are small flower buds from a Mediterranean plant that have been dried and pickled. Found near the olives in the supermarket, capers have a tangy, citrus-olive flavor that enhances many types of sauces, seafood, chicken and beef. Capers should be rinsed under cold water to remove excess salt before adding to recipes.

Chicken breast: Throughout the Eating *for* Life recipes, "chicken breast" refers to skinless, boneless chicken breasts, which is the most tender and lean part of the chicken. You can buy boneless, skinless chicken breasts or you can remove the skin and bone before cooking. Be sure to wash your hands, all utensils and any surfaces that have come in contact with raw chicken (or turkey) in hot soapy water. Always cook chicken until it is no longer pink in the center.

Chicken breast tenders: These are long strips of boneless, skinless chicken breast. You can usually buy them already sliced, or you can do it yourself by slicing a portion-size boneless, skinless chicken breast lengthwise into about four equal strips.

Chill: This means to place food in the refrigerator until it's thoroughly cold.

Chop: This is cutting food into small irregular-shaped pieces using a knife.

Coat: Used as a verb, this term means to cover food evenly, often with breadcrumbs, sauce or spices.

Combine: This means to mix two or more ingredients together.

Cooking spray: An oil, in aerosol form, that is often used to keep food from sticking to pots, pans, grills and utensils. It is available in different varieties, such as butter flavored or olive oil, and even one especially for grilling. Used sparingly, it adds very little fat and calories to cooked foods.

Cool: This cooking term means to let hot food or liquid stand at room temperature until it has "cooled" to the desired temperature.

Condiment: A sauce, relish or spice, such as ketchup, mustard or hot pepper sauce, that enhances the flavor of food.

Core: Removing the center of a fruit (i.e., apple, pear, pineapple). Cores contain small seeds, such as in an apple, or are tough and fibrous.

Couscous: This carbohydrate is coarsely ground durum wheat that is shaped into little beads and steamed. Couscous has a light texture and is often served in place of rice.

Crisp-tender: This term describes a point where vegetables are cooked until slightly tender yet still retaining some of their fresh, crisp texture.

Crushed: This basically means to "smash" an ingredient like a garlic clove with the side of a chef's knife before using it in a recipe.

Cube: Cutting the food into squares of $\frac{1}{2}$ inch or larger using a knife.

Dash: This is a small quantity, usually less than $\frac{1}{8}$ teaspoon for dry spices (such as pepper or cinnamon) or a couple of drops of liquid ingredients (such as hot pepper sauce or extracts).

Dice: Cutting food into cubes of $\frac{1}{2}$ inch or less using a knife.

Ditalini: Very small, short tubes of pasta often used in soups and salads.

Divided: When you see "divided" after an ingredient in an Eating *for* Life recipe, it means that you will be using that ingredient more than once in the preparation of the meal. The measurement for the ingredient is the total amount you will need. For example, an ingredient such as "2 Tbsp Parmesan cheese" may be "divided" and half used to coat chicken before it is cooked and the other half sprinkled on top of the finished meal.

Dollop: Here's where you top food with a spoonful of a soft food like whipped topping or sour cream.

Doneness: This is a point to which a food is cooked. For example, chicken baked until no longer pink in the center.

Drain: This is when you pour off liquid by putting the food, like pasta, into a strainer or colander that has been set in the sink.

Drizzle: This means to slowly pour a liquid, such as vinaigrette, in a fine stream, back and forth, over the food.

Dutch oven: This is a short, wide pot with handles and a lid that usually holds 5 quarts or more. It is often used for cooking soups, stews and pasta.

Egg noodles: These are short, flat pasta strips made with eggs (pasta is generally made with durum wheat flour and water). Noodles are available in several widths, including wide and extra wide, which are often used in soups or topped with thick sauces.

Fettuccine: These are long, flat "ribbons" of pasta, about $\frac{1}{4}$-inch wide. The difference between fettuccine and spaghetti is fettuccini is wider.

Filet/Fillet: This is a boneless piece of meat (chicken, fish, beef, etc.).

Five-spice powder: A pungent spice mixture often used in Chinese dishes. This blend of cinnamon, clove, fennel seed, star anise and Szechwan peppercorns can be found in most grocery stores in the Asian foods section.

Flake: This cooking term describes breaking a food into small pieces using a fork, for example canned tuna. Also, it is a way to test fresh fish for doneness. For example, fish should separate easily or "flake" when it is cooked through. You just insert a fork and gently twist to "flake."

Foil muffin liners: These foil cups are used to line muffin tins and can usually be found in the baking aisle. Lightly coat them with cooking spray before filling them with muffin batter. Be sure to remove the paper dividers between each foil cup before using them.

Fold: This is when you combine ingredients lightly using a rubber spatula. To "fold," you simply scrape across the bottom of a bowl and up the nearest side, then give the bowl a quarter turn and repeat until blended.

Fork-tender: This is a degree of doneness for cooked vegetables and meats where there is only slight resistance when pierced with a fork.

Freeze: This is when you place foods in the freezer until firm or for storage. The recommended temperature for your freezer is 0°F. Before storing cooked foods, divide them into portions, wrap them tightly in plastic wrap or bags made for freezing, heavy-duty foil or an airtight container. It is helpful to label foods and date them. Most foods will keep for two to four months when properly freezer stored. To reheat, bring soups and sauces to a boil, and heat other foods until they are steaming hot.

Garnish: Here's where you "decorate" food with small amounts of ingredients that add color and/or texture (i.e., parsley, fresh berries, cilantro).

Ginger: This is a brown-skinned root with a peppery, yet slightly sweet, taste that is often used in stir-fry meals. Ginger can be found in the produce section of most grocery stores. Remove the brown peel with a vegetable peeler or paring knife before using ginger in recipes.

Grate: To finely shred hard-textured foods like cheese, citrus peel or fresh ginger using a (you guessed it!) *grater*.

Grill: This is when you cook food outdoors on a rack over direct heat from either charcoal briquettes or propane. Grilling can also be done indoors with a "George Foreman-type" grill or on the stovetop with a cast-iron grill pan. Most foods that can be grilled can also be broiled.

Halved: To divide something into two equal portions or parts. For example, when a recipe calls for a "lemon, halved," that simply means you cut the lemon into two equal portions and use as indicated in the directions.

Hoisin sauce: This is a thick sauce with a sweet and slightly spicy flavor made from soybeans, vinegar, garlic, chilies and spices. It is often used in Asian-inspired meals and as a table condiment.

Hominy: This grain (also called "posole"; pronounced "pa-so-lee") is made of hulled corn kernels. Hominy has a firm texture and a mild, sweet taste and can be added to soups.

Hungarian paprika: This is a spice made from ground and dried sweet red peppers. This variety of paprika is known for having a rich, red-orange color as well as a unique and wonderful flavor.

Italian seasoning: This savory dried herb blend often contains oregano, basil, thyme and rosemary. It is used in Italian-inspired meals either during cooking or sprinkled on after cooking.

Jalapeño: Green or red chilis that range from hot to *very* hot. To "tame the fire," remove the seeds inside, wearing rubber gloves or covering your hands with plastic sandwich bags. When you're through, wash your hands thoroughly with soap and warm water as the oil can burn your eyes and skin. (Warning: Do *not* use the restroom after handling jalapeños before thoroughly washing your hands! This is a little free advice I can share with you, having learned the hard way not to do this!)

Julienne: This is when you cut vegetables into thin, uniform matchsticks about 2 inches long. (It's also the name of my hairstylist.)

Marinara sauce: This type of pasta sauce, often called "spaghetti sauce," is tomato based and may include onion, garlic, oregano and other Italian spices.

Marinate: Here is where you tenderize and flavor food by placing it in a seasoned liquid, called a "marinade." Marinades will often contain an acidic ingredient like vinegar or lemon juice. Use a large Ziploc bag or glass or plastic dish for best results and avoid marinating your food in metal pans. Refrigerate foods while they are marinating.

Microwave: Used as a verb, this means to cook, reheat or thaw food in a microwave oven. When reheating foods in the microwave, cook them until they are steaming hot.

Mince: This is chopping or cutting foods into tiny, irregular pieces using a knife.

Mix: This means to stir ingredients together, typically with a spoon or fork.

Napa cabbage: This variety of cabbage, also called Chinese cabbage, has long, light-green leaves and an oblong shape. Its mild flavor makes it a good choice for salads and stir-fries.

Olive oil: This is one of the healthiest oils and can be used for many purposes. A particular kind of olive oil, called "extra-virgin," is produced from the first pressing of olives, which is generally done without heat. It has a great flavor, high levels of fatty acids and polyphenols and low acidity. Extra-virgin, cold-pressed olive oil costs slightly more than lesser grades of olive oil, and it's worth it.

Parsnips: This vegetable looks like a white carrot and has a creamy texture and a sweet, nutty flavor. It's often used in soups and stews.

Pasta sauce: This is a universal term for a range of sauces—everything from creamy alfredo sauce to marinara. In Eating *for* Life recipes, the kind of pasta sauce referred to is tomato-based sauce, with minimal fat and low sugar content.

Penne: These are diagonally cut tubes of pasta. The outside is smooth or sometimes has ridges. Penne is good to use in pasta meals with sauces.

Pinch: The amount of powdery ingredients (i.e., cinnamon, pepper) you can hold between your thumb and forefinger—a pinch equals about $\frac{1}{16}$ of a teaspoon.

Poach: Cooking foods like eggs and salmon in hot water or broth just below the boiling point.

Preheat: To heat an oven, grill, broiler or other appliance to a specific temperature setting before using it.

Ramekin: This is a small (2 to 3 inches in diameter) straight-sided, white-porcelain dish that is often used for custards, soufflés or sauces.

Refrigerate: This is when you place food in the refrigerator to chill or store it. For proper food storage, set your refrigerator at 40°F or slightly lower. If covered tightly, most foods will keep in the refrigerator for three to four days. Be sure to refrigerate cooked foods within two hours of preparing them.

Rigatoni: Wide, large tubes of pasta with ridges that help hold sauce and seasonings. Rigatoni is good with hearty sauces and in oven-baked pasta meals.

Roast: This is when you cook meat or vegetables uncovered in the oven without adding liquid, usually until the exterior is crisp and the interior is cooked through. Most meats are suitable for roasting as are many vegetables, such as potatoes and peppers.

Rotini: This is pasta shaped like little corkscrews. It can be used in most any pasta meal, hot or cold.

Sauté: This means to cook food quickly in a small amount of oil, liquid or cooking spray in a skillet while stirring or turning frequently.

Score: As it pertains to cooking, "score" means to make shallow slices (parallel or crisscross) in the surface of meat or fish before cooking to help tenderize it and/or allow marinades to absorb more quickly.

Sear: Browning meat quickly over high heat to seal in the juices and enhance flavor.

Season: To enhance the flavor of foods with pepper, herbs, spices, etc.

Shallots: This vegetable is one of the mildest in the onion family. The cloves are covered in papery skin that ranges in color from beige to purple and should be removed before chopping. Shallots have a distinctive flavor that provide a subtle hint of both onion and garlic to sauces and salads.

Shiitake mushrooms: Brown Asian mushrooms with a flat cap and an almost meaty flavor. Be sure to remove and discard stems before using in recipes. If fresh shiitake mushrooms are not available, dried shiitake mushrooms can usually be found in the Asian food section of the grocery store. Soak dried mushrooms in hot water for 20 minutes, drain and rinse before using in recipes.

Shred: This is when you slice food into very narrow strips using a grater, knife or food processor. Cooked meat is shredded by pulling it apart with two forks.

Skewers: These are long, thin, pointed rods made of wood, bamboo or metal. They are used to hold meat and vegetables in place during cooking, often for kabobs. Before using wooden or bamboo skewers, soak them in water for about 15 minutes to keep them from burning on the grill or under the broiler.

Sift: Here's where you put dry ingredients, often flour, through a sifter, fine-mesh sieve or strainer. This adds air, reduces lumps and helps the ingredients combine more easily.

Simmer: Cooking liquid on the stovetop over low heat so it's just below the boiling point. A few small bubbles should be visible on the surface. Simmering is usually done after reducing heat from a boil.

Skim: Used as a verb, this means to remove the fat or foam from the surface of soups or broth with a spoon, ladle or skimmer (a flat utensil with holes in it).

Slices/Sliced: A thin piece cut from a larger food, normally uniform in size and width, such as tomato slices.

Slow cooker: An electrical appliance, also called a Crockpot, that cooks food with relatively low, steady heat for between five and 12 hours, depending on the heat setting you choose. It can help cook your dinners like pot roast or chili while you're at work.

Spaghetti: This is the most well known kind of pasta in America. It has long, round, thin strands of pasta and is made from a special kind of flour made from ground durum wheat.

Steam: This is when you cook food in a covered pan, with a small amount of boiling water. The vapor or "steam" cooks the food without adding fat or calories. To steam a vegetable like broccoli, for example, you fill a saucepan with about 1 inch of water and place it over high heat. Add the broccoli and bring it to a boil. Then, cover and steam until crisp-tender, about 7 minutes.

Stir: Combining ingredients with a circular or figure-eight motion using a spoon.

Stir-fry: An Asian method of cooking similar-sized pieces of food in a small amount of hot oil or cooking spray in a hot wok or skillet while stirring constantly. The keys to stir-frying are making sure your ingredients are chopped and prepared before you start and that your wok or skillet is hot and ready to go.

Stockpot: A tall, narrow pot with handles and a lid that comes in several sizes—8 quarts is a common and useful size. It is used for cooking soups, stews, pasta, potatoes, etc. It differs from a Crockpot in that it is used on the stovetop and is *not* an electrical appliance.

Tear: This means to break into pieces with your fingers. For example, you might tear romaine lettuce into small pieces for a salad.

Toast: Browning food lightly in a toaster, oven, broiler or skillet.

Toothpick test: Muffins (or other cakelike batters) are done when a wooden toothpick poked in the center comes out clean. If batter sticks to the toothpick, put the food back in the oven for a few more minutes. Then retest.

Toss: Mixing ingredients lightly with a lifting motion (i.e., salads, pasta with sauce) using a large spoon and fork.

Tuna, albacore: This "white meat" tuna is richer in heart-healthy omega-3 fatty acids than either dark or light meat tuna. Its mild flavor makes it a very popular canned tuna. (Tip: Be sure to use canned tuna packed in *water*, not oil. Okay?)

Tuna, yellow fin: This fresh tuna is also called Ahi and is an excellent "steak fish." Before cooking, it is dark red and looks almost like a beef steak. When cooked (rare, medium or well), it is light colored, flaky and flavorful.

Vinaigrette: This is simply an oil, vinegar and spice mixture used to dress salad greens or other cold foods like pasta salad.

Wasabi: A Japanese horseradish with a pale-green color and "head-clearing" heat. It is available in paste or powder form and is usually found in the Asian foods section of the grocery store.

Wedge: A slice of a fruit or other food, typically the result of cutting the whole food (like an orange) into several equal sections that are triangular in shape.

Whip: Combining ingredients (like egg whites) rapidly by hand or electric mixer to add air and increase volume so the ingredients are light and fluffy.

Whisk: Used as a verb, this means to beat liquid ingredients, such as eggs, sauces or pudding, with a fork or whisk to mix, blend or add air.

White pepper: This is a spice made from ripened black peppercorns with the hull removed. It has a slightly milder flavor than black pepper.

Zest: This is the grated peel of a lime or lemon. (It's also a term used in the heart of Italy to describe a special, vibrant quality—the spice of life. ☺)

Appendix D

Kitchen Essentials

Essential to your success is making sure your kitchen is properly equipped—that you have "set the table" for your success. You don't need to invest thousands of dollars in elaborate appliances, crystal and silver. However, in addition to the obvious essentials, which include plates, forks, spoons, knives, glasses and such, some accessories are needed to prepare the Eating *for* Life meal recipes featured in this book. Here's some of the kitchen essentials you may already own, or you may want to add to your kitchen. Most of these items are available at outlets ranging from Wal-Mart to Williams-Sonoma.

POTS AND PANS

Pots and pans come in a variety of materials. Stainless steel is a good choice. It is easy to clean, durable and does not react to acidic foods like tomato sauce. The higher-quality pots and pans have a layer of copper or aluminum on the bottom and sides or inside the steel for better heat conductivity. Look for pans with a thick base to guard against scorching and handles that are insulated so they don't get too hot.

- 1 Dutch oven or stockpot, with lid (5 quarts or more)
- 3 saucepans, with lids: small (1 quart),
  medium (2 quarts) and large (3 quarts)

Skillets with nonstick coating are easy to use, easy to clean and essential when you are cooking meals with small amounts of fat. Look for fairly heavy skillets that are moderately priced. With proper care, nonstick-coated cookware will last three to five years.

- 3 skillets: small (8 inches),
  medium (10 inches) and large (12 inches)

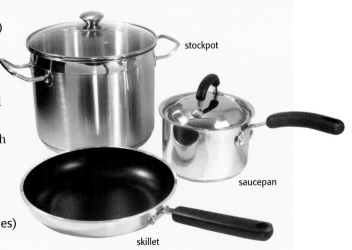

stockpot

saucepan

skillet

BAKEWARE

Throughout the Eating *for* Life meal recipes, the words **sheet**, **tin** and **pan** refer to *metal* pans. The words **dish** or **plate** refer to oven-safe *glass* or *ceramic*.

- 3 baking dishes, glass or ceramic, about 2 inches deep (8 inches x 8 inches / 11x7 / 9x13)
- 1 baking sheet or "cookie sheet" (18 inches x 12 inches x 1 inch)
- 1 loaf pan (9 inches x 5 inches)
- 1 muffin tin with 12 cups
- 2 pie plates, glass or ceramic (9-inch diameter)
- 1 broiler pan with slotted top

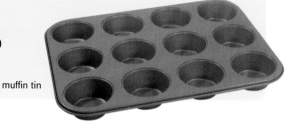

muffin tin

KNIVES

High-carbon, stainless-steel knives work well for chopping and slicing.

- 1 paring knife (3 to 4 inches)
- 1 chef's knife (8 to 10 inches)
- 1 serrated bread knife (8 inches)
- 1 knife sharpener
- 4 steak knives

paring knife   chef's knife   serrated bread knife

APPLIANCES

Here's the "big stuff" you'll need in your kitchen to prepare Eating *for* Life meals.

- 1 heavy-duty blender
- 1 microwave oven
- 1 grill (outdoor, indoor electric or stovetop grill pan)
- 1 slow cooker
- 1 toaster

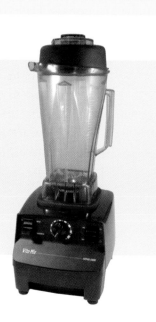

Vita-Mix blender

To prepare your Eating *for* Life meals efficiently, you'll need these kitchen basics.

- 1 can opener
- 1 colander
- 1 corkscrew
- 1 flour sifter or sieve
- 1 long-handled fork
- 1 4-sided grater
- 1 kitchen scissors
- 1 set of 3 nested mixing bowls
- 1 pastry brush
- 1 pepper grinder
- 1 potato masher
- 4 skewers (wood or metal), at least 6 inches long
- 1 soup ladle
- 1 metal spatula
- 2 long-handled spoons
- 1 long-handled, slotted spoon
- 1 rubber spatula
- 2 long-handled, wooden spoons
- 1 kitchen tongs
- 1 vegetable peeler
- 1 vegetable brush
- 1 whisk
- 2 hot pads
- 2 cutting boards, about 14 inches x 20 inches each (1 used only for raw meats, chicken and fish)
- Plastic or Tupperware freezer-safe, microwave-safe food storage containers

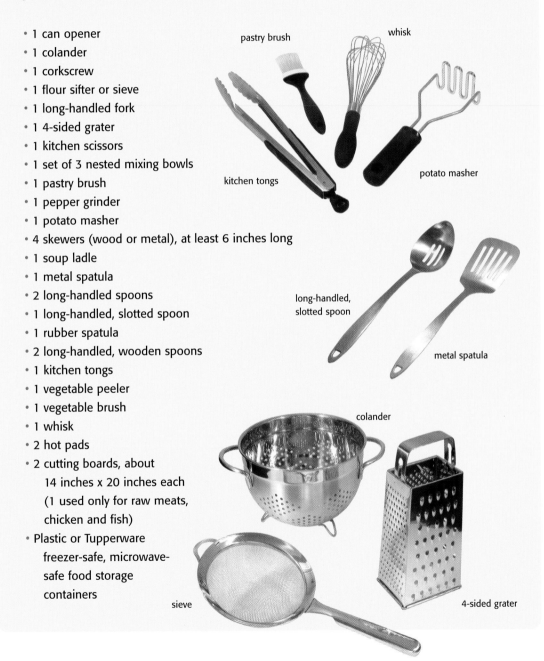

pastry brush

whisk

kitchen tongs

potato masher

long-handled, slotted spoon

metal spatula

colander

sieve

4-sided grater

Besides dishes and silverware, these items will help make serving easier and more appetizing.

- 4 dessert bowls
- 4 ramekins or custard cups
- 4 tall milk shake glasses

ramekins

MEASURING

A liquid measuring cup is clear glass or plastic with incremental markings. Read the measurement from eye level for accurate results.

liquid measuring cup

- 1 liquid measuring cup

Used to measure dry ingredients, graduated measuring cups are helpful. Your set should include $\frac{1}{4}$ cup, $\frac{1}{3}$ cup, $\frac{1}{2}$ cup and 1 cup.

measuring spoons

graduated measuring cups

- 1 set graduated measuring cups

Measuring spoons are used for measuring small amounts of liquid and dry ingredients. Sets usually include $\frac{1}{4}$ teaspoon, $\frac{1}{2}$ teaspoon, 1 teaspoon and 1 Tablespoon.

- 1 set measuring spoons

OPTIONALS

Once you have the basic essentials, here are a few more items you may want to add to your kitchen:

- 1 griddle (electric or stovetop)
- 1 toaster oven
- 1 wok
- 4 parfait glasses
- 1 popsicle mold
- 1 food processor

Conversion Charts

U.S. Equivalents

Large Volume

Cups	Fluid Ounces	Pints/Quarts
1 cup	8 fluid ounces	$\frac{1}{2}$ pint
2 cups	16 fluid ounces	1 pint
3 cups	24 fluid ounces	$1\frac{1}{2}$ pints = $\frac{3}{4}$ quart
4 cups	32 fluid ounces	2 pints = 1 quart
6 cups	48 fluid ounces	3 pints = $1\frac{1}{2}$ quarts
8 cups	64 fluid ounces	2 quarts = $\frac{1}{2}$ gallon
16 cups	128 fluid ounces	4 quarts = 1 gallon

Small Volume

Tablespoons	Cups	Fluid Ounces
1 tablespoon = 3 teaspoons	$\frac{1}{16}$ cup	$\frac{1}{2}$ fluid ounce
2 tablespoons	$\frac{1}{8}$ cup	1 fluid ounce
4 tablespoons	$\frac{1}{4}$ cup	2 fluid ounces
5 tablespoons + 1 teaspoon	$\frac{1}{3}$ cup	$2\frac{2}{3}$ fluid ounces
6 tablespoons	$\frac{3}{8}$ cup	3 fluid ounces
8 tablespoons	$\frac{1}{2}$ cup	4 fluid ounces
10 tablespoons + 2 teaspoons	$\frac{2}{3}$ cup	$5\frac{1}{3}$ fluid ounces
12 tablespoons	$\frac{3}{4}$ cup	6 fluid ounces
14 tablespoons	$\frac{7}{8}$ cup	7 fluid ounces
16 tablespoons	1 cup	8 fluid ounces

Metric Conversion Charts

These charts represent approximate equivalents, which are
easy to apply and precise enough for preparing meals.

Weight

1 ounce	=	30 grams
4 ounces	=	120 grams
8 ounces	=	240 grams
12 ounces	=	360 grams
1 pound	=	480 grams

Volume

1/4 teaspoon	=	1 milliliter
1/2 teaspoon	=	2 milliliters
1 teaspoon	=	5 milliliters
1 tablespoon	=	15 milliliters
2 tablespoons	=	30 milliliters
3 tablespoons	=	45 milliliters
1/4 cup	=	50 milliliters
1/3 cup	=	75 milliliters
1/2 cup	=	125 milliliters
2/3 cup	=	150 milliliters
3/4 cup	=	175 milliliters
1 cup	=	250 milliliters
1 quart	=	1 liter

Temperatures

32°F	=	0°C
250°F	=	120°C
275°F	=	140°C
300°F	=	150°C
325°F	=	160°C
350°F	=	180°C
375°F	=	190°C
400°F	=	200°C
425°F	=	220°C
450°F	=	230°C
475°F	=	250°C
500°F	=	260°C
525°F	=	270°C

Scientific References

Chapter 1

U.S. Department of Health and Human Services. *The Surgeon General's Call to Action to Prevent and Decrease Overweight and Obesity.*

Texas A&M research. In: D. Barboza, "If You Pitch It, They Will Eat," *New York Times*, August 3, 2003.

A.E. Gallo, "Food Advertising in the United States." In: E. Frazao, ed. *America's Eating Habits: Changes and Consequences.* Washington, D.C.: USDA, 1999: 173-180.

U.S. Census Bureau, United States Department of Commerce & U.S. Department of Health and Human Services.

U.S. Centers for Disease Control and Prevention.

Chapter 2

F.B. Hu, et al., "Diet and Risk of Type II Diabetes: The Role of Types of Fat and Carbohydrate," *Diabetologia* 44.7 (2001) : 805-817.

A.E. Kelley, et al., "Opioid Modulation of Taste Hedonics Within the Ventral Striatum," *Physiol. Behav.* 76.3 (2002) : 365-377.

L.H. Clemens, et al., "The Effect of Eating Out on Quality of Diet in Premenopausal Women," *J. Am. Diet. Assoc.* 99.4 (1999) : 442-444.

M.A. McCrory, et al., "Overeating in America: Association Between Restaurant Food Consumption and Body Fatness in Healthy Adult Men and Women Ages 19 to 80," *Obes. Res.* 7.6 (1999) : 564-571.

L. Cordain, et al., "Acne Vulgaris: A Disease of Western Civilization," *Arch. Dermatol.* 138.12 (2002) : 1584-1590.

L.R. Young and M. Nestle, "Expanding Portion Sizes in the U.S. Marketplace: Implications for Nutrition Counseling," *J. Am. Diet. Assoc.* 103.2 (2003) : 231-234.

U.S. Department of Health and Human Services. *The Surgeon General's Call to Action to Prevent and Decrease Overweight and Obesity.*

Chapter 3

Federal Trade Commission.

E. Cavallo, et al., "Resting Metabolic Rate, Body Composition and Thyroid Hormones. Short Term Effects of Very Low Calorie Diet," *Horm. Metab.* Res. 22.12 (1990) : 632-635.

F.L. Benoit, et al., "Changes in Body Composition During Weight Reduction in Obesity. Balance Studies Comparing Effects of Fasting and a Ketogenic Diet," *Ann. Intern. Med.* 63.3 (1965) : 604-612.

J. LaRosa, "Why the U.S. Weight Loss Industry Is Its Own Worst Enemy and What Can Be Done About It," Marketdata Enterprises, Inc.

Chapter 5

D.K. Layman, et al., "Increased Dietary Protein Modifies Glucose and Insulin Homeostasis in Adult Women During Weight Loss," *J. Nutr.* 133 (2003) : 405-410.

A. Cunliffe, et al., "Post-prandial Changes in Measures of Fatigue: Effect of a Mixed or Pure Carbohydrate or Pure Fat Meal," *Eur. J. Clin. Nutr.* 51.12 (1997) : 831-838.

R. Crovetti, et al., "The Influence of Thermic Effect of Food on Satiety," *Eur. J. Clin. Nutr.* 52 (1997) : 482-488.

M.J. Williams, et al., "Effects of Recovery Drinks After Prolonged Glycogen-Depletion Exercise," presented at the 1999 ACSM Annual Meeting.

Chapter 6

A.C. Guyton and J.E. Hall, *Textbook of Medical Physiology*, 1996.

S.M. Kleiner, "Water: An Essential But Overlooked Nutrient," *J. Am. Diet. Assoc.* 99.2 (1999) : 200-206.

A.P. Simopoulos, "n-3 Fatty Acids and Human Health: Defining Strategies for Public Policy," *Lipids* 36 (2001) : S83-S89.

"Patterns of Caloric Intake and Body Mass Index Among U.S. Adults," Economic Research Service, U.S. Department of Agriculture, 2002.

D.K. Layman, et al., "Increased Dietary Protein Modifies Glucose and Insulin Homeostasis in Adult Women During Weight Loss," *J. Nutr.* 133 (2003) : 405-410.

Chapter 6 (continued)

K. Fischer, et al., "Carbohydrate to Protein Ratio in Food and Cognitive Performance in the Morning," *Physiol. Behav.* 75.3 (2002) : 411-423.

A. Cunliffe, et al., "Post-prandial Changes in Measures of Fatigue: Effect of a Mixed or Pure Carbohydrate or Pure Fat Meal," *Eur. J. Clin. Nutr.* 51.12 (1997) : 831-838.

R.J. Bloomer, et al., "Alterations in Mood Following Acute Post-Exercise Feeding with Variance in Macronutrient Mix," *Med. Sci. Sports Exerc.* May 31, 2000 : S58.

R. Crovetti, et al., "The Influence of Thermic Effect of Food on Satiety," *Eur. J. Clin. Nutr.* 52 (1997) : 482-488.

W.P. Verboeket-van de Venne, et al., "Influence of the Feeding Frequency on Nutrient Utilization in Man: Consequences for Energy Metabolism," *Eur. J. Clin. Nutr.* 45.3 (1991) : 161-169.

R.C. Deutz, et al., "Relationship Between Energy Deficits and Body Composition in Elite Female Gymnasts and Runners," *Med. Sci. Sports Exerc.* 32.3 (2000) : 659-668.

J.M. Antoine, et al., "Feeding Frequency and Nitrogen Balance in Weight-Reducing Obese Women," *Hum. Nutr. Clin. Nutr.* 38.1 (1984) : 31-38.

S. Iwao, et al., "Effects of Meal Frequency on Body Composition During Weight Control in Boxers," *Scand. J. Med. Sci. Sports* 6.5 (1996) : 265-272.

J.S. Garrow, et al., "The Effect of Meal Frequency and Protein Concentration on the Composition of the Weight Lost by Obese Subjects," *Br. J. Nutr.* 45.1 (1981) : 5-15.

D.P. Speechly, et al., "Acute Appetite Reduction Associated with an Increased Frequency of Eating in Obese Males," *Int. J. Obes. Relat. Metab. Disord.* 23.11 (1999) : 1151-1159.

D.J. Jenkins, et al., "Nibbling Versus Gorging: Metabolic Advantages of Increased Meal Frequency," *N. Engl. J. Med.* 321.14 (1989) : 929-934.

Chapter 7

R.S. Ahima, et al., "Leptin Regulation of Neuroendocrine Systems," *Front. Neuroendocrinol.* 21.3 (2000) : 263-307.

G.R. Dubuc, et al., "Changes of Serum Leptin and Endocrine and Metabolic Parameters After 7 Days of Energy Restriction in Men and Women," *Metabolism* 47.4 (1998) : 429-434.

M. Dirlewanger, et al., "Effects of Short-Term Carbohydrate or Fat Overfeeding on Energy Expenditure and Plasma Leptin Concentrations in Healthy Female Subjects," *Int. J. Obes. Relat. Metab. Disord.* 24.11 (2000) : 1413-1418.

Chapter 8

E.F. Coyle, "Physical Activity as a Metabolic Stressor," *Am. J. Clin. Nutr.* 72.2 (2000) : 512S-520S.

M. Yoshioka, et al., "Impact of High-Intensity Exercise on Energy Expenditure, Lipid Oxidation and Body Fatness," *Int. J. Obes. Relat. Metab. Disord.* 25.3 (2001) : 332-339.

E.T. Poehlman, et al., "The Impact of Exercise and Diet Restriction on Daily Energy Expenditure," *Sports Med.* 11.2 (1991) : 78-101.

S.J. Long, et al., "The Ability of Habitual Exercise to Influence Appetite and Food Intake in Response to High- and Low-Energy Preloads in Man," *Br. J. Nutr.* 87.5 (2002) : 517-523.

R.G. McMurray, et al., "Diurnal Variations of Beta-Endorphin at Rest and After Moderate Intensity Exercise," *Chronobiol. Int.* 7.2 (1990) : 135-142.

R.G. McMurray, et al., "Exercise Intensity-Related Responses of Beta-Endorphin and Catecholamines," *Med. Sci. Sports Exerc.* 19.6 (1987) : 570-574.

M.F. McCarty, "Optimizing Exercise for Fat Loss," *Med. Hypotheses.* 44.5 (1995) : 325-330.

S.B. Roberts, "High-Glycemic Index Foods, Hunger, and Obesity: Is There a Connection?" *Nutr. Rev.* 58.6 (2000) : 163-169.

Chapter 9

A. Bendich, "Micronutrients in Women's Health and Immune Function," *Nutrition* 17.10 (2001) : 858-867.

R. Kingston and J.R. Hunt, "Dietary Supplements in Women: Responsible Strategies for Use," *J. Am. Pharm. Assoc. (Wash)* 40.5S1 (2000) : S34-S35.

L.R. Brilla and T.F. Haley, "Effect of Magnesium Supplementation on Strength Training in Humans," *J. Am. Coll. Nutr.* 11.3 (1992) : 326-329.

A.S. Prasad, et al., "Zinc Status and Serum Testosterone Levels of Healthy Adults," *Nutrition* 12.5 (1996) : 344-348.

Recipe Index

Tasteful Tip Index